A PRACTICAL MANUAL OF
Diabetic Foot Care

To our families: Audrey, Stephen and
Susie Edmonds; Julien, William and Dennis Foster
and Debra, Rebecca, Douglas and Lauren Sanders.

A PRACTICAL MANUAL OF
Diabetic Foot Care

Michael E. Edmonds
MD, FRCP

Professor of Diabetic Foot Medicine
Diabetic Foot Clinic
King's College Hospital
London, UK

Alethea V. M. Foster
PGCE, MChS, SRCh, Dip. Pod.M

Formerly Consultant Podiatrist
Diabetic Foot Clinic
King's College Hospital
London, UK

Lee J. Sanders
DPM

Chief, Podiatry Service
Department of Veterans Affairs Medical Center
Lebanon
Pennsylvania, USA

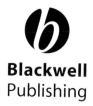

Blackwell
Publishing

© 2008 Michael E. Edmonds, Alethea V.M. Foster and Lee J. Sanders
Published by Blackwell Publishing
Blackwell Publishing, Inc., 350 Main Street, Malden, Massachusetts 02148-5020, USA
Blackwell Publishing Ltd, 9600 Garsington Road, Oxford OX4 2DQ, UK
Blackwell Publishing Asia Pty Ltd, 550 Swanston Street, Carlton, Victoria 3053, Australia

The right of the Authors to be identified as the Authors of this Work has been asserted in accordance with the Copyright, Designs and Patents Act 1988.

First published 2004
Second edition 2008

1   2008

Library of Congress Cataloging-in-Publication Data

Edmonds, M. E.
    A practical manual of diabetic foot care / Michael E. Edmonds, Alethea V.M. Foster,
Lee J. Sanders.— 2nd ed.
        p. ; cm.
    Includes bibliographical references and index.
    ISBN 978-1-4051-6147-3 (alk. paper)
    1. Foot—Diseases.   2. Diabetes—Complications.   I. Foster, Alethea V. M.
II. Sanders, Lee J., 1947–   III. Title.
    [DNLM: 1. Diabetic Foot—diagnosis—Case Reports.   2. Diabetic Foot—therapy—
Case Reports.   WK 835 E24p 2007]

RD563.E33 2008
617.5′85—dc22

                                                                                        2007031968

ISBN: 978-1-4051-6147-3

A catalogue record for this title is available from the British Library

Set in 9.25/11.5pt Minion by Graphicraft Limited, Hong Kong
Printed and bound in Singapore by Markono Print Media Pte Ltd

Commissioning Editor: Alison Brown
Development Editor: Rebecca Huxley
Editorial Assistant: Jennifer Seward
Production Controller: Debbie Wyer

For further information on Blackwell Publishing, visit our website:
http://www.blackwellpublishing.com

The publisher's policy is to use permanent paper from mills that operate a sustainable forestry policy, and which has been manufactured from pulp processed using acid-free and elementary chlorine-free practices. Furthermore, the publisher ensures that the text paper and cover board used have met acceptable environmental accreditation standards.

Contents

Acknowledgements

Ali Foster and Mike Edmonds offer special thanks first to their co-author, Lee Sanders, who contributed the updated chapter on surgical management of the diabetic foot and has again cast a critical and helpful eye over the other chapters giving an American perspective. His advice was invaluable.

For sections of the chapter on the management of diabetic major amputees we owe a great deal to Christian Pankhurst and Alan Tanner for details of prosthetic and orthotic management. We are also grateful to Rosalind Ham for sharing a physiotherapist's insights into the special problems faced by high-risk patients who lose a leg.

Lee Sanders would like to recognize the invaluable research assistance provided to him by Barbara E. Deaven, Medical Librarian, and Dorothy Melan, Library Technician, at VA Medical Center, Lebanon, Pennsylvania, USA.

We are grateful to colleagues past and present, who include: Simon Fraser, Huw Walters, Mary Blundell, Cathy Eaton, Mark Greenhill, Susie Spencer, Maureen McColgan-Bates, Mel Doxford, Sally Wilson, Adora Hatrapal, E. Maelor Thomas, Mick Morris, John Philpott-Howard, Jim Wade, Andrew Hay, Robert Lewis, Anne-Marie Ryan, Irina Mantey, Robert Hills, Rachel Ben-Salem, Muriel Buxton-Thomas, Mazin Al-Janabi, Dawn Hurley, Stephanie Amiel, Stephen Thomas, Daniela Pitei, Paul Baskerville, Anthony Giddings, Irving Benjamin, Mark Myerson, Paul Sidhu, Joydeep Sinha, Patricia Wallace, Gillian Cavell, Lesley Boys, Magdi Hanna, Sue Peat, Colin Roberts, David Goss, Colin Deane, Sue Snowdon, Ana Grenfell, Tim Cundy, Pat Ascott, Lindis Richards, Kate Spicer, Debbie Broome, Liz Hampton, Timothy Jemmott, Michelle Buckley, Rosalind Phelan, Maggie Boase, Maria Back, Avril Witherington, Daniel Rajan, Hisham Rashid, Ghulam Mufti, Karen Fairbairn, Ian Eltringham, Nina Petrova, Lindy Begg, Barbara Wall, Mark O'Brien, Sacha Andrews, Barry Pike, Jane Preece, Briony Sloper, Christian Pankhurst, Jim Beaumont, Matthew McShane, Cheryl Clark, Marcello Perez, Nicholas Cooley, Paul Bains, Patricia Yerbury, Charlotte Biggs, Anna Korzon Burakowska, David Ross, Jason Wilkins, David Evans, Carol Gayle, David Hopkins, Keith Jones, Bob Edmondson, Enid Joseph, Karen Reid, David Williams, Doris Agyemang-Duah, Jennifer Tremlett, Venu Kavarthapu, Om Lahoti, Mark Phillips, Paula Gardiner, and two great stalwarts of the Foot Clinic, Peter Watkins and the late David Pyke.

The Podiatry Managers and Community Podiatrists from Lambeth, Southwark and Lewisham have also contributed greatly to the work of the Foot Clinic at King's College Hospital over many years.

We are particularly grateful for the advice of the members of the Dermatology Department: Anthony du Vivier, Daniel Creamer, Claire Fuller, Elisabeth Higgins and Sarah MacFarlane.

We are also thankful to Audrey and Stephen Edmonds, and Nina Petrova for technical help with the production of the manuscript.

We give special thanks to Yvonne Bartlett, Alex Dionysiou, David Langdon, Lucy Wallace and Moira Lovell from the Department of Medical Photography at King's College Hospital, and the late lamented Chelsea School of Chiropody, London Foot Hospital, and to Barbara Wall for illustrations.

We are particularly grateful to our long-suffering editors, Alison Brown and Rebecca Huxley at Blackwell Publishing Ltd, and to our wives, Audrey Edmonds and Debra Sanders, and children for their patience and understanding.

We refer to patients throughout the book, when speaking generally, as 'he' simply because more men than women seem to develop diabetic foot ulcers.

This is a practical hands-on manual, uninterrupted by references. At the end of each chapter, we have given a classified reading list which should provide further information for our readers.

Prologue

O, let me teach you how to knit again
This scattered corn into one mutual sheaf,
These broken limbs again into one body.
(Titus Andronicus V, iii, William Shakespeare)

The first edition of 'A Practical Manual of Diabetic Foot Care' was named 'Medical Book of the Year 2004' by the British Medical Association, and we were pleased on behalf of all workers in this difficult field that the importance of the diabetic foot has been thus recognized and acknowledged as a major area of interest.

THE SCOPE OF THE PROBLEM

The scope of the problem of the diabetic foot is huge and is reflected by the fact that every thirty seconds a leg is lost to diabetes somewhere in the world. From the Arctic Circle to Australasia, diabetic foot disease is too commonly found. Fig. 1a shows a problem with the foot of a Hadj pilgrim in Saudi Arabia: the diabetic foot is the second most common emergency problem seen by surgeons among Hadj pilgrims. Fig. 1b portrays a lady with large ulcers on both feet who went on a beach holiday to the Mediterranean wearing cast protectors on her feet so that she could swim and sunbathe. Amputation rates vary throughout the world but are always increased in people with diabetes compared to those without diabetes, and amputations are still increasing in diabetic patients. In many parts of the world people with diabetes develop foot problems because of poverty: many neuropathic ulcers in developing countries are found on the feet of people who can only afford to wear home-made shoes made out of motor tyres (Fig. 2a). Injuries are very common when people wear sandals (Fig. 2b). Diabetic foot complications remain a major global public health problem, but we firmly believe that the problem is not insoluble, that most amputations can be prevented and that many ulcers can be healed when diabetes care is organized properly.

More and more we have come to believe that the key to successful management of the diabetic foot is the triad of early presentation, early diagnosis and early treatment, and we use the simple staging system as a framework for the care we offer. It is also important to remember three crucial points in the natural history of diabetic foot disease. It can initially present with minimal symptoms, but the pathology nevertheless proceeds rapidly and can quickly reach the point of no return. We also believe that optimal diabetic foot care to cope with such overwhelming pathology is multidisciplinary care, carefully organized by a team working together under the umbrella of a diabetic foot clinic (Fig. 3a,b). We are concerned that in many countries this multidisciplinary team approach is not available and we are also rendered anxious by the modern trend, in some countries, for diabetes care to be moved out of hospitals and into primary care. As foot lesions quickly reach the point of no return, it can be difficult to arrange prompt care sufficiently quickly outside a specialist multidisciplinary foot clinic.

We have always emphasized that infection is the great destroyer of the diabetic foot, and that patients with neuroischaemic feet and renal impairment are specially vulnerable. Another important lesson we have learned is that patients with peripheral vascular disease and sepsis often also have multiple comorbidities and are seriously ill, while the purely neuropathic foot is probably the easiest to treat. We think that all these are fundamental truths about the diabetic foot which have yet to be recognized by many countries and many health-care workers. Diabetic foot disease is a big problem but this book seeks to tell the reader how to solve it. We have learned valuable lessons about diabetic foot care from workers and teams from all over the world, striving in many different environments,

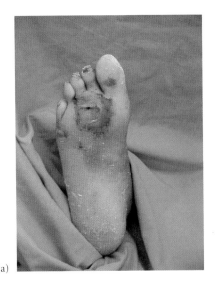

(a)

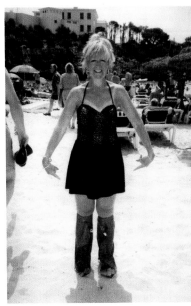

(b)

Fig. 1 (a) The foot of a Hadj pilgrim who walked barefoot round the mosque seven times and caused ulcers. (b) This lady wore cast protectors to cover her ulcerated feet on a beach holiday: note the leg oedema and severe sunburn.

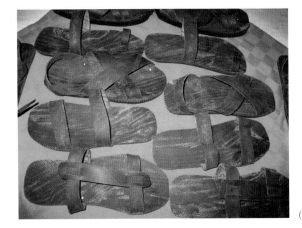

(a)

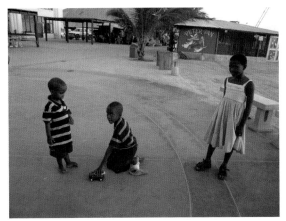

(b)

Fig. 2 (a) These shoes are made from worn-out motor tyres: they come in a variety of styles, all almost guaranteed to damage the neuropathic foot. (b) Even children have feet at risk when they wear sandals: this small boy has injured his foot.

often under great difficulties; these workers and teams have organized diabetic foot conferences (Fig. 4), set up successful diabetic foot clinics, and improved outcomes for their patients. Most of the systems we describe can be set up anywhere in the world and require only small adaptations to fit in with local customs.

The training available for health-care practitioners in diabetic foot care throughout the world remains inadequate. All too often, due to the inexperience of patients and health-care professionals, there are avoidable delays in accessing care which may cost the patient dear. A small break in the skin of a neuropathic foot which is deemed 'trivial' by an inexperienced health-care practitioner may lead to months of ulceration, destruction of fibrofatty padding and a problem foot which will lead to a lifetime of disability. Failure to recognize and treat infection early can lead to rapid destruction of a limb, or even to loss of life. Throughout the world there is an urgent need for extensive *practical* training for podiatrists, physicians, nurses, orthotists and surgeons, such as in Kerala, India, where Dr Arun Bal's surgical practice provides specialist

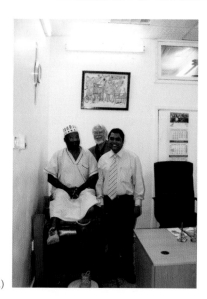

(a)

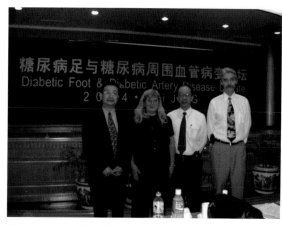

Fig. 4 A successful Diabetic Foot Conference held in Beijing by Dr Zhangrong Xu. International speakers seen here with Dr Xu included one of the authors, Professor Dennis Yue from Sydney Australia and Dr Robert Frykberg from Arizona, USA.

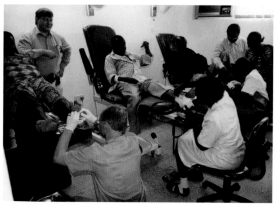

(b)

Fig. 3 (a) The multidisciplinary diabetic foot clinic in Dar es Salaam, Tanzania is run by Dr Gulam Abbas, seen here with Dr Karel Bakker, Chairman of the International Working Group for the Diabetic Foot. The patient in the chair painted the picture of diabetic foot patients which is hanging over the chair. (b) Shows a busy scene in this diabetic foot clinic with British podiatrist Neil Baker and the diabetic foot nurses treating diabetic feet. In the background is Dr Stefan Morbach, Chairman of the Diabetic Foot Study Group of the European Association for the Study of Diabetes. (Courtesy of Dr Karel Bakker.)

treatment for diabetic foot patients and trains young resident surgeons specifically in the surgical management of the diabetic foot. Dr Bal and his colleagues also run courses for podiatry assistants to train them in preventive foot care.

It is important to remember that the high-risk diabetic foot patient is always on a knife edge. Salvage of the foot in trouble requires rapid recognition and active and appropriate attempts to save the foot. . . . and not only the foot: the entire patient is at great risk. People with neuropathic or neuroischaemic feet can die quickly from a cascade of events initiated by their foot problem.

Catching an ulcer early and relieving the effects of high pressure and infection can lead to rapid healing without scarring and avoid a lifetime of disability. Everywhere in the world that triad of early presentation, early diagnosis and early treatment needs to be applied; this is a running principle throughout this book and in subsequent chapters we will elaborate on this.

Sadly, there are still too many areas of the world where people with diabetes are unable to obtain good foot care, where their foot problems are dismissed as trivial and they are turned away, or where the provision of foot care is dependent upon the patient being able to pay for it.

HISTORICAL BACKGROUND

Throughout this book we use case studies of real patients to illustrate important points and important problems. Case studies from the past may also help to illuminate current problems.

HISTORICAL CASE STUDY
Diabetic gangrene

A 55-year-old man with a much younger wife and two small children had developed weight loss, polyuria and polydypsia but refused to seek medical help, having convinced himself that he had cancer and nothing could be done for him. His wife contacted the general practitioner (GP) who was reluctant to visit, and the patient's symptoms were untreated for several years, during which time the entire family suffered from his depression and acerbic temper fits. It was not until 1941, when he developed black toes, pain, redness and swelling of his left foot and leg after stubbing his toe, that he agreed to see the doctor. His toes were black, red streaks were running up his leg, and diabetes was diagnosed. The presentation and diagnosis of diabetes was thus delayed for many years because of the patient's obduracy.

Even then, he was not immediately referred for specialist help but was treated at home by the GP, and it was not until several weeks later when he developed rigors and became extremely ill that he was finally referred to hospital. Ironically, his local hospital was a specialist centre, the renowned New England Deaconess Hospital in Boston, USA, run by Elliott Joslin; however, because of the delayed presentation they were unable to save the foot. The patient underwent an above-the-knee amputation and died one month later from a pulmonary embolus, having literally and figuratively turned his face to the wall and refused all rehabilitation or even to get out of bed. His life insurance payment was barely enough to cover the cost of the hospital fees and his funeral expenses.

Key points

There are many lessons to be learned from this case. Here are just a few of them:
- There is no such thing as 'mild diabetes'
- Even undiagnosed patients can develop severe foot problems
- Diabetic patients with ulcers should not be solely managed in the primary care setting
- Urgent referral to specialist centres is needed quickly for diabetic feet in trouble
- The patient does not always know what is best for him
- Patients about to undergo amputation need considerable help and support from an experienced rehabilitation team
- Diabetic foot problems are expensive and devastating to families.

The above described case is that of Dr Otto Emil Plath, the father of the American poet Sylvia Plath, former wife of the late Poet Laureate Ted Hughes, a feminist icon and a disturbed and unhappy woman who never got over the loss of her father when she was 8 years old. She described his diabetic foot problem seen through the eyes of a child:

Ghastly statue with one grey toe
Big as a 'Frisco seal . . .

Sylvia Plath committed suicide in 1962. In unpublished correspondence with one of the authors, Ted Hughes agreed that it was not so much her father's death but 'the manner of it' which led to her subsequent feelings of abandonment, psychological problems and suicidal tendencies. It is sometimes forgotten that it is not only the diabetic foot patient who suffers but also his family and friends who become involved in a tragic and life-shattering situation when a foot is neglected or not given specialist care sufficiently early.

It is depressing that cases of deferred presentation, inadequate investigations, paltry care and diabetic patients who lose their legs and die are still all too commonly seen, more than half a century after Dr Plath turned his face to the wall. However, the outlook for the diabetic foot is not entirely bleak. There are some hopeful trends, as the following section highlights.

ADVANCES IN DIABETIC FOOT CARE

Since the publication of the first edition of this book, the International Diabetes Federation (IDF) has collected valuable international diabetic foot data for an IDF publication, 'Time to Act'. Funds have been made available by the European Union for a multinational group, Eurodiale (a European study group for diabetes and the lower extremity), to run multicentre studies to compare outcomes in patients treated in 14 different European diabetic foot centres. The World Diabetes Foundation has funded a successful 'Step by Step' programme to improve diabetic foot care in developing countries, initially in India, Bangladesh, Sri Lanka, Nepal and Tanzania. The International Consensus Group on the Diabetic Foot has produced and updated simple and practical guidelines on diabetic foot care (Fig. 5) that have now been translated into 26 different languages: 80,000 copies have been distributed throughout the world. Robert Frykberg's team has updated new American guidelines.

As a result of these, and many other activities more multidisciplinary diabetic foot clinics than ever before are being established all over the world (Fig. 6) and a new generation of diabetic physicians is taking a real interest in the foot and regarding its management as an important area of their practice.

The work of the late Jacquie Lloyd Roberts, the UK podiatrist who established a successful group of diabetic foot clinics in Eastern Europe before her untimely death,

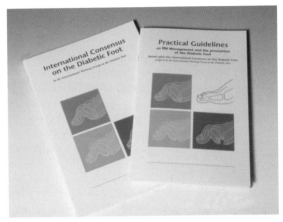

Fig. 5 The International Consensus and Practical Guidelines on the Diabetic Foot.

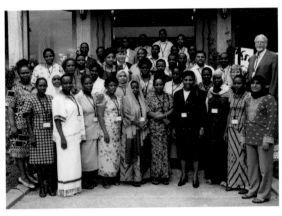

Fig. 7 The 'Step by Step' project in Tanzania: teams of physicians and nurses came from all over Tanzania to receive training in foot care. (Courtesy of Dr Karel Bakker.)

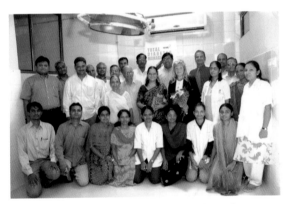

Fig. 6 A new diabetic foot clinic is inaugurated in India.

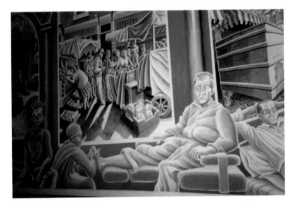

Fig. 8 'Only Connect': a painting of the King's diabetic foot clinic by Oscar Romp, our Artist in Residence.

is being continued by colleagues, and Dr Hermelinda Pedrosa continues to develop a chain of foot clinics in South America. Their work and the work of numerous other individuals and diabetic foot clinic teams, operating in many different parts of the world in very variable conditions, has clearly demonstrated the general principle that outcomes for diabetic foot patients improve when dedicated and enthusiastic individuals and teams organize a multidisciplinary diabetic foot service. With a flexible approach, many problems can be overcome. If key members of the team, such as podiatrists, are not available in certain countries, then doctors or nurses are taking on many aspects of the role of the podiatrist. In the 'Step by Step' project, health-care professionals from all over Tanzania (Fig. 7) were taught podiatry skills by using scalpels on sweet limes.

Successful interventions in the real world do not depend on the possession of high-technology equipment and vast financial budgets. Barriers to care which at first glance appear to be insurmountable can usually be overcome if we learn lessons from our own and other people's experiences, and, in the words of E. M. Forster, 'only connect' with each other (Fig. 8).

NEW AREAS COVERED IN THIS EDITION

A new edition is an opportunity to present revised and updated material, together with many new photographs and case studies and descriptions of fresh developments in the field. The reading lists at the end of each chapter have incorporated recent references. Older references have been retained when they have described fundamental work on the diabetic foot.

We have simplified our system for managing the infected foot and describe three distinct entities, of local infection, spreading infection and severe infection, together with up-to-date details of new antibiotics available for the diabetic foot. We give more information on commonly encountered organisms, and modern methods of diagnosis and management of infections. Infections with methicillin-resistant *Staphylococcus aureus* (MRSA) and other 'resistant' organisms, vancomycin-resistant enterococcus (VRE) and bacteria producing extended-spectrum beta-lactamases (ESBLs) are discussed. The table of antibiotics with reduction of dosage in renal impairment has been updated. Diabetic foot problems in pregnancy are very rare: we describe a case, and include new tables of antibiotics that can safely be taken in pregnancy and by breastfeeding mothers. Infection with *Clostridium difficile*, as a complication of antibiotic therapy, is also considered.

We have also updated the management of painful neuropathy. In addition, we have revised the section on Charcot's osteoarthropathy, describing specific risk factors in type 1 patients compared with type 2 diabetes, and Lee Sanders discusses the latest techniques to reconstruct the unstable or deformed Charcot foot. Always mindful of the importance of the ischaemic foot, particularly when complicated by infection, we have described a fast-track service to deliver immediate vascular assessment and intervention on a day-case basis, where appropriate. We give up-to-date advice on smoking cessation and discuss the impact of Vacuum-assisted Closure (VAC) therapy which has improved outcomes in patients with ischaemic feet.

Following in the footsteps of the late Roger Pecararo, we have described common pathways to amputation in our chapter on the unsalvageable foot (Chapter 7). Emphasis has been placed on preventing and managing the comorbidities of the diabetic foot patient, which all healthcare professionals should recognize.

For the first time we give an illustrated description of the partial nail avulsion procedure, the permanent solution to a recurrent ingrowing toe nail. Nail problems are very common in people with diabetes in all countries of the world and we are frequently asked for details of management. We have also added some illustrations to the descriptions of total-contact cast and Scotchcast boot manufacture.

We hope that all diabetic foot enthusiasts will enjoy this new edition of our Practical Manual, and will find it as useful, practical and easy to use as its predecessor.

PRACTICE POINTS

- The multidisciplinary diabetic foot service has been developed as a successful model of care throughout the world
- The triad of early presentation, early diagnosis and early treatment is the key to success
- Diabetic foot problems are frequently underestimated: there is no such thing as a trivial lesion of the diabetic foot
- Diabetic foot patients may not know what is best for them once neuropathy and ischaemia develop
- Increased interest in the diabetic foot over the last 25 years has resulted in major advances in the care of the diabetic foot patient but expensive, high-tech methods are not always needed.

FURTHER READING

The scope of the problem

Al-Salamah SM. General surgical problems encountered in the Hadj pilgrims. *Saudi Med J* 2005; **26**: 1055–7.

Boulton AJ, Vileikyte L, Ragnarson-Tennvall G, Apelqvist J. The global burden of diabetic foot disease. *Lancet* 2005; **366**: 1719–24.

Chin MH, Cook S, Jin L *et al.* Barriers to providing diabetes care in community health centers. *Diabetes Care* 2001; **24**: 268–74.

Jeffcoate W, Bakker K. World Diabetes Day: footing the bill. *Lancet* 2005; **365**: 1527.

Thompson L, Nester C, Stuart L, Wiles P. Interclinician variation in diabetes foot assessment—a national lottery? *Diabet Med* 2005; **22**: 196–9.

van Houtum WH. Barriers to the delivery of diabetic foot care. *Lancet* 2005; **366**: 1678–9.

Viswanathan V. The diabetic foot: perspectives from Chennai, South India. *Int J Low Extrem Wounds* 2007; **6**: 34–6.

Winocour PH, Morgan J, Ainsworth A, Williams DR. Association of British Clinical Diabetologists (ABCD): survey of specialist diabetes care services in the UK, 2000. 3 Podiatry services and related foot care issues. *Diabet Med* 2002; **19** Suppl 4: 32–8.

Historical background

Joslin EP. The menace of diabetic gangrene. *N Engl J Med* 1934; **211**: 16–20.

Lawrence RD. *The Diabetic Life.* JA Churchill, London, UK, 1925.

Foster A, Edmonds M. The Roots of Ariel; Sylvia Plath and her Father's Foot. *Diabet Med* 1995; **12**: 580–4

Advances in diabetic foot care

Anichini R, Zecchini E, Cerretini I *et al*. Improvement of diabetic foot care after the Implementation of the International Consensus on the Diabetic Foot (ICDF): results of a 5-year prospective study. *Diabetes Res Clin Pract* 2007; **75**: 153–8.

Bakker K, van Houtum WH, Riley PC. The International Diabetes Federation focuses on the diabetic foot. *Curr Diab Rep* 2005; **5**: 436–40.

Bal A. Diabetic foot: magnitude of the problem. *J Indian Med Assoc* 2002; **100**: 155–7.

Boulton AJM, Cavanagh PR, Rayman G (eds). *The Foot in Diabetes*, 4th edn. Wiley and Sons Ltd, Chichester, UK, 2006.

Das AK, Joshi SR. 'Put Feet First, Prevent Amputations'—diabetes and feet. *J Assoc Physicians India* 2005; **53**: 929–30.

Edmonds ME, Blundell MP, Morris ME *et al*. Improved survival of the diabetic foot: the role of a specialised foot clinic. *Q J Med* 1986; **232**: 763–71.

El Sakka K, Fassiadis N, Gambhir RP, Halawa M. An integrated care pathway to save the critically ischaemic diabetic foot. *Int J Clin Pract* 2006; **60**: 667–9.

Frykberg RG, Zgonis T, Armstrong DG *et al*. Diabetic Foot Disorders: a clinical practice guideline (2006 revision). *J Foot Ankle Surg* 2006; **45** (5 Suppl): S1–S66.

Lavery LA, Wunderlich RPO, Tredwell JL. Disease management for the diabetic foot: effectiveness of a diabetic foot prevention program to reduce amputations and hospitalizations. *Diabetes Res Clin Pract* 2005; **70**: 31–7.

Merriman LM, Turner W. *Clinical Skills in Treating the Foot*, 2nd edn. Churchill Livingstone, Edinburgh, UK, 2007.

Orieno CF, Nyamu PM, Atieno-Jalango G. Focus on delay as a strategy for care designs and evaluation of diabetic foot ulcers in developing countries: a review. *East Afr Med J* 2005; **82** (12 Suppl): S204–8.

Prompers L, Huijberts M, Apelqvist J *et al*. High prevalence of ischaemia, infection and serious comorbidity in patients with diabetic foot disease in Europe. Baseline results from the Eurodiale study. *Diabetologia* 2007; **50**: 18–25.

Schraer CD, Weaver D, Naylor JL *et al*. Reduction of amputation rates among Alaska Natives with diabetes following the development of a high-risk foot program. *Int J Circumpolar Health* 2004; **63** Suppl 2: 114–9.

The International Working Group on the Diabetic Foot. *International Consensus on the Diabetic Foot*. The International Working Group on the Diabetic Foot, Amsterdam, The Netherlands, 1999.

Wong M, Haswell-Elkins M, Tamwoy E *et al*. Perspectives on clinic attendance, medication and foot-care among people with diabetes in the Torres Strait Islands and Northern Peninsula Area. *Aust J Rural Health* 2005; **13**: 172–7.

Introduction

**Beseech you, tenderly apply
Some remedies for life.**
(A Winter's Tale III, ii, William Shakespeare)

In this second edition, we still emphasize the importance of the simple staging system (fully described below), as a fundamental part of our approach to the management of the diabetic foot. By applying the staging process to all diabetic foot patients it is possible, through one simple assessment, to detect the conditions that need addressing and plan their treatment using simple but fundamental principles.

- Where there are high plantar pressures in the neuropathic foot leading to callus, or abnormal mechanical forces on the margins of the neuroischaemic foot, then the pressure must be relieved
- The ulcer is a pivotal event on the road to amputation and needs specialist treatment
- Ischaemia and infection are the greatest dangers faced by the diabetic foot patient
- When significant ischaemia is found in conjunction with a foot ulcer then urgent vascular intervention should be sought
- If infection is present it must be eradicated
- Good control of diabetes helps to prevent complications and heal foot problems
- Patients and health-care professionals who have been educated effectively are safer than patients and health-care professionals who are ignorant.

The importance of all the above points is reflected in the structure of the simple staging system.

We prefer to make the assessment simple, and *treatment-based*. We omit any non-essential aspects, which sometimes form a part of other assessment systems and make them unnecessarily complicated. For example, when examining ulcers we feel that the differences between a superficial ulcer and a deep ulcer do not really change the treatment and small shallow ulcers which go wrong can destroy the foot.

The simple staging system has therefore been developed as a practical, treatment-based tool that provides a framework for diagnosing and managing the diabetic foot, and this chapter describes the application of this system through:

- Practical assessment, which consists of history-taking, examination and investigations
- Classification of the diabetic foot into the neuropathic and neuroischaemic foot
- Staging the foot. The six specific stages in the natural history of the diabetic foot (Table 1.1) are described in this chapter
- Management plan for each stage.

The clinical assessment we describe is quick and simple, but will enable the practitioner to make a basic classification and staging and the foot can then be placed into the correct stage, which has specific implications for treatment. Investigations will be needed to assess severity so as to determine treatment.

Following this system will enable the practitioner to make rapid, effective decisions that will detect problems early, organize rapid treatment and prevent deterioration and progression.

Table 1.1 Stages of the diabetic foot

Stage 1	Normal foot
Stage 2	High-risk foot
Stage 3	Ulcerated foot
Stage 4	Infected foot
Stage 5	Necrotic foot
Stage 6	Unsalvageable foot

A Practical Manual of Diabetic Foot Care, 2nd edition, Edmonds, Foster and Sanders.
Published 2008 Blackwell Publishing. ISBN 978-1-4051-61473

PRACTICAL ASSESSMENT

This can be divided into three parts:
- History-taking
- Examination
- Investigations.

History

Patients should be encouraged to be open and non-defensive. The history can be divided into the following sections:
- Presenting complaint
- Past foot history
- Diabetic history
- Past medical history
- Drug history
- Family history
- Psychosocial history.

Presenting complaint
Be aware that some patients may be asymptomatic due to neuropathy.

The presenting complaint is usually one or more of the following:
- Skin breakdown
- Oedema
- Colour change
- Pain, discomfort and abnormal sensations.

For skin breakdown, oedema and colour change or any other presenting complaints, the following questions may be helpful:
- Where is the problem?
- When did it start?
- How did it start?
- What makes it better?
- What makes it worse?
- How has it been treated?

As regards pain, this may be a specific complaint alone or it may accompany the above problems. Pain is always a significant symptom in the diabetic foot and should be taken very seriously. Pain may arise locally or it may be diffuse. Local sources may originate from bone, joint and soft tissue including skin and subcutaneous tissue. Generalized pain in both feet suggests neuropathy. Diffuse pain in a single foot suggests ischaemia. However, pain in the ischaemic foot should not always be blamed on reduced arterial perfusion because it may be caused by infection, and infection in the ischaemic patient will rapidly destroy the foot unless quickly treated.

In the neuropathic foot, severe infections can cause pain or throbbing. Pain around an ulcer suggests infection or ischaemia. Throbbing suggests infection. The following questions should be asked about pain:
- When did it start?
- How did it start?
- Was there an injury? Neuropathic patients are often unaware of injury
- Where is the pain?
- What is its nature?
- What aggravates the pain?
- What relieves the pain?
- When does it occur?
- Is it related to time of day or activity?
- What treatments have been given so far?

Clinical tips to diagnose pain due to neuropathy and ischaemia are shown in Table 1.2.

Patients may not complain of pain itself but of other abnormal sensations which would suggest neuropathy:
- Pins and needles (paraesthesiae)
- Unpleasant tingling (dysaesthesiae)
- Tightness (as if a constricting band is around the foot)
- A subjective feeling of coldness (which the patient may erroneously attribute to ischaemia) even though the temperature of the feet is warm
- A burning sensation
- Heaviness
- Numbness ('my feet feel as if they don't belong to me').

After discussing the presenting complaint, the rest of

Table 1.2 Clinical tips on pain

Pain due to neuropathy
- Burning pain with contact discomfort in both feet and lower legs which may also involve the thighs
- Sharp shooting (lancinating) or lightning pains like electric shocks, lasting a few seconds
- Pain relieved by cold
- Pain worse during periods of rest
- Unilateral burning pain in the leg with muscle wasting suggests a focal neuropathy, commonly a femoral neuropathy

Pain due to ischaemia
- Persistent pain, worse on elevation and relieved by dependency (hanging the leg out of bed)
- Pain in the calf on exercise relieved by rest (claudication). However, claudication is often absent in ischaemia because of concurrent neuropathy and the distal distribution of the arterial disease
- Feet with severe ischaemia may have little pain because of neuropathy

the history-taking is devoted to gathering important relevant information about the patient to aid diagnosis and management. This information can be acquired from various sources including direct questioning of the patient or his family, the patient's medical notes and the referral letter.

Past foot history
- Previous ulcers and treatment; other foot problems such as Charcot's osteoarthropathy, etc.
- Amputations:
  Major
  Minor
- Peripheral angioplasties
- Peripheral arterial bypasses.

Diabetic history
- Type of diabetes
- Duration of diabetes
- Treatment of diabetes:
  Insulin
  Oral hypoglycaemics.

Complications of diabetes
Retinopathy
- Background
- Proliferative
- Previous laser therapy
- Vitrectomy
- Cataract.

Nephropathy
- Proteinuria
- Severe renal impairment (estimated glomerular filtration rate [eGFR] ≤ 30 mL/min)
- Renal replacement therapy:
  Continuous ambulatory peritoneal dialysis (CAPD)
  Haemodialysis
  Renal transplant.

Cardiovascular
- Angina
- Heart failure
- Myocardial infarction
- Coronary artery angioplasty
- Coronary artery bypass.

Cerebrovascular
- Transient ischaemic attack
- Stroke.

Past medical history
- Serious illness (e.g. cancer, rheumatoid arthritis, etc.)
- Accidents
- Injuries
- Hospital admissions
- Operations.

Drug history
- Present medication
- Known allergies.

Family history
- Diabetes
- Other serious illness
- Cause of death of near relatives.

Psychosocial history
- Occupation
- Number of cigarettes smoked per day
- Number of units of alcohol per day
- Psychiatric illness; drug or alcohol dependency, etc.
- Home circumstances:
  Type of accommodation
  Lives alone
  Lives with friends or relatives.

Examination

There is a need for sensitivity on the part of the examiner. Many elderly patients find it difficult to describe their symptoms accurately and extreme patience is needed to draw out the required information. Many people will be fearful and anxious at their first visit. If, rarely, they have ischaemia but no neuropathy, or they have a severely infected foot, then they will be afraid that the examination will be painful. Other patients may be embarrassed about their feet, or may have very sensitive and ticklish feet. Before the feet are handled the patient should be reassured that the examination will not be painful and that everything will be explained. The feet should be grasped gently but firmly, and poking, prodding and tickling should be avoided. The toes should be separated gently: if they are pulled apart violently the skin between the toes may split.

The examination should be performed systematically. It consists of five parts:
- Inspection
- Palpation
- Neurological assessment
- Footwear assessment
- General examination.

Inspection

The feet should be fully examined in a systematic fashion: first the right and then the left, including dorsum, sole, medial border, lateral border, back of the heel, malleoli and interdigital areas, with a full assessment of the following:

- Skin
- Corns and callus
- Nails
- Oedema
- Deformity
- Limited joint mobility
- Colour
- Necrosis.

Skin

The general features of the skin should be assessed, especially looking for signs of skin breakdown.

In the neuropathic foot, the skin is dry and fissured and prominent dilated veins secondary to autonomic neuropathy may be visible. Hair loss can be a sign of neuropathy as well as ischaemia. Atrophy of the subcutaneous layer with a thin, shiny, wrinkled skin may indicate ischaemia.

The classical sign of skin breakdown is the foot ulcer. Ulcer assessment is described in Chapter 4. Abrasions, bullae and fissures also represent breakdown of the skin. Bullae are often the first sign of skin breakdown in the ischaemic foot. They are also a feature of fungal skin infections (tinea pedis), as is webspace maceration. Dry skin around the heel will form deep fissures unless an emollient is applied regularly (Fig. 1.1).

Look for other skin lesions, on the leg as well as the foot, including:

- Necrobiosis lipoidica diabeticorum
- Shin spots (diabetic dermopathy).

Necrobiosis lipoidica diabeticorum (NLD) is characterized as well-circumscribed red papules that extend radially with waxy atrophic telangiectatic centres (Fig. 1.2a,b). NLD evolves to ulceration in about one-third of cases and a case has been reported of association with malignancy.

The round or oval macular hyperpigmented lesions of diabetic dermopathy (Fig. 1.3) are found in the anterior tibial region.

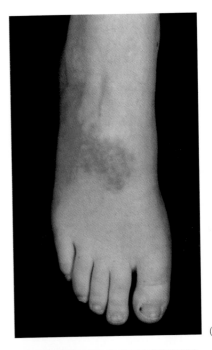

(a)

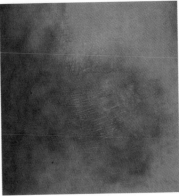

(b)

Fig. 1.2 (a) Necrobiosis lipoidica diabeticorum (NLD) on dorsum of foot. (b) Close-up of NLD.

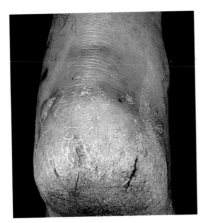

Fig. 1.1 Fissures are a portal of entry for infection and can lead to severe ulceration.

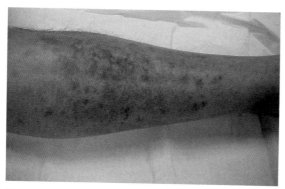

Fig. 1.3 Diabetic dermopathy.

As well as skin lesions specific to the diabetic foot, it is important to recognize inflammatory skin disease such as psoriasis, eczema and dermatitis, which also occur in non-diabetic patients but may complicate the diabetic foot and leg.

Corns and callus

These are thickened areas of keratosis which develop at sites of high pressure and friction (Fig. 1.4). Corns are discrete areas, usually not more than 1 cm in diameter, and can extend to a depth of several millimetres. Callus forms diffuse plaques. Neither should be allowed to become excessive as this is a common forerunner of ulceration (usually in the presence of neuropathy) and urgent action should be taken to deflect pressure from the area. Haemorrhage within callus is an important precursor of ulceration.

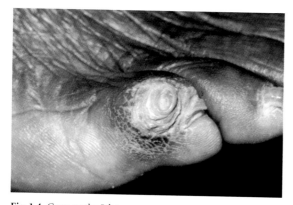

Fig. 1.4 Corn on the 5th toe.

Nails

It is important to inspect the nails closely as the nail bed and periungual tissues may become the site of ulceration. (Problems with nails are discussed fully in Chapter 2). The following should be assessed:

- Structure of the nails
- Colour of the nail bed
- Abnormalities under the nail
- Signs of nail infections.

Structure of the nails

Thickened nails are common in the population at large. If the shoes press on thickened nails they may cause bleeding under the nail. Eventually this may lead to ulceration. Atrophic nails may be present in patients with neuropathy and ischaemia.

Ingrowing toe nail (onychocryptosis) arises when the nail plate is excessively wide and thin, or develops a convex deformity, putting pressure on the tissues at the nail edge. Callus builds up in response to pressure and inflammation. Eventually, usually after incorrect nail cutting (when the nail is cut incompletely leaving behind a splinter of nail at the side which grows into the sulcus) or trauma, the nail penetrates the flesh.

Colour of nail bed

Red, brown or black discolouration of the nails may indicate subungual haematoma. The cause may be acute trauma or chronic trauma such as pressure from ill-fitting shoes (Fig. 1.5a).

In acute ischaemia the nail beds are very pale (Fig. 1.5b).

Abnormalities under the nail

Discharge of fluid from beneath or around the nail, and any maceration or softness of the nail plate, may reveal the presence of a subungual ulcer or infection.

Nail infections

Fungal infection of the nail usually invades the nail plate dorsally causing onycholysis, where the nail comes away from the nail bed and is often thickened. The hallux nail is most commonly affected. Infection starts in one corner and over a period of years it spreads to involve the entire toe nail and may affect other nails.

Paronychia is associated with a nail that has a convex nail bed with tendency to incurve in the corners. Repetitive pressure in the insensitive foot can cause microtrauma in the nail groove, causing the nail to act as a foreign body thus creating a foreign body inflammatory response with secondary inflammation and localized infection (Fig. 1.6).

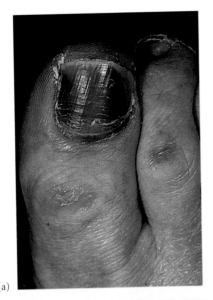

(a)

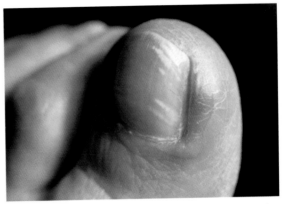

Fig. 1.6 Pressure on the sulcus from a convex nail has resulted in inflammation with secondary infection.

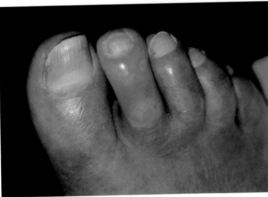

(b)

Fig. 1.5 (a) Subungual haematoma and red marks on toes resulting from wearing tight shoes. (b) Acute ischaemia—pale nail beds.

Oedema

Oedema is a major factor in predisposing patients to ulceration and delaying healing, and often exacerbates a tight fit inside poorly fitting shoes. The cause of oedema in the foot must be vigorously pursued and treated appropriately.

In patients on dialysis, oedema often fluctuates and becomes most marked just before dialysis. Appropriate arrangements need to be made for provision of adjustable footwear.

Oedema also impedes healing of established ulcers. It may be bilateral or unilateral and may involve the foot or be limited to the toes.

Causes of bilateral foot oedema include:
- Cardiac failure
- Renal impairment secondary to diabetic nephropathy
- Chronic venous insufficiency (sometimes unilateral)
- Rarely, neuropathic oedema secondary to diabetic neuropathy, when it is related to increased arterial blood flow and arteriovenous shunting
- Primary lymphoedema
- Secondary lymphoedema related to previous recurrent bilateral foot infections
- Severe ischaemia associated with dependency (often unilateral).

Causes of unilateral foot oedema are usually associated with local pathology in the foot or leg. These include:
- Infection, when it is usually associated with erythema and a break in the skin
- Charcot foot (a unilateral hot, red, oedematous foot; sometimes the oedema can extend to the knee)
- Gout, which may also present as a painful, hot, red, oedematous foot
- Trauma, fracture, muscle or tendon rupture, often associated with bruising
- Deep vein thrombosis
- Venous insufficiency
- Secondary lymphoedema due to malignancy or previous infection in the lower limb
- Common peroneal nerve palsy
- Localized collection of blood or pus in the foot, which may present as a fluctuant swelling
- In the early postoperative phase of revascularization of a limb.

In the tropics, filaria may be the cause of lymphoedema.

Chronic post-phlebitic limbs develop lymphoedema

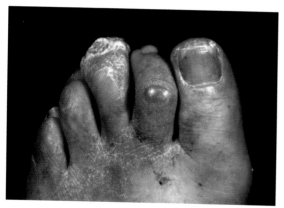

Fig. 1.7 Gout with tophi on second toe.

following repeated deep vein thromboses, with ligneous changes to the soft tissues.

Oedema of the toe can be due to:

* Trauma
* Fracture
* Soft tissue infection
* Osteomyelitis
* Gout (Fig. 1.7)
* Charcot toe.

Deformity

Common deformities include:

* Pes cavus
* Fibrofatty padding depletion (FFPD) or displacement
* Hammer toes
* Claw toes
* Hallux valgus
* Charcot foot
* Deformities related to previous trauma and surgery.

Pes cavus

Normally the dorsum of the foot is domed due to the medial longitudinal arch, which extends between the first metatarsal head and the calcaneus. When it is abnormally high, the deformity is called pes cavus and leads to reduction of the area of the foot in contact with the ground during walking. Resulting abnormal distribution of pressure leads to excessive callus formation and ulceration under the metatarsal heads. This deformity is a sign of a motor neuropathy but may be idiopathic. It is often associated with clawing of lesser toes or a trigger first toe.

Fibrofatty padding depletion (FFPD) or displacement

A common complication is reduction of the thickness of the fibrofatty padding over the metatarsal heads (Fig. 1.8a,b).

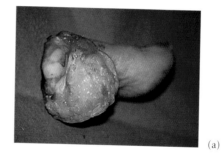

(a)

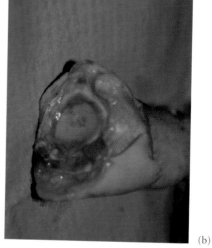

(b)

Fig. 1.8 (a) Amputation specimen from 29-year-old non-diabetic patient showing thick fibrofatty padding. (b) Amputation specimen from 29-year-old diabetic patient with history of neuropathy and ulceration showing great reduction in fibrofatty padding.

Normal feet contain cushions of fibrofatty padding over the metatarsal heads which absorb plantar pressures. In diabetic neuropathy the fibrofatty padding may be pushed forward or depleted by previous ulceration, rendering the plantar metatarsophalangeal area a site of abnormally high pressures and prone to ulceration.

Hammer toes

A hammer toe is a flexible or rigid deformity characterized by buckling of the toe. The toe takes on the configuration of a swan's neck. In people with diabetic neuropathy, hammer toes are commonly caused by weakness of the small intrinsic muscles (interossei and lumbricals) of the foot, which can no longer stabilize the toes on the ground. Muscle imbalance results in the affected toes sitting slightly back and up on the metatarsal head.

This deformity results in increased pressure over the metatarsal head, over the prominent interphalangeal joint and at the tip of the toe.

Claw toes

Claw toes are similar to hammer toes, but with more buckling and greater deformity. There is fixed flexion deformity at the interphalangeal joint, associated with callus and ulceration of the apex and dorsal aspect of the interphalangeal joint. Although claw toes may be related to neuropathy, they are often unrelated, especially when the clawing is unilateral and associated with trauma or surgery of the forefoot. Claw toes may rarely result from acute rupture of the plantar fascia.

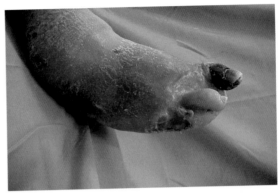

Fig. 1.9 Inversion deformity following surgical debridement.

Hallux valgus

Hallux valgus is a deformity of the first metatarsophalangeal joint with lateral deviation of the hallux and a medial prominence on the margin of the foot. This site is particularly vulnerable in the neuroischaemic foot and frequently breaks down under pressure from a tight shoe.

Charcot foot

Bone and joint damage in the tarsometatarsal joints and mid-tarsal joints leads to two classical deformities: the rocker-bottom deformity, in which there is displacement and subluxation of the tarsus downwards, and the medial convexity, which results from displacement of the talonavicular joint or from tarsometatarsal dislocation. Both are often associated with a bony prominence which is very prone to ulceration and healing is notoriously difficult.

When the ankle and subtalar joints are involved, instability of the hindfoot can result. These patients with hindfoot Charcot's osteoarthropathy are far more difficult to manage than patients with Charcot joints in the forefoot or mid-foot.

Deformities related to previous trauma and surgery

Deformities of the hip and fractures of the tibia or fibula lead to shortening of the leg and abnormal gait, which predisposes to foot ulceration. Ray amputations remove the toe together with part of the metatarsal. They are usually very successful but disturb the biomechanics of the foot leading to high pressure under the adjacent metatarsal heads. After amputation of a toe, deformities are often seen in adjoining toes. We have seen three cases of development of a grossly inverted foot following 5th ray amputation where tendon attachments of the peroneal muscles to the base of the 5th metatarsal were destroyed (Fig. 1.9).

Limited joint mobility (including hallux rigidus)

Limited joint mobility can affect the feet as well as the hands and involves the ankle, subtalar, mid-tarsal and toe joints. The range of movements in these joints will partially depend on the age of the patient but can be reduced by diabetes itself. In the diabetic foot, the two main joints to test are the ankle and the first metatarsophalangeal joint. For both of these joints the range of dorsiflexion and plantarflexion should be tested. Limited joint mobility of the first metatarsophalangeal joint results in excessive forces on the plantar surface of the first toe, which is unable to dorsiflex at the toe-off phase of the gait cycle, causing callus formation and ulceration on the underside of the hallux. It is common in barefooted and sandal-wearing populations. A plantar-flexed foot, with limitation of movement at the ankle joint commonly leads to plantar forefoot ulceration.

Colour

It is important to observe the colour of the foot including the toes. Colour changes may be localized or diffuse. Common colour changes are red, blue, white or black (Fig. 1.10).

Causes of the red foot

- Cellulitis
- Critical ischaemia, especially on dependency (dependent rubor)
- Charcot foot
- Gout
- Burn or scald.

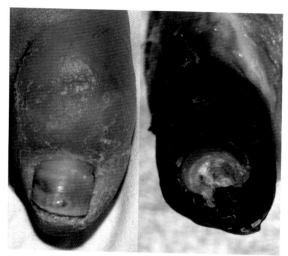

Fig. 1.10 Toes; red, and black. The red toe has cellulitis, and the black toe is gangrenous.

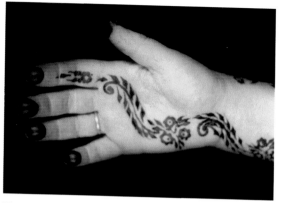

Fig. 1.11 Henna has been applied to this hand. Note the black fingertips. This can be mistaken for gangrene.

Causes of the red toe
- Cellulitis
- Osteomyelitis
- Ischaemia
- Gout
- Chilblains
- Dermatitis/eczema.

Causes of the blue foot
- Cardiac failure
- Chronic pulmonary disease
- Venous insufficency (often with brownish pigmentation—haemosiderosis).

Causes of the blue toe
- Severe infection
- Ischaemia.

The foot may have a pale white appearance in severe ischaemia, especially on elevation. In acute ischaemia, the foot is pale, often with purplish mottling. Emboli to the digital arteries can also result in a blue toe. In Raynaud's disease if there is acute vasospasm the toe becomes white.

Necrosis

Areas of necrosis and gangrene can be identified by the presence of black or brown devitalized tissue. Such tissue may be wet (usually related to infection) or dry.

Causes of the black toe
- Severe chronic ischaemia
- Acute ischaemia
- Emboli
- Bruise
- Blood blister
- Shoe dye
- Dirt
- Application of henna (Fig. 1.11)
- Tumour (melanoma).

Palpation

Palpation should take place to assess:
- Pulses
- Temperature of the foot
- Oedema
- Crepitus.

Pulses

The most important manoeuvre to detect ischaemia is the palpation of foot pulses, an examination which is often undervalued.
- The dorsalis pedis pulse is palpated, using the index, middle and ring fingertips together, lateral to the extensor hallucis longus tendon on the dorsum of the foot (Fig. 1.12)
- The posterior tibial pulse is palpated below and behind the medial malleolus (Fig. 1.13).

If either of these foot pulses can be felt then it is highly unlikely that there is significant ischaemia in the foot.

If both pulses are absent, the patient should undergo Doppler examination to measure the ankle brachial pressure index and to record the blood velocity profile or sonogram. This is described under Investigations, below.

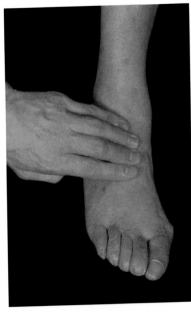

Fig. 1.12 Palpation of the dorsalis pedis pulse.

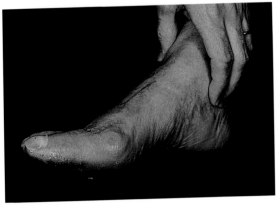

Fig. 1.13 Palpating the posterior tibial pulse.

Classically, in the neuropathic foot, the pulses are bounding, with a high volume.

Temperature of the foot

Skin temperature is compared between both feet with the back of the examining hand. Normally any one area on a foot will be within 2°C of the corresponding area on the other foot. Warm areas or hot spots outside this range indicate inflammation which may be due to infection, fracture, Charcot's osteoarthropathy or soft tissue trauma. An increase in unilateral pedal temperature, especially in the absence of ulceration, is best presumed to be Charcot's osteoarthropathy.

The temperature gradient is checked by using the back of the hands and gently moving them from the pretibial region of the leg distally over the dorsum of the foot to the toes while keeping in contact with the patient's skin. An asymmetric gradient may indicate either unilateral ischaemia on the colder side or unilateral inflammatory response such as Charcot's osteoarthropathy or infection on the warmer side.

In the neuroischaemic foot, coexisting autonomic neuropathy may keep the foot relatively warm, although an ice-cold foot is indicative of acute ischaemia.

Patients with neuropathy frequently complain of having cold feet when their feet are in fact warm.

Causes of the hot foot
- Soft tissue injury or fracture
- Cellulitis
- Charcot foot
- Gout
- Deep vein thrombosis.

Causes of the cold foot
- Chronic ischaemia
- Acute ischaemia
- Cardiac failure.

Patients on a very cold day may present with cold feet which merely reflect a severe vasoconstriction in response to a cold environment. It is sometimes difficult to differentiate this from the ice-cold ischaemic foot; however, the latter will remain cold in the clinic whereas the former will gradually warm up.

Oedema

Oedema already suspected on inspection can be confirmed by gentle digital pressure applied for a few seconds.

Crepitus

Very occasionally palpation may reveal gas in tissues as a fine crackling sensation.

Neurological assessment

Simple inspection will usually reveal signs of motor and autonomic neuropathy but sensory neuropathy must be detected by a sensory screening test or a simple sensory examination.

Motor neuropathy

The classical sign of a motor neuropathy is a high medial longitudinal arch, leading to prominent metatarsal heads and pressure points over the plantar forefoot.

Complicated assessment of motor power in the foot or leg is not usually necessary, but it is advisable to test dorsiflexion of the foot to detect a foot drop secondary to a common peroneal nerve palsy, which is usually unilateral and will affect the patient's gait. If pain is present in one leg only, a more detailed neurological examination is indicated to rule out compressive lesions of nerve roots supplying the lower limb—see under Painful neuropathy in Chapter 3.

Autonomic neuropathy

Signs of an autonomic neuropathy include a dry skin with fissuring and distended veins over the dorsum of the foot.

The dry skin is secondary to decreased sweating. The sweating loss normally occurs in a stocking distribution, which can extend up to the knee. The distended veins are secondary to arteriovenous shunting associated with autonomic neuropathy (Fig. 1.14).

Sensory neuropathy

An important indication of neuropathy will be a patient who has no pain even when significant foot lesions are present. Painless ulceration is definite evidence of a peripheral neuropathy. It is important to detect patients who have sufficient neuropathy to render them susceptible to foot ulceration. This can be carried out using a monofilament which, when applied perpendicular to the foot, buckles at a given force of 10 g. Ability to feel that level of pressure provides protective sensation against foot

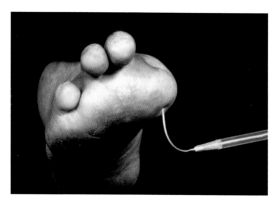

Fig. 1.15 A monofilament is applied perpendicular to the foot and pressed until it buckles at a given force of 10 g.

ulceration. It is helpful first to demonstrate the technique on the patient's forearm.

The number of sites tested varies according to different protocols. Sites examined include the plantar aspects of the first toe, the first, third and fifth metatarsal heads, the plantar surface of the heel and the dorsum of the foot. The filament should not be applied at any site until callus has been removed. If the patient cannot feel the filament at any of the tested areas, then protective pain sensation is lost, indicating susceptibility to foot ulceration (Fig. 1.15). The 10-g monofilament may become overstrained and inaccurate after use on numerous occasions and should be replaced regularly. A study has assessed differences in the performance of commercially available 10-g monofilaments. Monofilaments were tested using a calibrated load cell. Each monofilament was subjected to 10 mechanical bucklings of 10 mm while the load cell detected the maximal buckling force. Longevity testing was performed on a subset of the monofilaments by subjecting them to continuous compression until the buckling force was less than 9 g. Longevity and recovery testing suggest that each monofilament would survive usage on 10 patients before needing a recovery time of 24 hours before further usage.

If filaments are not available, then a simple clinical examination detecting sensation to light touch using a cotton wisp and vibration using a 128 Hz tuning fork will suffice. A recent study showed that the tuning fork is a valid and reliable test in screening for polyneuropathy and was superior to the monofilament. When using the tuning fork, it is best to compare a proximal site with a distal site to confirm a symmetrical stocking-like distribution of the neuropathy. The use of 'pin-prick' to detect sensory loss should be avoided.

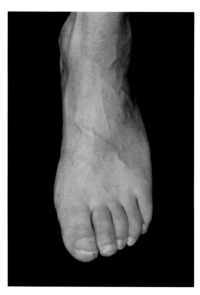

Fig. 1.14 Distended veins secondary to autonomic neuropathy.

Other useful but simple and practical tests for detecting neuropathy, if health-care practitioners have no access to formal equipment, include the Achilles tendon pinch, and the application of vertical pressure onto the nail plate. In practice, any patient who walks on a foot with ulceration or heavy plantar callus without concern has significant neuropathy.

Footwear assessment

It is important to examine both shoes and socks.

Examination of patient's footwear

- Is the shoe long enough?
- Is the toe box broad and deep enough?
- Are the heels low (below 5 cm)?
- Does the shoe fasten with a lace or strap to prevent friction? Slip-ons are unsuitable for everyday wear.
- Is the sole thick enough to provide protection from puncture wounds?
- Is the shoe lining worn, with rough areas that may prove irritating and warrant replacement?
- Are there foreign bodies within the shoes?
- Is there excessive wear under hallux suggesting a hallux rigidus?
- Is there wear across the whole of the tread suggesting pes cavus?
- Does the shoe avoid pressure points over the toes or margins of the feet?
- Does the heel cup fit snugly round the heel?
- What other types of shoes does the patient wear and when? Patients should be advised not to wear slippers around the house.

Examination of patient's socks

- Are the socks large enough?
- Are the seams too prominent?
- Is there a tight band at the top?
- Are the socks in good repair—no holes or lumpy darns?
- Are the socks made of absorbent material?
- Are the socks very thick, taking up too much space in the shoe?

General examination

As part of the diabetic foot assessment, and indeed the diabetic assessment, all patients should have a physical examination including the following systems:

- Cardiovascular
- Respiratory
- Abdomen

- Eyes:
  Visual acuity
  Fundi.

(A patient lacking necessary visual acuity to give himself a daily foot examination is a patient at risk, and his family or caregiver should help him.)

Investigations

Investigations include:
- Neurological
- Vascular
- Skin temperature
- Laboratory
- Radiological
- Foot pressures.

Neurological

The degree of neuropathy can be quantified by the use of the neurothesiometer (Fig. 1.16). When applied to the foot, it delivers a vibratory stimulus that increases as the voltage is raised. The vibration threshold increases with age, and, for practical purposes, any patient unable to feel a vibratory stimulus of ≥ 25 volts is at risk of ulceration.

A small number of patients have a small-fibre neuropathy with impaired pain and temperature perception but with intact touch and vibration. They are prone to ulceration and thermal traumas but test normally with filaments and neurothesiometer, and a clinical assessment of light touch and vibration is normal. As yet, there is no simple inexpensive method of detecting and quantifying small-fibre neuropathy. However, a simple temperature assessment of cold sensation can be made by placing a cold tuning fork on the patient's foot and leg.

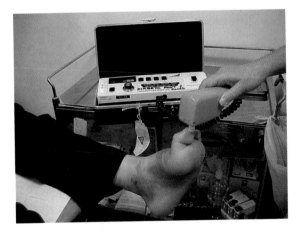

Fig. 1.16 The neurothesiometer.

Vascular

A small hand-held Doppler can be used to quantify the vascular status.

Used together with a sphygmomanometer, the brachial systolic pressure and ankle systolic pressure can be measured, and the pressure index, which is the ratio of ankle systolic pressure to brachial systolic pressure, can be calculated. In normal subjects, the pressure index is usually > 1, but in the presence of ischaemia is < 1. Thus, absent pulses and a pressure index of < 1 confirms ischaemia. Conversely, the presence of pulses and a pressure index of > 1 rules out ischaemia; this has important implications for management, namely that macrovascular disease is not an important factor and further vascular investigations are not necessary.

Many diabetic patients have medial arterial calcification, giving an artificially elevated systolic pressure, even in the presence of ischaemia. It is thus difficult to assess the diabetic foot when the pulses are not palpable, but the pressure index is > 1. There are two explanations:

- The examiner may have missed the pulses, particularly in an oedematous foot, and should go back to palpate the foot after the arteries have been located by Doppler ultrasound
- If the pulses remain impalpable, then ischaemia probably exists in the presence of medial wall calcification. It is then necessary to use other methods to assess flow in the arteries of the foot, such as examining the pattern of the Doppler arterial waveform or measuring transcutaneous oxygen tension or toe systolic pressures. Furthermore, absence of foot pulses would be an indication to investigate popliteal and femoral arteries.

Skin temperature

It is helpful to follow-up the clinical assessment of skin temperature with the use of a digital skin thermometer. An infrared thermometer is ideal and skin temperatures are compared between similar areas on each foot. This is particularly helpful in the management of the Charcot foot.

Laboratory

Laboratory investigations are determined by clinical findings, but the following investigations are useful as a baseline in most patients:

- Full blood count (to detect anaemia or polycythaemia), and white blood cell count (to reflect the presence of infection)
- Serum electrolytes, urea and creatinine (to assess baseline renal function)
- Serum bilirubin, alkaline phosphatase, gamma glutamyl transferase, aspartate transaminase (to assess baseline liver function)
- Blood glucose and HbA_{1c} (to assess diabetic control)
- Serum cholesterol and triglycerides (to assess arterial disease risk factors)
- C-reactive protein (as an acute inflammatory marker).

Radiological

These will be determined by the clinical presentation, and may not always be necessary. However, in most cases, an X-ray of the foot will be required to detect:

- Osteomyelitis
- Fracture/dislocation
- Charcot foot
- Gas in soft tissues
- Foreign body.

CASE STUDY
Foreign body

A 45-year-old woman with type 2 diabetes of 8 years' duration trod on a nail whilst decorating her house. She removed the nail and was seen in a casualty department and given tetanus prophylaxis. Subsequently she noticed a discomfort at the site of penetration of the nail, which was associated with a focal swelling of the soft tissues. This persisted for several months and she eventually presented at the diabetic foot clinic, where an X-ray showed a possible radio-opaque body adjacent to the head of the first metatarsal (Fig. 1.17a,b). An MRI showed increased signal from a possibly metallic object, and during the MRI she reported increased pain and burning in her foot which may have been related to movement of the metallic fragment within the magnetic field. An ultrasound showed a 4 × 5 mm hypoechoic area of granulomatous tissue just below the skin. There was a ring-down type artefact within it suggestive of focal dense material. The patient underwent surgery and a metallic fragment was removed.

Key points
- Persistent discomfort after a puncture injury may indicate a persisting foreign body
- It is important to X-ray the foot even though the foreign body has apparently been removed
- An ultrasound is a useful means of investigating foreign bodies.

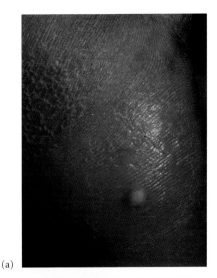

(a)

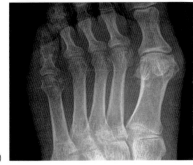

(b)

Fig. 1.17 (a) Focal swelling of the soft tissues at site of penetration of nail. (b) A radio-opaque foreign body adjacent to 5th metatarsal head.

Foot pressures

These techniques measure the pressure distribution on the plantar surface of the foot. There are two main methods: 'out-of-shoe' and 'in-shoe'. The introduction of the optical pedobarograph considerably improved the accuracy of out-of-shoe pressure measurements. Developments in computer technology have led to microprocessor-like recording devices to quantify in-shoe foot pressures and these include the EMED system and the F-Scan system. These systems have the possibility of identifying patients at risk of plantar neuropathic ulceration and give a basis for the implementation of footwear adjustments or surgical intervention. We have found that they are also useful educational tools as described in Chapter 3.

CLASSIFICATION AND STAGING

After completing this basic assessment, it will now be possible to classify the diabetic foot and distinguish between the neuropathic foot and the neuroischaemic foot, as for practical purposes, the diabetic foot can be divided into these two distinct entities. Neuropathy is nearly always found in association with ischaemia, so the ischaemic foot is best called the neuroischaemic foot. In rare cases the foot may clinically be ischaemic without signs of neuropathy, but in practice, the diabetic ischaemic foot is treated in the same way as the neuroischaemic foot.

It is essential to classify the diabetic foot in this way by differentiating between the neuropathic and the neuroischaemic foot as their management will differ in many respects, and the particular vulnerability of the ischaemic foot renders recognition essential, ischaemia being a most important factor on the pathway to major amputation.

Usually there will be no doubt as to which category the foot should be placed in. However, if the examiner has any doubt as to the correct classification, then the foot should be regarded as neuroischaemic, because if a neuroischaemic foot is wrongly classified as neuropathic, with resulting failure to do further tests to confirm ischaemia and adapt the care plan accordingly, this may lead to preventable catastrophe and loss of the foot.

With the passage of time, nearly every neuropathic foot will become ischaemic. Thus it is very important to reassess diabetic feet annually so as to detect patients who drift from the neuropathic to the neuroischaemic foot.

Neuropathic foot

- The neuropathic foot is a warm, well-perfused foot with bounding pulses and distended dorsal veins due to arteriovenous shunting
- Sweating is diminished so skin and any callus tend to be hard and dry and prone to fissuring
- Toes are clawed and the arch of the foot may be raised
- Ulceration commonly develops on the sole of the foot, associated with neglected callus and high plantar pressures
- Despite the good circulation, necrosis can develop secondary to severe infection
- The neuropathic foot is also prone to bone and joint problems which we refer to as Charcot's osteoarthropathy.

Neuroischaemic foot

- The neuroischaemic foot is a cool, pulseless foot with poor perfusion and almost invariably also has neuropathy

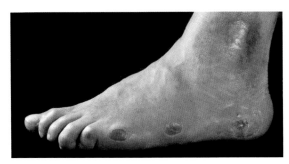

Fig. 1.18 Neuroischaemic foot with ulceration on the margins.

- The colour of the severely ischaemic foot can be a deceptively healthy pink or red caused by dilatation of capillaries in an attempt to improve perfusion
- The neuroischaemic foot may be complicated by oedema, often secondary to cardiac failure or renal impairment
- Ischaemic ulcers are commonly seen around the edges of the foot, including the apices of the toes and the back of the heel, and are associated with trauma or wearing unsuitable shoes (Fig. 1.18)
- The neuroischaemic foot develops necrosis in the presence of infection or if tissue perfusion is critically diminished
- Even if neuropathy is present and plantar pressures are high, plantar ulceration is rare. This is probably because the foot does not develop heavy callus, which requires good blood flow.

After classification of the diabetic foot, it is necessary to make the appropriate staging in its natural history.

The natural history of the diabetic foot can be divided into six stages as shown:

- Stage 1: Normal foot
- Stage 2: High-risk foot
- Stage 3: Ulcerated foot
- Stage 4: Infected foot
- Stage 5: Necrotic foot
- Stage 6: Unsalvageable foot.

The simple staging system covers the entire spectrum of diabetic foot disease but it emphasizes the development of the foot ulcer in stage 3 as a pivotal event demanding urgent and aggressive management. However, each stage demands specific treatment.

Other classifications of the diabetic foot are essentially classifications of ulcers and do not cover the whole natural history of the diabetic foot: they may be useful for researchers who want to compare like with like, but are not a practical framework on which treatments can be based.

The simple staging system used in this book has been created to allow all practitioners, whether experienced in diabetic foot care or not, to make an initial assessment of the diabetic foot at whatever stage in the natural history it might be. The stage sets the place in the natural history and also determines treatment. The aim is to keep all diabetic feet at as low a stage as possible.

Stage 1

At this stage, the patient does not have the risk factors of neuropathy, ischaemia, deformity, callus and oedema. The patient is not vulnerable to foot ulcers. The patient's foot is free of diabetic complications but may be affected by other foot pathologies that occur in the general population. The foot is usually asymptomatic and any problems, including pain, are non-diabetic in nature.

Stage 2

The patient has developed one or more of the risk factors for foot ulceration including neuropathy, ischaemia, deformity, callus and oedema. The major risk factors are neuropathy and ischaemia and it is rare for the other three to cause problems when neuropathy and ischaemia are absent. When they are present, however, all these risk factors need addressing to reduce susceptibility to ulceration.

Patients without current active foot ulceration but with a history of previous ulceration should be regarded as at risk.

Within stage 2, there are specific conditions which are non-ulcerative but require treatment. These include:

- Severe chronic ischaemia
- Acute ischaemia.

There are also specific complications of neuropathy:

- Charcot's osteoarthropathy, including neuropathic fractures
- Painful neuropathy.

Stage 3

The foot has a skin breakdown. Although this is usually an ulcer, it is important not to underestimate apparently minor injuries such as blisters, skin fissures or grazes, all of which have a propensity to become ulcers if they are not treated correctly and fail to heal quickly. Ulceration is usually on the plantar surface in the neuropathic foot and on the margins in the neuroischaemic foot (Fig. 1.19).

Stage 4

The foot has developed infection, which can complicate both the neuropathic foot (Fig. 1.19) and the neuroischaemic foot (Fig. 1.19).

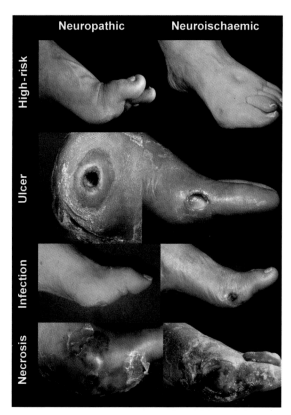

Fig. 1.19 Composite picture to show the natural history of the neuropathic and neuroischaemic foot as it passes from high-risk through ulceration, infection and necrosis.

Stage 5

Necrosis has supervened. In the neuropathic foot, infection is usually the cause. In the neuroischaemic foot, infection is still the most common reason for tissue destruction although ischaemia contributes (Fig. 1.19). In some cases ischaemia alone can lead to necrosis of a previously intact foot, with slow onset of dry necrosis and necrotic toes which appear shrivelled (Fig. 1.20). The diabetic foot in the patient with renal failure (the so-called renal foot) is very prone to develop necrosis, even in the absence of infection: for management see Chapter 6.

Stage 6

The foot cannot be saved and will need a major amputation.

Reasons for major amputation:
- Extensive necrosis which has destroyed the foot
- Severe infection which puts the patient's life at risk
- Agonizing ischaemic pain which cannot be relieved

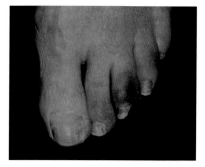

Fig. 1.20 Dry necrosis in a neuroischaemic foot.

- Unstable foot and ankle, usually secondary to Charcot's osteoarthropathy, which does not respond to external or internal fixation.

MULTIDISCIPLINARY MANAGEMENT

The aim in managing the diabetic foot is always to keep the patient at as low a stage as possible. At each stage of the diabetic foot it is necessary to take control of the foot to prevent further progression, and management will be considered under the headings shown in Table 1.3. The cornerstone of this approach to the diabetic foot is to encourage early presentation to allow early diagnosis and early intervention within the multidisciplinary diabetic foot clinic.

Multidisciplinary teams are essential for optimal management of the high-risk diabetic foot and there is no room for inter-professional rivalry. Over the years we have seen a healthy and welcome move towards the development of considerable mutual respect between team members from different specialties in many countries. We will describe the makeup and organization of the Diabetic Foot Clinic as it has evolved at King's College Hospital. While the situation we describe is not (of course) the only way of organizing patients with diabetic foot problems, it has proved to be successful in reducing amputations and improving outcomes for diabetic patients with foot problems.

Table 1.3 Multidisciplinary management

Mechanical control
Wound control
Microbiological control
Vascular control
Metabolic control
Educational control

No one person can take control of the diabetic foot. Successful management needs the expertise of a multidisciplinary team including the following:
- Podiatrist
- Physician
- Nurse
- Orthotist
- Surgeon
- Radiologist.

It is helpful if the multidisciplinary team works closely together, within the focus of a diabetic foot clinic, which ideally is situated in a hospital. It is extremely important that there is a geographical focus of diabetic foot care to serve the diabetic patients in a defined geographical area. This will be vital for patients who know where exactly to come for their routine and emergency appointments, and also vital for local health-care professionals who will know where to seek help and where to obtain advice and education. Busy diabetic foot clinics will need to be open and available to patients throughout the working week and suitable arrangements need to be made with their associated casualty departments to see patients out of office hours. This overall umbrella of care focused within a definite place is vital for the diabetic foot patient who often has multiple comorbidities and complications and needs urgent investigations and help.

The diabetic foot team should be based in such a diabetic foot clinic, and should meet regularly for joint consultations as well as for ward rounds and X-ray conferences and clinical sessions.

Some roles of team members may overlap, depending on local expertise and interest. At King's College Hospital the roles have evolved in the following ways as discussed below.

Roles of the members of the multidisciplinary diabetic foot team

Podiatrists
The podiatrists man the clinic's emergency service throughout the week, and undertake specialist wound care of ulcers, including debridement, and plaster casting for indolent ulcers and Charcot's osteoarthropathy. The podiatrists play a part in diagnosing problems, call in other members of the team, as appropriate, and also educate patients, their families and friends and other health-care professionals. They also provide routine preventive foot care.

One of the extended roles of the podiatrist in the UK is as a diabetic foot practitioner who specializes in looking after inpatients on the hospital wards. Podiatrists in the USA have become surgical specialists. Many podiatrists are now involved in clinical research. There is an urgent need for podiatry training in developing countries.

Physician
The physician plays a key role in the diagnosis of foot complications and is also crucial in the diagnosis and management of infection, working closely with the medical microbiologists. The physician also decides on the need for admission and organizes the admission, liaises with all members of the foot team and is responsible for the medical care of patients, including the management of diabetes and its complications.

Nurses
Nurses are also involved in ensuring optimal care of diabetes and its complications and in addition play an important role in the investigation of ischaemic patients, using Doppler sonography and transcutaneous oxygen and also in the assessment and management of the patient with neuropathy, including those with painful neuropathy. The health-care assistant prepares the dressing trolleys and also assists in dressing the ulcers.

Orthotists
Orthotists measure and take casts for the manufacture of insoles, shoes, orthotics and braces: they also deliver footwear education to patients and staff. The orthotists carry out joint consultations in the podiatry rooms and then measure and cast the patients in the orthotists' rooms, which are adjacent to the foot clinic.

Surgeons
Surgeons take part in joint consultations when the foot is infected to decide on the need for incision and drainage, surgical debridement and digital or ray amputation. Historically, in our Diabetic Foot Clinic, the orthopaedic surgeon works with the neuropathic patients, and one of their important roles is to assess the patient's suitability for surgical treatment of osteomyelitis. The vascular surgeon works with patients who have acute and chronic ischaemia and performs distal bypasses.

Radiologists
The interventional radiologists work in conjunction with the vascular surgeons to assess those patients suitable for revascularization of the ischaemic foot. The radiologists interpret X-rays and scans and perform angiograms and angioplasties.

Other members of the multidisciplinary team include microbiologists, physiotherapists, the rehabilitation physician and team, and the psychiatrists. The roles of all these people are very important but they do not usually work within the diabetic foot clinic.

The multidisciplinary team approach has reaped benefits both for patients and for staff in terms of expansion of traditional roles, increasing opportunities to learn from people in other disciplines, rapid access to patients and reducing numbers of hospital visits.

It is not possible for the entire team to be working together throughout the week as most people have additional responsibilities outside of the diabetic foot clinic. However, it is useful if all members of the team are accessible in an emergency in addition to having a formal commitment to work within the diabetic foot clinic with other team members at certain times. The podiatrist should be based within the diabetic foot centre throughout the entire working week, if at all possible, to maintain an emergency diabetic foot service, where walk-in patients can be seen immediately. Other members of the team will combine to see special problems under the umbrella of the diabetic foot clinic. As well as the basic day-to-day service for patients with emergency and follow-up appointments, the King's College Hospital Diabetic Foot Clinic has evolved fresh approaches to deal efficiently with an ever-increasing workload. These approaches may include:
- Joint fast-track services
- Joint ward rounds and X-ray conferences
- Specialized clinics.

Fast-track services

Joint vascular fast-track services
A joint vascular clinic can be organized to offer rapid investigations and priority treatment and regular follow-up. Many angiograms and angioplasties can now be performed on a day-case basis.

Joint orthopaedic clinics
At these clinics, selected patients with problems that may be amenable to orthopaedic surgical intervention are selected and seen at a joint clinic. Patients suitable for surgery are admitted, operated on and followed long-term.

Inpatient care

Joint ward rounds
Patients are also admitted as emergencies from the diabetic foot clinic. They are usually admitted to the medical wards under the care of the diabetologist, but when there is an overt vascular problem they are admitted directly under the vascular surgeons. While they are inpatients they are cared for by the admitting team but there is a joint ward round weekly when patients are seen together, both on the medical and surgical wards. On these rounds, the ward staff and the diabetic foot practitioner are joined by a pharmacist and the diabetic foot clinic team. They see every inpatient and discuss their medication and other aspects of their care, with a view to avoiding any delays and achieving discharge as quickly as possible.

Joint X-ray conferences
These are held weekly and are attended by the vascular surgeon and his team, the interventional radiologist, the diabetic foot practitioner and the diabetic foot team. Individual cases are discussed and treatments planned.

Other associated foot clinics have arisen within the King's College Hospital Diabetic Foot Clinic to fulfil very specialized functions within diabetic foot care. These include those discussed below.

Joint renal/foot clinic
Ideally, a podiatrist from the diabetic foot clinic should attend the renal unit for one morning a week, assessing and treating diabetic patients on dialysis or with renal transplants, and working with the renal physician and renal nurses. The feet of every patient with diabetes should be inspected at each clinic visit and additional appointments arranged as necessary. With this programme, outcomes in renal patients with diabetes were as good as those seen in diabetic patients.

Painful neuropathy clinics
At King's College Hospital these are currently run by a diabetes foot specialist nurse and a physician. Patients with painful neuropathy need considerable support and reassurance. There is a large armamentarium of different treatments which are covered in Chapter 3.

Clinics to rehabilitate diabetic amputees
Diabetic patients who have undergone a major amputation are at very high risk of developing problems in their remaining foot. Ideally they will be seen regularly by the rehabilitation physician and the physiotherapists and orthotists, together with a podiatrist who provides regular foot care and rapid referral to the diabetic foot clinic if problems develop.

Defined pathways and timescales for treatment and follow-up

Patients in stages 1 and 2 can be seen in primary care. Patients in stages 3–5 are best seen in the multidisciplinary diabetic foot clinic, which takes early referrals from a primary care service. However, there should be very rapid referral pathways between the primary care service and the hospital.

- Stage 1—Annual review with basic foot education
- Stage 2—It is difficult to stratify the risk of ulceration within this group. Any patient with one or more of the following—neuropathy, ischaemia, deformity, callus, oedema—should be referred for education and podiatry, receiving 3-monthly or more frequent treatment.

Patients with specific problems will need the following referrals:

Severe chronic ischaemia to diabetic foot clinic or vascular clinic within 1 week.

Acute ischaemia to diabetic foot clinic or vascular clinic same day.

Any neuropathic fracture/acute Charcot's osteoarthropathy to diabetic foot clinic within 24 hours. Patients with history of Charcot's osteoarthropathy are always best managed by the hospital team as problems frequently develop in other joints. Renal patients should also be seen by the hospital team.

Painful neuropathy to diabetic foot clinic within 2 weeks. This is a singularly disagreeable condition and patients should not feel abandoned

- Stage 3—To diabetic foot clinic within 1 week. Maximum treatment interval 2 weeks with provision for emergency access in case of deterioration
- Stage 4—To diabetic foot clinic same day (may need admission for intravenous antibiotics or outpatient treatment with oral or intramuscular antibiotics). Maximum treatment interval 1 week
- Stage 5—To diabetic foot clinic same day for admission: after discharge, maximum treatment interval 1 week until any remaining necrosis is dry and well demarcated, then every 2 weeks until fully healed
- Stage 6—To diabetic foot clinic same day for admission. Remaining foot should be inspected daily during perioperative and rehabilitation period. After discharge from hospital, should be followed up with maximum interval between treatments of 6 weeks.

PRACTICE POINTS

- The basic approach to the diabetic foot is assessment, classification, staging and multidisciplinary management using the simple staging system as a treatment-based system
- Diabetic feet should be classified into neuropathic and neuroischaemic feet to ensure that ischaemia is never missed
- The natural history of the diabetic foot falls into six stages: normal, high-risk, ulcerated, infected, necrotic and unsalvageable
- Multidisciplinary management consists of mechanical, wound, microbiological, vascular, metabolic and educational control
- The multidisciplinary foot care service should include podiatrist, physician, orthotist, nurse, surgeon and radiologist
- Joint clinics help to provide improved care to diabetic foot patients.

FURTHER READING

Practical assessment

Wu S, Armstrong DG, Lavery LA, Harkless LB. Clinical examination of the diabetic foot and identification of the at-risk patient. In Veves A, Giurini JM, LoGerfo FW (eds). *The Diabetic Foot*, 2nd edn. Humana Press, New Jersey, USA, 2006, pp. 201–26.

Booth J, Young MJ. Differences in the performance of commercially available 10-g monofilaments. *Diabetes Care* 2000; **23**: 984–88.

Cavanagh PR, Ulbrecht JS. What the practising clinician should know about foot biomechanics. In Boulton AJM, Cavanagh PR, Rayman G (eds). *The Foot in Diabetes*, 4th edn, John Wiley and Sons Ltd., Chichester, UK, 2006, pp. 68–91.

Crawford F, Inkster M, Kleijnen J, Fahey T. Predicting foot ulcers in patients with diabetes: a systematic review and meta-analysis. *QJM* 2007; **100**: 65–86.

Lyons TE, Rich J, Veves A. Foot pressure abnormalities in the diabetic foot. In Veves A, Giurini JM, Logerfo FW (eds). *The Diabetic Foot*, 2nd edn. Humana Press, New Jersey, USA, 2006, pp. 163–184.

Meijer JW, Smit AJ, Lefrandt JD et al. Back to basics in diagnosing diabetic polyneuropathy with the tuning fork! *Diabetes Care* 2005; **28**: 2201–5.

Merriman LM, Turner W. *Clinical Skills in Treating the Foot*, 2nd edn. Churchill Livingstone, Edinburgh, UK, 2007.

Shaw KM, Cummings MH (eds) *Diabetes Chronic Complications*, 2nd edn. John Wiley & Sons Ltd, 2005.

Van Schie CHM, Boulton AJM. Biomechanics of the diabetic foot. In *The Diabetic Foot*, 2nd edn. Veves A, Giurini JM and Logerfo FW (eds), Humana Press, New Jersey, USA, 2006.

Winkler AS, Ejskjaer N, Edmonds M, Watkins PJ. Dissociated sensory loss in diabetic autonomic neuropathy. *Diabet Med* 2000; **17**: 457–62.

Classification and staging

Armstrong DG, Lavery LA, Harkless LB. Validation of a diabetic wound classification system. The contribution of depth, infection, and ischemia to risk of amputation. *Diabetes Care* 1998; **21**: 855–9.

Foster A, Edmonds M. Simple Staging System: a tool for diagnosis and management. *Diabetic Foot* 2000; **3**: 56–62.

Multidisciplinary management

Edmonds M, Foster AVM. Reduction of major amputations in the diabetic ischaemic foot: a strategy to 'take control' with conservative care as well as revascularization. *VASA* 2001; **58**: 6–14.

Faglia E, Favales F, Aldeghi A *et al.* Change in major amputation rate in a center dedicated to diabetic foot care during the 1980s: prognostic determinants for major amputation. *J Diab Comp* 1998; **12**: 96–102.

Holstein P, Ellitsgaard N, Olsen BB, Ellitsgaard V. Decreasing incidence of major amputations in people with diabetes. *Diabetologia* 2000; **43**: 844–7.

Larsson J, Apelqvist J, Stanstrom A *et al.* Decreasing incidence of major amputations in diabetic patients: a consequence of a multi-disciplinary foot care team approach? *Diabetic Medicine* 1995; **12**: 770–6.

Plank J, Haas W, Rakovac I *et al.* Evaluation of the impact of chiropodist care in the secondary prevention of foot ulcerations in diabetic subjects. *Diabetes Care* 2003; **26**: 1691–5.

Strauss MB. The orthopaedic surgeon's role in the treatment and prevention of diabetic foot wounds. *Foot Ankle Int* 2005; **26**: 5–14.

2

Stage 1: the normal foot

There is a sickness
Which puts some of us in distemper.
(A Winter's Tale *I, ii, William Shakespeare*)

PRESENTATION AND DIAGNOSIS

The stage 1 foot has no risk factors for diabetic foot problems and is a normal foot. Neither neuropathy nor ischaemia, nor the other major risk factors which would make ulceration more likely, namely deformity, callus and oedema, are present. These five factors have to be excluded in order to diagnose a foot at stage 1.

In the Introduction (Chapter 1) we have described the full foot assessment consisting of history-taking, examination and simple investigations. Ideally this should be carried out on the first presentation of a patient. The assessment will need to be adapted when it is used for a screening examination as part of the annual review. It is possible for the foot screening to be carried out by any suitably trained health-care professional. We have compared results of screening by groups of nurses, medical students and podiatrists, all of whom had received brief training in application of the simple staging system and the results from each group did not differ significantly.

The screening assessment consists of five parts:

- Enquiring as to any previous history of ulceration or other serious foot problems
- Testing for neuropathy (we use 10 g monofilament or a tuning fork)
- Palpation of foot pulses to ensure that ischaemia is not missed. (It is so important not to miss ischaemia that we perform palpation of pulses on every diabetic patient at every clinic visit)
- Inspection of the foot to look for the following abnormalities:
  Deformity
  Callus
  Oedema
  Ulceration
  Signs of infection
  Necrosis
- Limited joint mobility can be assessed by a simple biomechanical assessment to detect hallux rigidus and a reduced range of movement at the ankle joint.

If any of these are found the patient must be staged above stage 1. Patients with none of these problems are classified as stage 1. However, the screening of stage 1 patients should be repeated at yearly intervals to ensure that patients who develop risk factors or foot problems are restaged and offered treatment as appropriate.

Although stage 1 patients are at low risk compared with any other stage of diabetic foot, they should still be regarded as vulnerable patients when compared with the non-diabetic population. It should never be forgotten, moreover, that the most high-risk diabetic foot patients begin their diabetic lives as stage 1 patients. Things are rarely static in the world of the diabetic foot and poorly controlled patients deteriorate and develop complications and foot problems. Health-care workers dealing with diabetic feet can never relax even when the patient's feet are at stage 1.

MANAGEMENT

The aims of management are to ensure that:
- The development of patients' risk factors for diabetic foot ulceration is prevented or delayed
- If risk factors do develop, they are detected early and patients placed in stage 2
- Common foot problems that can occur in the general population are efficiently treated and do not lead to

A Practical Manual of Diabetic Foot Care, 2nd edition, Edmonds, Foster and Sanders.
Published 2008 Blackwell Publishing. ISBN 978-1-4051-61473

tissue breakdown even in the absence of neuropathy and vascular disease.

The following components of multidisciplinary management are important for stage 1 patients.

Mechanical control

- To encourage the use of suitable footwear, discourage inadequate footwear and thus prevent subsequent deformity and callus formation
- To keep the foot intact by treatment of non-ulcerative pathologies. There is no such thing as a trivial lesion of the diabetic foot; all foot problems need early diagnosis and appropriate intervention.

Metabolic control

To prevent or delay the development of neuropathy, microvascular and macrovascular complications.

Educational control

- To encourage healthy foot care/footwear habits and detect ignorance or non-compliance early
- To make provision for intellectual deficit and psychological and social problems. Behaviour modification is an important component of care (Fig. 2.1a,b).

Because stage 1 patients have no ulcers, infection, gangrene or ischaemia, there is no need for wound, microbiological or vascular control to be addressed.

Mechanical control

Mechanical control is achieved by wearing the correct footwear and also by the recognition and treatment of common foot problems.

Footwear
Advice on buying shoes

Stage 1 patients may obtain their shoes from shoe shops or mail-order catalogues, though it is probably best for the foot to be measured and the shoes sized and tried on, or bought 'on approval' and checked by a health-care professional. Staff of shoe shops can be taught which footwear is suitable for diabetic feet. Normal feet swell when the patient has been on his feet a lot, so shoes are best bought towards the end of the day.

For everyday wear, house shoes and for when the patient is on his feet a lot, selection should be made according to the following principles (Fig. 2.2):

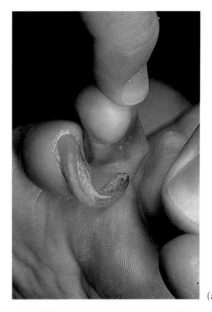
(a)

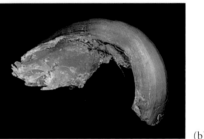
(b)

Fig. 2.1 Neglected nail (a) before and (b) after cutting.

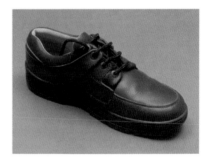

Fig. 2.2 A high-street man's shoe.

- The shoe should be 'foot-shaped'
- Toe box should be roomy to avoid pressure on toes and borders of foot
- Heel cup should fit snugly
- Heels should be low (under 5 cm high)
- Shoe lining should be smooth

- Sole should be sufficiently thick to prevent puncture wounds
- Shoe should fasten with lace or strap to hold foot back in shoe
- Court or slip-on shoes should be avoided except for special occasions
- Trainers are useful if they are sufficiently long, broad and deep, with cushioned soles and a built-in rocker, and are worn with the laces fastened. However, there are many inadequate trainers and deck shoes on sale which have thin soles, a lack of cushioning, and no rocker built in
- Wearing socks reduces friction within shoes
- Socks should be non-constricting with no tight band around ankle or calf
- Socks with prominent seams should be worn turned inside-out
- Socks should be made of absorbent materials such as cotton
- If shoes cause pain, callus, red marks or blisters then they do not fit properly and should be discarded (Fig. 2.3a,b)
- In hot climates, sandals may be worn; however, they give little protection against trauma and the foot is not held firmly in place, resulting in excessive shear. Fig. 2.4

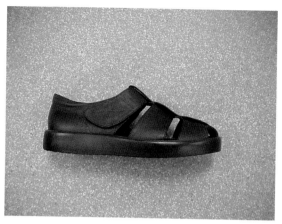

Fig. 2.4 The Singapore sandal, designed for diabetic patients in hot, humid tropical countries.

shows a sandal designed for use in Singapore by the local podiatry service which avoids these problems and is suitable for wear in tropical countries.

Wearing 'good' shoes will prevent or delay the onset of footwear-related deformity, and prevent callus from developing by reducing the mechanical forces applied to the feet.

Features of a bad shoe include:
- Slip on style, which causes pressure on the forefoot
- High heels, which reduce the range of toe dorsiflexion and can lead to hallux rigidus
- Thin-soled shoes, which make the foot sensitive to any unevenness of the ground and vulnerable to penetration by sharp objects.

If shoes are the wrong size or wrong style, they can cause permanent damage to the feet, resulting in deformity and callus. Elderly people may be reluctant to discard worn-out or ill-fitting shoes.

Even when shoes are of the correct style and fitting it is wise to 'wear them in' gradually by walking for a few minutes around the house in the new shoes for several days before wearing them for protracted periods outside. The reason for this is that even a shoe which is apparently a suitable style and a good fit may cause problems, and unless it is tested out in the home there is a danger that it will cause blisters.

Common foot problems

In maintaining mechanical control, it is important to diagnose foot problems including:
- Nail problems
- Fungal infections
- Corynebacteria infections

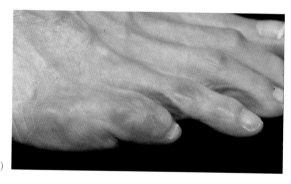

(a)

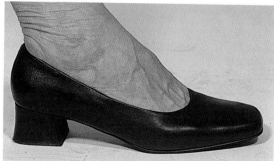

(b)

Fig. 2.3 (a) Red marks on toes after (b) wearing unsuitable shoes with no proper fastening and narrow toe box.

- Fissures
- Verrucae
- Bullae
- Chilblains (perniosis)
- Malignancy
- Inflammatory skin diseases
- Hyperhydrosis and bromodrosis
- Insect bites
- Traumas
- Fractures
- Gout.

Nail problems

Many people in stage 1 will be able to cut their own nails (Table 2.1). They should be taught the correct techniques for cutting normal nails as follows:

- Nails should be cut straight across or in a gentle curve
- The corners should not be cut out: a piece may be left behind and lead to an ingrowing toenail
- The nail plate should not be cut in one piece: a gentle 'nibbling' technique should be used to avoid splitting the nail plate
- The nail should not be cut so short that the seal between nail and nail bed is broken
- The nails should not be left so long that they can catch on the socks, risking trauma
- The nails should be cut regularly: even normal nails can cause problems if neglected
- The nails should be cut after the bath, when the nail plate will be softer, more flexible and easy to cut
- If nail cutting is difficult or painful, patients should seek professional help.

There is no reason why any health-care professional should not cut normal nails in diabetic stage 1 feet, but proper nail nippers should be provided for staff, who should be taught correct techniques as explained above.

Onychauxis

Onychauxis is thickening of the nail without deformity. It follows an insult to the nail bed and is common. Regular filing will reduce the thickness of the nail. Without regular reduction onychogryphosis will develop.

Table 2.1 Patients who can safely cut their own toe nails

Patients who can safely cut their own toe nails
Have pain-free normal nails with no pathology
Can see feet clearly
Can reach feet
Have been taught correct nail cutting techniques

Onychogryphosis (ram's horn nail)

This is thickening of the nail with deformity. The cause is an insult to the nail bed. Treatment can be palliative or surgical. Palliative treatment consists of regularly cutting and thinning the nail plate at 3-monthly treatment intervals and can result in a normal appearance of the nail.

If only one nail is affected and the patient dislikes the need for regular treatment, the nail plate can be removed under ring block local anaesthesia. If the exposed nail bed is treated with topical phenol the nail will be replaced by a fibrous plate which does not need regular reduction and has a cosmetically acceptable appearance. However, this procedure is invasive and should not be carried out on ischaemic feet.

CASE STUDY
Schizophrenia and neglected nails

A 35-year-old man with type 2 diabetes of 5 years' duration had schizophrenia and was reluctant to attend the diabetic foot clinic for help with his nail care. At an annual appointment the nurse in the diabetes clinic persuaded him to remove his shoes and socks and found that his nails were overgrown, deformed and neglected (Fig. 2.5). He was asked to attend the foot clinic regularly and agreed as long as he did not have to wait after he arrived, and could be seen without making a prior appointment.

Key points

- Even normal nails will become deformed if they are neglected
- People with concurrent psychiatric disease will need help in cutting their nails

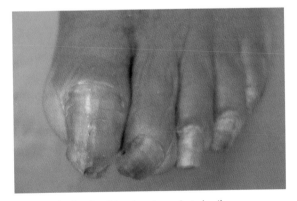

Fig. 2.5 The foot in schizophrenia: neglected nails.

• It may be hard to persuade them to accept care and it may be necessary to relax the usual rules.

Onychocryptosis (ingrowing toe nail)
This is frequently caused by improper nail-cutting technique, when a spike of nail is left behind at the side of the nail. As the nail plate grows forward the spike is pushed laterally into the nail sulcus (the groove of flesh at the side of the nail) and penetrates the soft tissues. Other causes of onychocryptosis include pressure on the side of the nail from tight shoes or tight socks, antithrombotic stockings or support hose, a trauma to the side of the nail, as when the toe is stubbed, and a patient who pulls and picks at the nail. Some teenagers with a very thin nail plate and a fleshy nail sulcus are particularly prone to onychocryptosis. Hypergranulation tissue is often present but resolves after treatment.

Treatment of onychocryptosis involves removal of the offending splinter (nail spicule) (Fig. 2.6a,b), and the ragged edge of the nail is then filed smooth with a Black's file (a small file specially designed to fit into the sulcus and under the nail). Unless the splinter is removed quickly, the spike of nail will penetrate the flesh, and in these circumstances infection rapidly supervenes. Proprietory remedies are useless unless the nail splinter is removed. Where onychocryptosis is recurring or chronic it can be treated very successfully with partial nail avulsion under local anaesthetic (without adrenaline). This procedure should not be performed on ischaemic feet. Unless revascularization is possible, palliative care is best. The partial nail avulsion procedure is described below.

Fig. 2.7a–e shows the partial nail avulsion procedure. Lidocaine is injected into both sides of the toe to achieve a ring block. It may be necessary to loosen the tissues at the nail sulcus with a fine ointment spatula if they are fibrosed and closely adherent to the nail plate. A pair of Thwaites nippers (English Anvil) is then used to split the nail by inserting the blunt-edged piece under the nail plate and cutting down on it with the upper blade. The split in the nail is then extended proximally with a Beaver chisel passed under the eponychium (cuticle). The already loosened nail wedge is then lifted away using a pair of artery forceps. It is essential to remove all of the feather edge of the nail wedge. Phenolization of the exposed area of nail bed to prevent regrowth of the troublesome side of the nail prevents recurrence of the problem. Phenol is applied on a Black's file and rubbed into the wound for three minutes. The wound is then dressed with paraffin gauze and outer dressings. Healing is protracted because of the chemical burn. Postoperative pain is less than with surgical incision and removal of the nail bed (nail wedge resection). Patients should be reviewed regularly until full healing is achieved.

When the nail is irreparably damaged or a partial nail avulsion would leave an unacceptably narrow nail, then total nail avulsion is an option.

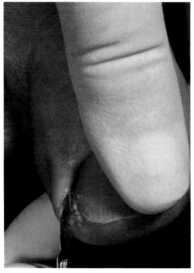 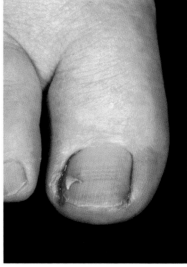

Fig. 2.6 (a) Onychocryptosis: a spike of nail has been left behind after cutting. (b) The offending spike has been removed and lies on the nail plate.

(a)　　　　　　　　　　(b)

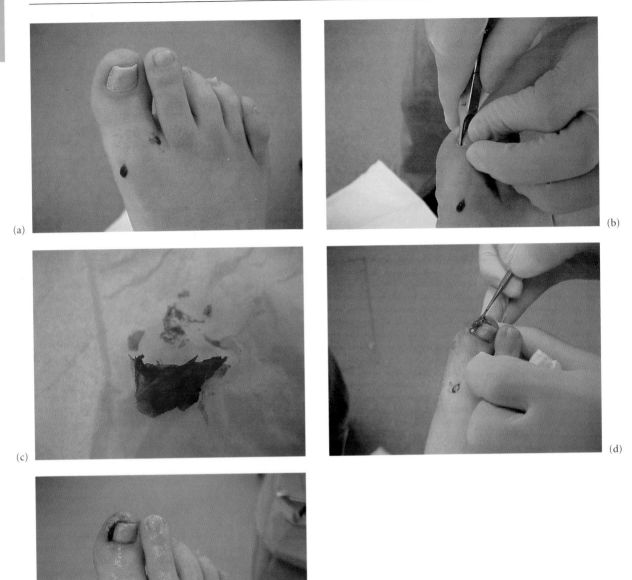

(a)

(b)

(c)

(d)

(e)

Fig. 2.7 Partial nail avulsion. (a) Lidocaine has been injected into the toe to complete a ring block. (b) Thwaites nippers (English Anvil) are used to split the nail. (c) The splinter of nail has been removed. (d) Liquid phenol is applied to the nail using a Black's file dipped in phenol as applicator. (e) The procedure is completed: the offending part of the nail bed has been chemically ablated.

STAGE 1

CASE STUDY
Acute onychocryptosis

A 26-year-old man with type 1 diabetes of 20 years' duration had acute onychocryptosis (Fig. 2.8a) which had not responded to palliative care and underwent total nail avulsion. His toe healed in 5 weeks (Fig. 2.8b–d).

Key points
- For acute onychocryptosis which does not respond to palliative care, surgery can be a permanent solution
- A partial or total nail avulsion with phenolization can take several weeks to heal.

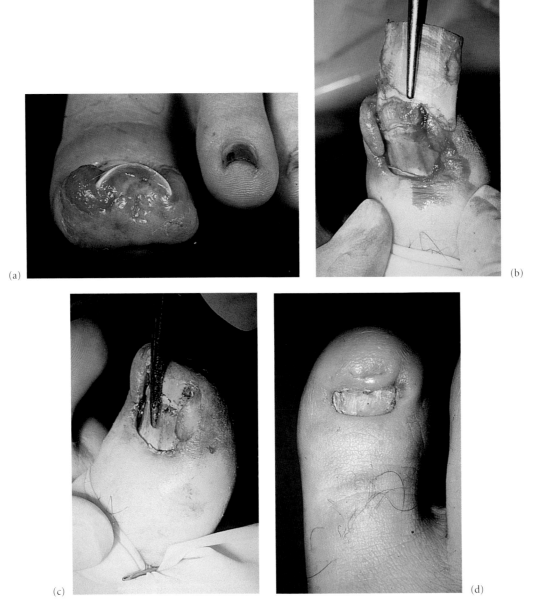

(a)

(b)

(c)

(d)

Fig. 2.8 (a) Acute onychocryptosis. (b) The nail plate is lifted off the nail bed with artery forceps. A tourniquet ensures a bloodless field. (c) Phenol is applied to the nail bed to prevent regrowth. (d) A fibrous plate has replaced the troublesome nail 6 months later.

Involuted toe nail

This is excessive lateral curvature of the nail plate. If epithelial cells become trapped as they are shed in the sulcus, they can accumulate, causing pain and pressure. The nail sulcus is gently cleared with a Black's file. In severe cases, nail avulsion with phenolization of the nail bed, as shown in Fig. 2.8, can provide a permanent solution.

Nail infections

Onychomycosis (fungal nail). When fungal infection invades the nail plate it first causes white or yellowish discolouration of a patch of nail, which subsequently becomes thickened and friable. The majority of infections are caused by moulds called dermatophytes, or by yeasts, notably *Candida albicans*. There are four distinct types of onychomycosis:

- Distal and lateral subungual onychomycosis, which affects toe nails twice as commonly as finger nails. This is commonly caused by dermatophyte infection. The nail becomes detached from the bed (onycholysis) changing to a creamy white opaque colour (Fig. 2.9)
- Proximal subungual onychomycosis which is secondary to chronic paronychia caused by infection with yeasts of *Candida* species and is often associated with interdigital candidiasis
- Superficial white onychomycosis which is caused by *Trichophyton mentagrophytes* and is relatively uncommon
- Total dystrophic onychomycosis—where the whole of the nail plate is destroyed—is a consequence of any of the first three types.

Onychomycosis can cause chronic pain, physical disability and secondary bacterial infection. Patients may be concerned about the cosmetic appearance. Eradication of the fungal infection in the toe nails is not easy, and some patients will opt for palliative care if they are not concerned by the cosmetic effect and the infection is not spreading.

Diagnosis can be confirmed by culture of nail clippings taken from the most proximal part of the affected nail to obtain crumbly material; however, many infections are treated without laboratory confirmation. Treatment can be palliative or active. Palliative care involves regular debulking and thinning of the nail, which can be done with a scalpel by a podiatrist. This approach is usually sufficient for most fungal nail infections and active treatment should only be considered when the infection is causing unpleasant symptoms or distress.

Active treatment involves topical or systemic agents.

The thickness of the nail is reduced with a scalpel and an antifungal agent applied directly to the remnants. Agents available include topical amorolfine nail lacquer and strong iodine BP. Treatment should continue until a new nail has formed, which may take up to 12 months.

If systemic treatment is undertaken it is important to be aware of the possible side-effects of therapy.

- Terbinafine 250 mg daily for 3 months is the drug of choice for fungal nail infections. It is especially active against dermatophytes. Rarely, it can cause liver toxicity
- Itraconazole 200 mg daily for 3 months or as Sporanox Pulse 200 mg bd for 7 days and subsequent courses repeated after a 21-day interval. It is active against a broad spectrum of fungi including dematophytes and yeasts. Itraconazole has been associated with liver damage and should not be given to patients with a history of liver disease.

Inflammation of the nail fold. Inflammation of the nail fold, or paronychia, can be acute or chronic.

Acute paronychia due to bacterial infection is painful, points and discharges pus. If the margin of the nail plate is pressing on the inflamed area it should be cut back, and if a splinter of nail has penetrated the sulcus it must be removed. Collections of pus should be drained. A swab is sent for microscopy and culture, and appropriate systemic antibiotics prescribed.

Chronic paronychia results in the periungual tissues appearing erythematous and oedematous. The infection extends to the nail plate which may develop yellowish-green or yellowish-brown pigmentation.

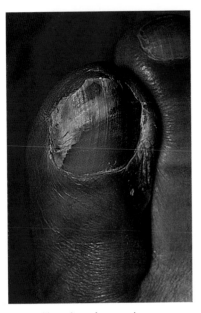

Fig. 2.9 Distal and lateral onychomycosis.

Chronic paronychia is frequently caused by infection with *Candida albicans* and the treatment is with itraconazole, as described above. The feet should be kept dry.

Lesions under the nail
These can be due to:
• Haematoma
• Necrosis
• Melanoma
• Exostosis.

Subungual haematoma. This follows a trauma to the nail, when blood collects under the nail plate causing red, purple or black discolouration. Pain can be agonizing. The patient should be reassured that drainage will relieve pain and reduce damage to the nail bed. The blood is evacuated through a small hole made in the nail plate by paring with a scalpel or with a chiropodist's nail drill. If the nail plate is loose it should be cut back as far as possible to prevent the loose area from catching on the hose and causing further injury, and also to assist inspection of the nail bed.

Subungual necrosis. This can be due to trauma, infection or hydrostatic pressure from a haematoma under the nail bed which is not evacuated in time to prevent local ischaemia and tissue death.

CASE STUDY
Subungual necrosis

A 79-year-old man with type 2 diabetes of 7 years' duration dropped the family bible on his left great hallux. The toe was exquisitely painful and rapidly developed discolouration beneath the nail plate. After 4 days he visited his general practitioner who diagnosed a subungual haematoma and referred him to the diabetic foot clinic and he was seen the same day (Fig. 2.10a,b). The pedal pulses were palpable. There was no fracture on X-ray. The nail plate was cut back to reveal an area of necrosis involving the nail bed. Differential diagnosis was necrosis caused by infection or purely by hydrostatic pressure from a collection of blood under the nail plate. Systemic antibiotics were prescribed. The necrotic area gradually dried, demarcated and healed. When the new nail plate grew back it was onychogryphotic.

Key points
• It is impossible to assess a nail bed lesion properly without removing the overlying nail plate

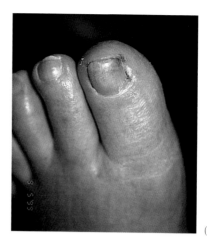

(a)

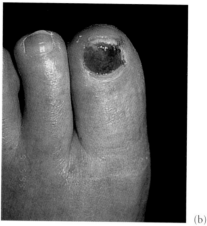

(b)

Fig. 2.10 (a) Apparent subungual haematoma. (b) The nail bed is necrotic.

• All painful subungual haematomas should be drained without delay by cutting back the nail plate.

Subungual melanoma. Malignant melanoma may also present as a discoloured area under the nail plate. Irregular discolouration of the nail bed and plate and progressive destruction of nail are seen. Some melanomas are not associated with pigment (Fig. 2.11).

Patients should be referred urgently to the dermatology clinic. Failure to diagnose malignant melanoma can lead to early metastatic spread. The diabetic foot clinic team should develop close links with the dermatology clinic so that cases of suspected malignant melanoma can be seen urgently.

Subungual exostosis. An acutely painful cherry red spot develops under the nail plate. A lateral X-ray reveals

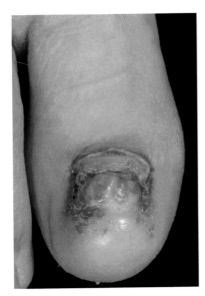

Fig 2.11 Amelanotic melanoma.

bony outgrowth of the distal phalanx. The treatment is surgical.

Fungal infections (tinea pedis)

Tinea pedis infection is caused by a dermatophyte fungus. It can present in several ways:

- Dry, scaly, often in a 'moccasin-like' distribution on the sole and borders of the foot
- Acute vesicular
- Interdigital, with moist, cracked areas which may be sore, itchy and sometimes malodorous, and are associated with whitish, rubbery, macerated skin, and can undergo erosion and cracking.

Scrapings can be taken and sent to the laboratory for identification of the infective organism but usually a clinical diagnosis is made.

Treatment of tinea pedis

Topical anti-fungal cream is usually sufficient. Canesten spray (clotrimazole 1% in isopropyl alcohol) applied topically is best for interdigital areas. For other parts of the foot Canesten cream can be applied. Treatment should be continued for at least 2 weeks after resolution of symptoms to avoid relapse. Nystatin cream, terbinafine cream and Whitfield's ointment (benzoic acid) may also be useful. Preparations containing tolnaftate or chlorphenesin can be bought over the counter in formulations including powder and cream.

Patients with fungal infections should receive precise instructions regarding duration of therapy and preventative measures for the future.

Patients should be advised to continue using their anti-fungal agent until 2 weeks after the symptoms have resolved, and then to apply surgical spirit to the previously affected areas after washing them daily and drying them carefully. They can also be advised to wear clean socks every day.

CASE STUDY
Interdigital tinea pedis

A 37-year-old woman with type 2 diabetes of 2 years' duration complained of severe itching between the 4th and 5th toes of her right foot. She had purchased a proprietary powder and a cream for athlete's foot and had used them for 2 weeks with no improvement. She said that the cream 'got all over the place' and the powder formed lumps which made her toes all the more sore. Between her toes was an area of thickened rubbery white skin (Fig. 2.12) which was gently debrided away: the underlying tissue was intact, but macerated and inflamed. We prescribed Canesten spray and advised her to desist from using her proprietary remedies. When she returned to the clinic 3 weeks later the foot was healed and the problem did not recur.

Key point

- For interdigital application a spray may be more effective than a cream or powder.

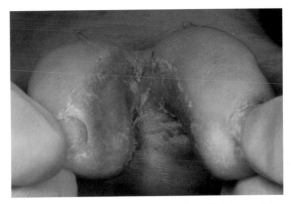

Fig. 2.12 An area of thickened rubbery white skin between the toes (tinea pedis).

Corynebacterium infections

CASE STUDY
Pitted keratolysis (superficial corynebacteria infection) masquerading as tinea pedis

A 40-year-old man with type 2 diabetes of 11 years' duration developed a rash on the border of the right foot (Fig. 2.13a) and the left foot (Fig. 2.13b). On the plantar surfaces of the forefeet the skin has become white with clusters of punched out pits (Fig. 2.13c). Note the skin is macerated on the plantar aspect (Fig. 2.13d).

Key points
- Superficial corynebacteria infection may be mistaken for tinea pedis
- Pitted keratolysis is caused by a cutaneous infection with *Micrococcus sedentarius* (now renamed *Kytococcus sedentarius*), *Dermatophilus congolensis*, or species of *Corynebacterium* and *Actinomyces*.

Limit the use of occlusive footwear and reduce foot friction with properly fitting footwear. Absorbent cotton socks must be changed frequently to prevent excessive foot moisture.

Fissures
Fissures are moist or dry cracks in epidermis at sites where skin is under tension. Deep fissures may involve dermis.

Fissures can occur in dry skin, when the treatment is an emollient, such as Doublebase, E45 cream, olive oil or cocoa butter, or in wet skin, where an astringent or antiperspirant such as aluminium chloride is helpful. Where the skin is consistently very dry, Calmurid, which contains urea, is helpful.

Verrucae
Warts may occur anywhere on the foot and may be single or multiple, and appear as round flattened papules or plaques. They are whitish or grey in colour with a rough surface.

If they are on the plantar surface and thus subjected to pressure from walking, they may be difficult to distinguish from corns. However, warts are painful when they

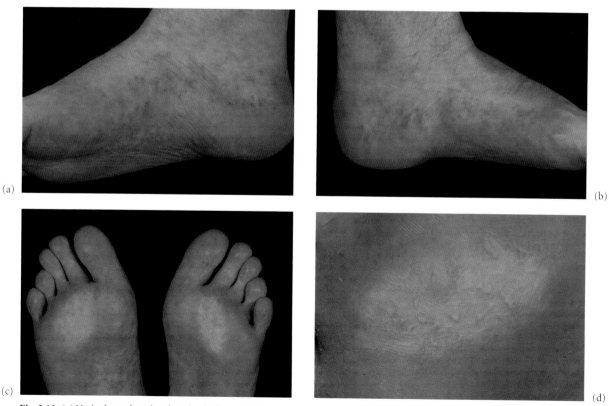

(a)

(b)

(c)

(d)

Fig. 2.13 (a) Vesicular rash on border of right foot. (b) Vesicular rash on border of left foot. (c) Coalescence of vesicles. (d) Maceration with exudate.

are squeezed while corns are painful when they are pressed. Skin striations are interrupted by warts but not by corns. Removal of a verruca by scalpel debridement reveals tiny reddish brown dots. Dots are not visible following removal of corns.

Small speckles of black (thrombosed blood vessels) can be a sign that the verruca is resolving spontaneously.

Accumulation of hyperkeratosis may cause pain on walking: excess keratin can be pared with a scalpel by the podiatrist or the patient may use a pumice stone. However, warts do not need to be treated unless they are painful or spreading: most will resolve within 2 years without treatment and they are less infectious than is commonly thought.

Some swimming pools require people with verrucae to wear verruca socks to avoid cross-infection.

The recommended treatment for ablation of painful or spreading verrucae in people with diabetes is cryotherapy with liquid nitrogen. The resulting breakdown of tissue should be kept clean and covered with a dressing. However, treatment with liquid nitrogen can cause severe pain and ulceration and should only be used on stage 1 feet in patients with diabetes. Treatment with strong acids or silver nitrate is not recommended in diabetic patients. Sometimes surgical treatment with excision of the wart is required. Patients should be warned not to self-diagnose or self-treat warts. Some foot malignancies present as wart-like lesions.

CASE STUDY
Verruca pedis

A 28-year-old woman with type 1 diabetes of 14 years' duration presented with multiple verrucae. The appearances were typical of warts (Fig. 2.14a–d). Although they were not painful she was concerned that she might infect her family. She was reassured that even without treatment the warts would almost certainly resolve within 2 years. She was advised not to walk with bare feet, to wear plastic sandals in the shower and to purchase verruca socks from the chemist for use when she went swimming with her children.

Key points
- Fig. 2.14b shows the breaks in the skin striae which are typical of warts
- Warts that are not painful do not require treatment. If they become painful then cryotherapy with liquid nitrogen is the treatment of choice, but only in the absence of ischaemia
- Very basic precautions prevent spread of warts.

Bullae (blisters)
These are superficial accumulations of clear fluid within or under the epidermis which develop following trauma to the skin. Common causes include unsuitable shoes, failure to wear socks and walking in wet footwear. Pedal bullae are sometimes associated with hypoglycaemic episodes.

Several serious lesions, including early neuropathic and early ischaemic ulcers, pressure ulcers, burns, puncture wounds and infections complicating ulceration, may first present as a bulla.

Unless bullae are small, superficial and containing clear fluid, they should be regarded as stage 3 lesions.

Small, flaccid bullae can be cleaned and covered with a sterile non-adherent dressing. Large bullae (over 1 cm in diameter) and all tense bullae should be lanced with a scalpel and drained before dressing. Aspiration with a syringe is less useful because the hole frequently seals, fluid accumulates again and unrelieved hydrostatic pressure causes extension of the blister.

The cause of blisters should always be ascertained and addressed. Bullosis diabeticorum is a rare condition where diabetic patients present with intraepidermal blisters which are not associated with trauma and heal without scarring. Treatment of bullosis diabeticorum is as for bullae.

Chilblains (perniosis)
These are localized inflammatory lesions, provoked by cold and injudicious reheating. Chilblains are frequently found on the toes. Initially they are white due to vasoconstriction, but usually present as dusky red swellings which are intensely pruritic in the acute stages. When they become chronic they present as purplish lesions. They are best managed by taking preventative measures. Patients should avoid standing in the cold and damp, and should refrain from toasting their toes in front of the fire when their feet are chilled. In the cyanotic phase compound tincture of benzoin BP may be used.

Malignancy
Although skin malignancy is rare in the foot, the diagnosis should be considered, especially in unusual and non-responsive conditions.

It is important to be aware that squamous cell carcinoma, malignant melanoma and, very rarely, basal cell carcinoma, may present in the foot and that missing an early diagnosis of malignant melanoma or squamous cell carcinoma may lead to the patient's death. Early presentation, early diagnosis and early treatment can save the patient's life.

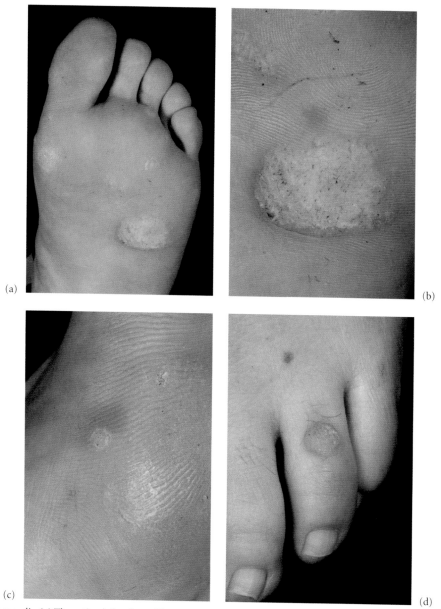

Fig. 2.14 Verruca pedis. (a) The patient's forefoot with numerous verrucae. (b) Close-up view of a large plantar wart: note that the skin striations are broken which is an important diagnostic feature. (c) Thrombosed papilli are evident as small blackish red speckles and can be a sign of impending resolution of the verruca. (d) Dorsal verruca on the 4th toe.

Squamous cell carcinoma

It may present as a reddish plaque, warty lesion, nodule or as an ulcer with undermined ragged edges. Squamous cell carcinomas are likely to arise at the site of a scar or an existing lesion such as venous ulcer or subungual ulcer.

Most squamous cell carcinomas are locally aggressive and can spread to draining lymph nodes. Suspicious lesions should be biopsied. Repeated biopsies may be needed to establish the diagnosis. We have seen a number of patients where the first and even the second biopsy was regarded as clear of malignancy and only later biopsies were positive. Treatment is surgical excision.

Basal cell carcinoma

Although the most common skin tumour overall, it is very rare on feet, especially on the plantar surface, and even rarer as subungual ulcer. These are usually ulcerated lesions with raised 'pearly' margins. They are treated by cryotherapy or surgery.

Malignant melanoma

Malignant melanomas arise from existing moles or spontaneously from no apparent pre-existing lesion. Some melanomas produce little or no pigmentation and are termed hypo- or amelanotic melanomas. Melanomas are usually pigmented lesions on the foot which are irregular in outline and border, and variable in colour. They may be painful. It is wise to refer without delay to the dermatologist all pigmented lesions that develop *de novo*, change in size, shape or colour, or develop inflammation, ulceration and bleeding, because delayed diagnosis is likely to lead to local and systemic spread and the death of the patient. We have seen one patient with a small crusted lesion on the cheek who resisted referral to the dermatology clinic for several weeks. The lesion was a malignant melanoma and she died 2 years later from metastatic spread.

CASE STUDY
Squamous cell carcinoma

A 50-year-old woman with undiagnosed type 2 diabetes, applied Bazooka, a proprietary wart remedy, to a small brown tender papule over her right third metatarsal head. Within a few days she developed a cutaneous erosion which failed to heal for 9 months and became increasingly painful (Fig. 2.15a,b). Diabetes was diagnosed by her general practitioner and she was referred to the diabetic foot clinic. She was referred on to the dermatologist because her plantar ulcer was unusually painful. The ulcer was biopsied and proved to be a squamous cell carcinoma. She underwent wide excision, but already had pulmonary, pelvic and lymph node metastases. She underwent chemotherapy and radiotherapy but died 18 months later.

Key points

- It is important to have a high index of suspicion for plantar lesions which initially appear as papules and then break down to ulcers
- A full history should be taken of all foot lesions
- Diagnosis of skin lesions that have been treated with proprietary remedies is difficult as the morphology may be altered by the topical application of acids
- Lesions with abnormal appearance should always be referred to the dermatology clinic without delay.

Inflammatory skin diseases

Practitioners treating diabetic patients may encounter dermatological conditions that first manifest themselves on the foot, including:
- Dermatitis/eczema
- Psoriasis.

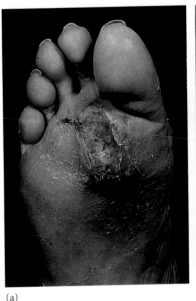
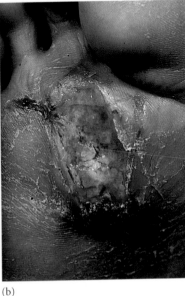

(a)   (b)

Fig. 2.15 (a) Ulcer following application of a proprietary wart remedy to a lesion which subsequently proved to be a squamous cell carcinoma. (b) Close-up of lesion.

It is important to be aware of these conditions so that an early diagnosis can be made and appropriate referral to the dermatology clinic arranged.

Dermatitis/eczema

Dermatitis is an inflammatory skin disease caused by different factors. Eczema and dermatitis are essentially interchangeable terms. Acute dermatitis presents as redness and scaling with vesiculation. Chronic dermatitis is recognized by thickening of the skin and excoriation. Dry, fissured, scaly lesions are treated with bland emollients.

Contact dermatitis, in which there is a hypersensitivity reaction to specific allergens, is a notable manifestation of dermatitis of the feet. Some patients become sensitized to shoes or socks or common household products (Fig. 2.16). Contact dermatitis can also be caused by an inflammatory reaction to dressings (Fig. 2.17).

Where possible the cause of contact dermatitis should be established and removed.

Varicose eczema is associated with venous hypertension. There may be a history of varicose veins or deep vein thrombosis, and haemosiderin deposition leading to brown discolouration of patches of skin. Areas of varicose eczema may break down and develop into venous leg ulcers.

Psoriasis

Psoriasis usually affects the sole rather than the dorsum of the foot, with epidermal thickening and erythematous scaling lesions. Pustular psoriasis presents with recurrent

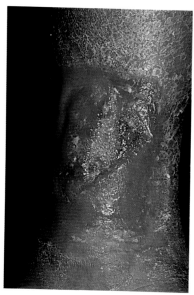

Fig. 2.17 Dermatitis caused by allergy to a dressing.

crops of sterile pustules with erythema distributed on the sole and lateral border of the foot.

CASE STUDY
Pustular psoriasis

A 31-year-old man with type 1 diabetes of 16 years' duration presented with red and scaly plaques on both feet (Fig. 2.18a–c). The differential diagnosis was pustular psoriasis, fungal infection or keratoderma blenorrhagicum. On close examination pustules were seen and the dermatology clinic confirmed a diagnosis of pustular psoriasis. He was treated with Dermovate ointment to good effect.

Key points

- In a scaly rash presenting on the feet it is important to look for pustules which, in the absence of surrounding erythema or other signs of infection, can indicate a diagnosis of pustular psoriasis
- In this condition the pustules are sterile and antibiotics are not needed unless there is tissue breakdown and discharge
- Keratoderma blenorrhagicum is a pustular rash associated with Reiter's syndrome. It can mimic pustular psoriasis.

Psoriasis is associated with nail lesions including lifting of nail plate with onycholysis.

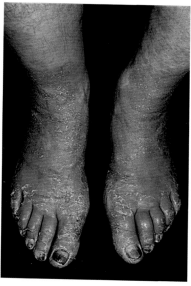

Fig. 2.16 This patient became sensitized to his socks.

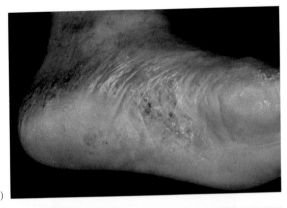

(a)

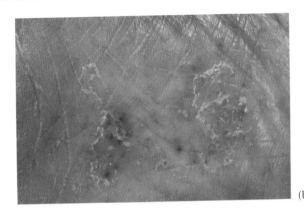

(b)

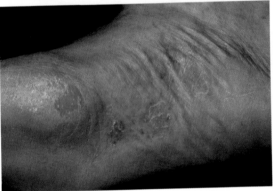

(c)

Fig. 2.18 Pustular psoriasis (a) Left foot of patient showing pustular eruption. (b) Close-up view of lesions reveals pustules. (c) Similar eruption on right foot of same patient.

Hyperhydrosis and bromodrosis

Hyperhydrosis is excessive sweating of the feet, and may be a particular problem in teenagers and in patients who live in tropical climates with high humidity. The skin becomes white, macerated and rubbery in texture and prone to blistering and fungal infections. It may be due to hyperthyroidism or anxiety. There may be an exceedingly unpleasant associated odour (bromodrosis).

The following procedures may help both conditions:
- Patients should avoid closed-in shoes made of plastic or other synthetic materials. Trainer-style shoes may exacerbate the problem
- Instead, patients should wear shoes made of leather or modern materials which can 'breathe' and allow moisture to evaporate
- Shoes should be changed regularly
- Insoles should be removed at the end of the day to dry out
- Absorbent cotton or acrylic fibre socks should be worn
- The patient should wear clean socks every day
- The feet should be washed every day, dried carefully and swabbed with surgical spirit including the interdigital area
- Talcum powder should be used in moderation

- Charcoal soles may be useful for patients with bromodrosis.

Insect bites

Insect bites can cause unpleasant cutaneous reactions.

CASE STUDY
Insect bite

A 35-year-old woman with type 1 diabetes of 9 years' duration, no neuropathy or ischaemia, and poorly controlled diabetes, was bitten on the lateral border of her left foot by a mosquito. The lesion was intensely pruritic and she scratched the foot. The next day she had developed swelling of the foot and cellulitis and lymphangitis spreading up the foot (Fig. 2.19a,b). She was treated with antihistamine and systemic antibiotics and the foot improved after 3 days.

Key points
- Insect bites may cause severe cutaneous reactions, leading to severe swelling and erythema of the foot

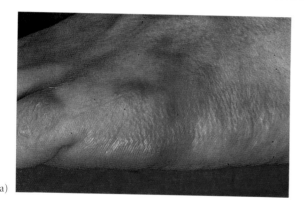

(a)

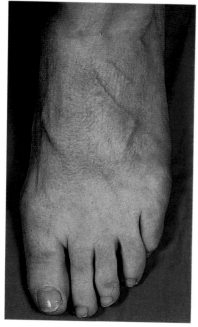

(b)

Fig. 2.19 (a) Insect bite on lateral border. (b) Spreading lymphangitis.

- Patients should be warned to use mosquito repellent and cover up if sitting outside in summer in areas where biting or stinging insects are troublesome.

Traumas

Superficial traumas to the feet are extremely common, particularly if patients walk barefoot or wear unsuitable shoes. The cause of the trauma should always be identified to prevent recurrence.

Superficial cuts or grazes may be cleaned with normal saline (which can be easily made up by adding two teaspoons of salt to previously boiled water and allowing the solution to cool). Lesions should then be covered with a sterile dressing or plaster. All diabetic patients should be advised to keep a first aid box at home to treat accidental injuries.

Fractures

These follow a significant trauma to the stage 1 foot, and are usually very painful and associated with severe bruising. A commonly seen fracture in patients who walk barefoot is fracture of the 5th toe caused by catching the toe on a piece of furniture and everting the toe forcefully. Intra-articular fracture of the hallux can lead to hallux rigidus, with subsequent overloading of the plantar surface and development of callus and ulceration.

Patients in stage 1 have protective pain sensation, and fractures are treated as for non-diabetic patients. Minor fractures of a toe are usually treated by using the adjoining toe as a splint and strapping the two toes together. Metatarsal fractures may be treated in a cast or brace.

Gout

Gout may present as acute gouty arthritis or as painful gouty tophi in the feet. Patients usually complain of redness, warmth, swelling and severe pain.

CASE STUDY
Relapsed case of acute gouty arthritis

A 42-year-old man with type 2 diabetes of 7 years' duration presented with acute pain and swelling of the right forefoot (Fig. 2.20a,b). He gave a previous history of gout but was not on allopurinol therapy. The differential diagnosis was cellulitis, an exacerbation of his gout or Charcot's osteoarthropathy. He was given amoxicillin 500 mg tds and flucloxacillin 500 mg qds and colchicine 0.6 mg every hour for 3 hours. His renal function was normal but his serum uric acid was raised, at 0.45 mmol/L and a diagnosis of exacerbation of his gout was made and his antibiotics were stopped. His discomfort and erythema quickly resolved and he was given long-term therapy with allopurinol after he had recovered from the present exacerbation.

Key points
- The differential diagnosis of a hot painful, swollen foot in diabetes is cellulitis, gout or Charcot's osteoarthropathy
- Diabetic patients with redness, warmth and swelling of the foot should be given antibiotic treatment if infection is suspected

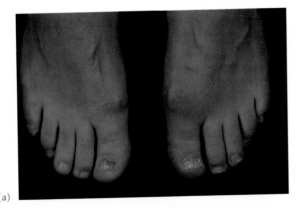

(a)

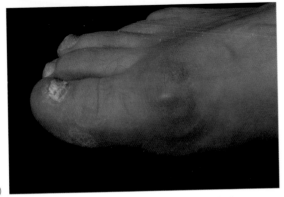

(b)

Fig. 2.20 (a) Relapsed case of acute gout of the right foot. (b) Close-up view.

- If the patient gives a history of previous gout, then a hot swollen foot may represent a further attack, but other possibilities, particularly infection, should be considered
- A serum uric acid is helpful in diagnosing acute gout but may be normal in some cases of gout
- Nonsteroidal anti-inflammatory drugs should be used with caution in diabetic patients especially those with nephropathy.

CASE STUDY
Gouty tophus

A 67-year-old man with type 2 diabetes of 2 years' duration presented with a painful right foot (Fig. 2.21a,b). On examination a gouty tophus was suspected and the diagnosis was confirmed when his blood results revealed elevated serum uric acid. Initially, the toe was debrided and the patient was given amoxicillin 500 mg tds and flucloxacillin 500 mg qds. The toe improved rapidly and healed within 4 weeks. He was then given long-term allopurinol therapy.

Key points
- Ulceration in the diabetic foot can rarely be caused by a gouty tophus. This should be suspected when deposits of whitish crystalline material are noted within an ulcer or beneath the skin of an intact foot

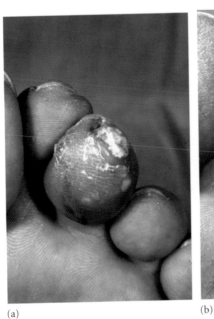

(a)

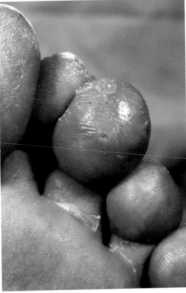

(b)

Fig. 2.21 (a) Gouty tophus before debridement. (b) Much improved after debridement.

- The diagnosis can be confirmed by measuring serum uric acid, although in rare cases this can be normal. Diagnosis should then be confirmed by identifying urate crystals in synovial fluid on microscopy
- Gouty tophus is an indication for life-long allopurinol therapy
- Differential diagnosis of gouty tophus includes pseudo gout and calcium deposits from scleroderma.

Metabolic control

This should follow principles of modern diabetic management. Tight control of blood glucose, blood pressure, blood cholesterol and triglycerides, as well as stopping smoking and giving antiplatelet therapy when indicated, is extremely important at stage 1 in order to preserve neurological and cardiovascular function. Diabetic patients are at a high risk of developing atherosclerotic disease and it is appropriate to manage such patients to the same targets of blood glucose, blood pressure and serum lipids as those patients with established cardiovascular disease. Furthermore, the incidence of neuropathy is associated with potentially modifiable cardiovascular risk factors, including a raised triglyceride level, body mass index, smoking, and hypertension.

Hypoglycaemia is an important metabolic complication of diabetic treatment. It is defined as blood glucose less than 3.5 mmol/L (63 mg/dL). The incidence of hypoglycaemia is 10% per year in type 1 diabetes on twice daily insulin and 30% in those with multiple injections. There is less risk in type 2 diabetes: 0.5% per year if taking sulphonylureas and 2–3% in those taking insulin. All healthcare professionals managing diabetic foot patients should be confident in diagnosing and treating hypoglycaemia.

Blood glucose control

The results of the Diabetes Control and Complications Trial (DCCT) and the UK Prospective Diabetes Study demonstrated the value of tight control of blood glucose with sustained decreased rates of retinopathy, nephropathy and neuropathy. Treatment regimens that reduced average HbA_{1c} to ~7% (~1% above the upper limits of normal) were associated with fewer long-term microvascular complications.

In DCCT, people with type 1 diabetes who achieved near-normal glycaemic control experienced a 69% reduction in subclinical neuropathy and a 57% reduction in clinical neuropathy, as compared with the control subjects who received the usual treatment and who had higher levels of glycaemia.

The value of tight blood glucose control in preventing macrovascular complications is not yet firmly established, but lowering HbA_{1c} may reduce the risk of myocardial infarction and cardiovascular death.

Poorly controlled stage 1 patients may be more prone to develop sepsis than well-controlled patients.

Patients may injure their feet if they become hypoglycaemic. One of our patients damaged his feet on three separate occasions during severe hypoglycaemic episodes.

Blood pressure control

Hypertension (blood pressure greater than 140/90 mmHg) is a common comorbidity of diabetes, affecting 20–60% of people with diabetes, depending on age, obesity and ethnicity. Hypertension is also a major risk factor for cardiovascular disease and microvascular complications, including retinopathy, nephropathy and neuropathy. In type 1 diabetes, hypertension is often the result of underlying nephropathy. In type 2 diabetes, hypertension is likely to be present as part of the metabolic syndrome (i.e. obesity, hyperglycaemia, dyslipidaemia) that is accompanied by high rates of cardiovascular disease.

Randomized clinical trials have demonstrated the clear benefit of lowering blood pressure to 130 mmHg systolic and 80 mmHg diastolic and this should be the target blood pressure for patients with type 1 and type 2 diabetes.

Blood lipid control

Patients with diabetes have an increased prevalence of lipid abnormalities which contribute to high rates of cardiovascular disease, especially in type 2 diabetes, and are also associated with neuropathy. Lipid management aimed at lowering low-density lipoprotein (LDL) cholesterol, raising high-density lipoprotein (HDL) cholesterol and lowering triglycerides has been shown to reduce macrovascular disease and mortality in patients with type 2 diabetes, particularly those who have had prior cardiovascular events. Reduction of saturated fat and cholesterol intake, weight loss and increased physical activity has been shown to improve the lipid profile in patients with diabetes.

Statins have been used as first-line pharmacological therapy for LDL lowering. Indeed, statins are now recommended for all diabetic patients greater than 40-years-old (or younger if there is evidence of cardiovascular disease) and for all patients with microalbuminuria above 20-years-old. High serum triglycerides should be treated with improved glycaemic control, statins and, if necessary, fibrates to achieve recommended targets.

In type 2 diabetes, modern targets are LDL cholesterol < 2.5 mmol/L, HDL cholesterol > 1.0 mmol/L and fasting triglycerides < 1.5 mmol/L. These are also applicable to patients with type 1 diabetes in view of their high morbidity from cardiovascular disease.

Reduction of smoking

Smoking is a very significant risk factor for peripheral vascular disease and is also associated with peripheral neuropathy. Clear, unequivocal advice should be given to stop smoking, but it is a very difficult habit to break.

Patients may be helped by the prescription of nicotine replacement therapy or the administration of smoking cessation drugs such as bupropion, an antidepressant, or more recently varenicline. Enrolment in a smokers' clinic programme may help the patient to give up. Health-care professionals cannot afford to ignore the problem of smoking in diabetic patients and should strongly encourage them to stop. Treatment should still be offered to patients who continue to smoke, but advice to stop or reduce the amount of tobacco consumed should be frequent and unequivocal.

Antiplatelet therapy

Patients with diabetes who are 50 years of age or more, or who are younger but have had diabetes for more than 10 years, should take aspirin 75 mg daily. If aspirin cannot be tolerated, then clopidogrel 75 mg daily should be prescribed.

Hypoglycaemia

Health-care professionals looking after diabetic foot patients should be aware of the symptoms and signs of hypoglycaemia. However, many patients attending the clinic will have neuropathy and also long-standing diabetes. This may result in the patient not experiencing the typical symptoms of hypoglycaemia. Thus it is important to have a high index of suspicion for hypoglycaemia when patients do not seem to be their usual selves.

Hypoglycaemic unawareness

Sympathetic responses decrease with increasing duration of diabetes, and patients may become unaware that they are hypoglycaemic: they develop hypoglycaemic unawareness. It occurs in 25% of patients with type 1 diabetes and in about 50% of patients who have had type 1 diabetes for more than 20 years. There is a change in the glucose threshold for activation of physiological responses to low glucose. The threshold is reduced to 2.5 mmol/L (45 mg/dL) from 4.0 mmol/L (72 mg/dL). Warning signs develop late and the brain does not recognize them because cognitive function diminishes below a glucose level of 3.0 mmol/L (54 mg/dL).

Capillary blood glucose measurement should be available as well as first aid treatment. A stock of glucose drink and biscuits should be available together with Glucogel formerly known as Hypostop Gel, glucagon and intravenous glucose.

Patients with foot problems should be aware that their treatment and investigations may be time consuming and should bring snacks or sandwiches.

Warning signs of hypoglycaemia are due to sympathetic overactivity and cerebral impairment because of reduced glucose availability.

Sympathetic overactivity

- Trembling
- Paraesthesiae around the mouth
- Shakiness
- Anxiety
- Hunger
- Sweating.

Cerebral dysfunction

- Confusion or altered behaviour
- Slurred speech
- Irritability
- Loss of consciousness.

Protocol for treating hypoglycaemia within the diabetic foot clinic

Non-medical reception staff should be trained to keep a close eye on patients who are waiting for treatment, and organize sandwiches, drinks or lunch as appropriate.

Reception staff should be familiar with signs and symptoms of hypoglycaemia and call a health-care professional if they suspect hypoglycaemia.

If the patient reports symptoms of hypoglycaemia or staff suspect hypoglycaemia, a capillary blood glucose should be measured. If below 3.5 mmol/L (63 mg/dL), hypoglycaemia is confirmed.

- If the patient is not drowsy and can swallow, give 130 mL Lucozade or 200 mL fresh orange juice
- On recovery give 20 g of starchy carbohydrate such as a slice of bread or two digestive biscuits
- If patient cannot swallow, give Hypostop Gel around gums or glucagon 1 mg intramuscularly
- Check capillary blood glucose again after 15 minutes
- Give another glass of Lucozade sparkling glucose drink if blood glucose is still below 3.5 mmol/L (63 mg/dL).

However, if blood gucose is below 2.5 mmol/L, consider giving glucagon 1 mg intramuscularly if not given previously.
- If very drowsy give 75 mL of 20% glucose intravenously into a large vein through a large-gauge needle or give 1 mg glucagon intramuscularly
- Patient should not be left alone
- Check blood glucose again before they go home. If the patient has become hypoglycaemic from sulphonylurea therapy he should be admitted for at least 24 hours and may need intravenous glucose therapy (5–20% as required)
- Give advice on hypoglycaemia prevention.

Educational control

General principles

It is never too soon to educate diabetic patients in the care of their feet, and even patients at stage 1 will need to be taught how to look after their feet, how to inspect their feet, how to detect foot problems and what to do and where to go when problems arise. As an absolute minimum, all people with diabetes need to know:
- What constitutes good foot care
- What makes footwear suitable
- What to do and where to go if they develop a foot problem
- Simple first aid self-treatment for the foot
- The importance of the annual review examination.

We also believe that all people with diabetes should be taught about the possibility of neuropathy and ischaemia and related foot problems developing in the future, and the implications of these complications for their future wellbeing. If possible, this should be done without alarming the patient, who should never be made to feel that foot complications are inevitable.

Modes of communication in the education of patients will include one-to-one discussion during the foot treatment, group discussions and distribution of written material or audiovisual material. Pictorial and cartoon materials for patients who cannot read or write have been produced by the World Diabetes Foundation as part of their 'Step by Step' programme for developing countries.

It is also possible to ask patients to advise and help other patients. Different patients respond to different modalities and different approaches: there is no one correct way of approaching education.

Teaching patients good foot care and footwear habits, and addressing barriers to care is an important aspect of gaining long-term improvements in outcomes. However, newly diagnosed patients may feel overwhelmed and inundated with information. For this reason, it may be best to delay foot care and footwear education for a few weeks, until the patient is feeling less upset and confused, and has digested the myriad of other pieces of information he has been given. However, the feet should always be checked at diagnosis since some type 2 patients, undiagnosed for some time, may already have diabetic foot problems. Diabetes foot care education should always be individualized and tailored according to a specific patient's needs, lifestyle and psyche, and frequently adapted as necessary. The reasons for requests being made to the patient to adapt his lifestyle should always be explained. It is cruel to tell a young, fashion-conscious diabetic patient that she should spend the rest of her life in lace-up shoes, or the parents of a small diabetic child that he should never go barefoot. As in all areas of diabetes education, compromises sometimes have to be agreed upon. Advice should be practical and relevant to the patient's lifestyle. However, if the patient's behaviour or lifestyle renders him likely to develop future problems he should be warned.

Patients with a history of severe diabetic complications in near relatives, some of whom may have lost a limb, may be particularly vulnerable, both because of genetic factors and because of fear and loss of hope which makes them deny the efficacy of preventative treatment and fail to appreciate the long-term rewards of good control and foot care. These patients need extra support and education. For some patients the complications of diabetes seem inexorable. They believe that no matter what they do, the outcome will be the same—amputation. This hopeless attitude needs to be corrected by education.

The approach must always be flexible. Some patients want a lot of information in order to feel safe: others will 'switch off' if given more than very simple basic information. Verbal education is best issued in small 'digestible' chunks, and reinforced by written material, including diagrams and pictures. Some patients will wish to have quite extensive information about the foot in diabetes and they can be taught about neuropathy and ischaemia, the implications of these conditions, the ways in which their onset can be delayed or prevented and the terminology used to describe diabetic foot problems. Verbal education should be reinforced with written and pictorial education and vice versa.

If group education sessions are held, the patients' families should be invited to attend and everybody should be taught how to check the feet. Group education may help lonely or isolated people with diabetes, especially the newly diagnosed. Patients from ethnic minorities and their families can be seen in a group with an interpreter.

We ask patients to remove their shoes at education group sessions as this is a good 'ice-breaker' and also leads to detection of previously unsuspected problems.

Some clinics have used patients as educators and we have found this approach helpful. Reformed reprobates can have great insight into barriers to care! Some of our patients have worked as volunteers, giving advice and encouragement to other patients. We also find that our 'open plan' clinic, where individual treatment areas are not walled or curtained off, enables patients and health-care professionals to learn from each other.

CASE STUDY
Poorly controlled diabetes

A 17-year-old girl with type 1 diabetes of 4 years' duration was referred to the diabetic foot clinic for education. A paternal uncle had type 1 diabetes and neuropathic ulceration. Her background was a chaotic one of great poverty and social deprivation with a history of truanting and running away from home. Her HbA_{1c} was 14%. She had frequent admissions to hospital for ketotic episodes and traumatic lesions to her heels and her navel which became infected. She was educated in foot care and footwear but continued to wear unsuitable shoes; she also frequently missed appointments at the diabetic clinic and diabetic foot clinic. However, she agreed to attend the clinic in emergency and to take antibiotics if her foot lesions became infected. She had no more admissions for foot problems, but subsequently developed severe neuropathy, proliferative retinopathy and end-stage renal failure and is currently on dialysis.

Key points
- A flexible, friendly approach in education is important to achieve cooperation and a positive outcome
- Sympathetic support and a safe haven may encourage patients to seek help early and avoid hospital admissions for foot problems.

Educational programmes for stage 1 patients should be based on the following.

Routine foot care
- Wash your feet every day in the bath or shower or a bowl of warm water. Dry gently between toes
- Use mild, domestic soap and rinse the feet well after washing (and when cleaning the area between the toes try not to jerk them apart: this can split the skin and make a sore place)
- Do not soak feet for too long: this makes them drier as it removes oil from the skin

- If skin is dry, rub some moisturizing cream (hand cream, peanut oil, olive oil and cocoa butter are all good) into dry areas, but not between the toes
- If feet are moist and sweaty, apply surgical spirit to them twice daily, including the area between toes
- Avoid walking barefoot
- Apart from simple first aid to injuries, do not try to treat foot problems yourself. See your diabetic foot team
- Do not buy proprietary remedies from the chemist
- If you want to try 'alternative medicines' for your diabetes or for your feet, please discuss this with your health-care team first.

Daily foot check
Get into the habit of keeping a close eye on your feet and nails.

Remember the four danger signs of foot problems:
- Redness or other colour changes in a foot or part of a foot (red, blue, black, purple or pale)
- Swelling
- Pain or throbbing
- Breaks in the skin.

If any of these develops you should seek help via your diabetic foot service, which should make clear the procedure for obtaining urgent help.

Check feet regularly for unusual lumps, bumps, splits, cracks, athlete's foot, rashes or verrucae (warts). If you find them, seek help as above.

Remember
- That neglected hard skin and callus can cause ulceration
- That if your foot changes shape or becomes infected you need help
- Check shoes daily for penetrating nails or sharp objects
- Check your feet every day for these danger signs or for anything else unusual about your feet
- If you have difficulty getting down to your feet, you can use a mirror to see the soles
- Ask your family to help you to check your feet if you have problems with your eyesight
- Always ask for advice if you notice anything unusual about your feet.

Nail care
It is quite safe for you to cut your own toe nails if:
- Nails are a normal shape and free of pain
- You can see your feet clearly
- You can reach your feet easily
- You have been taught correct nail cutting techniques.

Correct nail cutting techniques
- Cut nails after bath or shower: the water will soften them and make it easier
- Special nail nippers are better than ordinary scissors
- Do not cut a nail in one piece: nibble away at it. File your nails to reduce length and thickness. Rub the file in one direction only, towards the end of your toe, to avoid rocking the nail
- Do not let your toe nails grow beyond the length of the toe: they may catch on shoes and socks and become damaged
- Do not cut your nails too short: if you break the seal between the nail and the flesh you may get an infection
- Never dig or cut down the side of your nails: you risk leaving a spike of nail behind and causing an ingrowing toe nail
- Use a soft nail brush in the bath or shower to remove dirt or debris from around or under nails
- Never pick or pull off pieces of nail or skin
- Nails need regular cutting: even normal nails will give trouble if they become too long
- If you have problems getting down to your feet or cannot see clearly, please ask for help cutting your nails from a family member or friend
- If your nails are painful or an unusual shape, change colour, or become thickened or ingrowing, or if you injure your nails, seek help from a health-care professional.

First aid information
Keep a small first aid box at home (and also take it on holiday) containing:
- Sterile dressings
- Plasters
- Bandages
- Hypoallergenic tape (sticky tape with special backing to prevent skin irritation)
- Antiseptic cream
- Tweezers
- Scissors.

Any wound which breaks the skin should be carefully cleaned under a running tap or with saline solution. (Make your own saline solution with half a pint of previously boiled water and two teaspoons of salt.)

Liquid antiseptics should be diluted according to the manufacturer's instructions before applying them to a sore place. (Never apply full-strength antiseptic to your foot: it will burn the flesh.) Then tape or bandage a clean dressing over the wound.

If the following occurs:
- Wound does not heal within a few days
- Foot becomes painful
- Foot becomes swollen
- Foot becomes red or discoloured

seek help from your health-care professional as your foot may be infected.

Never stop taking your diabetic medication, even if your blood glucose is high and you cannot eat.

Footwear guide
- Choose a shoe which is long, broad and deep. There should be half an inch of space between the end of the foot and the end of the shoe when you are standing
- Shoes which fasten with a lace or strap are better than slip-ons
- Heels should be under 5 cm high
- The inner lining should be smooth
- Buy shoes in the afternoon—feet swell during the day.
- New shoes should be worn in gradually and one pair of shoes should not be worn for days on end
- Wear stockings or socks to avoid blisters
- If socks have prominent seams wear them inside out
- Break shoes in gently.

Background to diabetic foot problems
People with diabetes whose diabetic control is poor may develop nerve damage (called neuropathy) which causes numbness of the feet. The blood vessels may also be damaged leading to a poor blood supply (ischaemia). Both of these problems can cause foot ulcers. It is important for all people with diabetes to give their feet special care and attention, as described above, to prevent foot problems.

PRACTICE POINTS

- All diabetic patients should have their feet screened annually
- Although stage 1 patients are at low risk compared with any other stage of diabetic foot, they should still be regarded as vulnerable patients when compared with the non-diabetic population.
- Diabetic patients should be advised to wear suitable footwear so as to prevent subsequent deformity
- Common foot problems should be diagnosed early and treated appropriately
- It is important to achieve good metabolic care with control of blood glucose, blood pressure, blood lipids, smoking cessation and taking antiplatelet therapy when indicated
- All diabetic patients should be educated in good foot care, told why good diabetes control is important and warned about foot complications.

FURTHER READING

General background

Boulton AJM, Cavanagh PR, Rayman G (eds). *The Foot in Diabetes*, 4th edn. John Wiley & Sons, Ltd., Chichester, UK, 2006.

Edmonds ME, Foster AVM. *Managing the Diabetic Foot*, 2nd edn. Blackwell Science, Oxford, UK, 2005.

Foster AVM. *Podiatric Assessment and Management of the Diabetic Foot*. Churchill Livingstone, London, UK, 2006.

Foster AVM, Edmonds ME. *Colour Atlas of Foot and Ankle Disorders*. Churchill Livingstone, Oxford, UK, 2007.

Pfeifer MA, Bowker J (eds). *Levin and O'Neal's The Diabetic Foot*, 7th edn. Elsevier, Philadelphia, USA, 2007.

McGill M, Molyneaux L, Yue DK. Which diabetic patients should receive podiatry care? An objective analysis. *Intern Med J* 2005; **35**: 451–6.

Shaw KM and Cummings MH (eds). *Diabetes Chronic Complications*, 2nd edn. John Wiley & Sons, Ltd., Chichester, UK, 2006.

Tesfaye S, Chaturvedi N, Eaton SEM *et al*, for the EURODIAB Prospective Complications Study Group. Vascular risk factors and diabetic neuropathy. *N Eng J Med* 2005; **352**: 341–50.

Veves A, Giurini JM, LoGerfo FW (eds). *The Diabetic Foot*, 2nd edn. Humana Press, New Jersey, USA, 2006.

Mechanical control

Burns SL, Leese GP, McMurdo ME. Older people and ill fitting shoes. *Postgrad Med J* 2002; **78**: 344–6.

Espensen EH, Nixon BP, Armstrong DC. Chemical matrixectomy for ingrown toenails: Is there an evidence basis to guide therapy? *J Am Podiatr Med Assoc* 2002; **92**: 287–95.

Robbins JM. Treatment of onychomycosis in the diabetic patient population. *J Diabetes Complications* 2003; **17**: 98–104.

Metabolic control

CAPRIE Steering Committee. A randomized, blinded trial of clopidogrel versus aspirin in patients at risk of ischaemic events (CAPRIE). *Lancet* 1996; **348**: 1329–39.

Diabetes Control and Complications Trial Research Group. The effect of intensive treatment of diabetes on the development and progression of long-term complications in insulin dependent diabetes mellitus. *N Engl J Med* 1993; **329**: 977–86.

Fox C, MacKinnon M. *Vital Diabetes: Your essential reference for diabetes management in primary care*. Class Health, London, UK, 2002.

Heller S. Diabetic hypoglycaemia. *Baillieres Best Pract Res Clin Endocrinol Metab* 1999; **13**: 279–94.

IDF Clinical Guidelines Task Force Global guidelines for type 2 diabetes. Recommendations for standard, comprehensive and minimal care. *Diabetic Medicine* 2006; **23**: 579–93.

Joint British Societies. Guidelines on prevention of cardiovascular disease in clinical practice. *Heart* 2005; **91**: 1–52.

Sheehan P. Introduction to diabetes: Principles of care in the surgical patient with diabetes. In Veves A, Giurini JM, LoGerfo FW (eds). *The Diabetic Foot*, 2nd edn. Humana Press, New Jersey, USA, 2006, pp. 1–38.

UK Prospective Diabetes Study Group. Intensive blood-glucose control with sulphonylureas or insulin compared with conventional treatment and risk of complications in patients with type 2 diabetes (UKPDS 33). *Lancet* 1998; **352**: 837–53.

UK Prospective Diabetes Study Group. Tight blood pressure control and risk of macrovascular and microvascular complications in type 2 diabetes. (UKPDS 38). *Br Med J* 1998; **317**: 703–13.

Watkins PJ, Amiel SA, Howell SL, Turner E. *Diabetes and its Management*, 6th edn. Blackwell Publishing, Oxford, UK, 2003.

Educational control

Assal JP, Muhlhauser I, Pernet A *et al*. Patient education as the basis for diabetes care in clinical practice and research. *Diabetologia* 1985; **28**: 602–13.

Batista F, Pinzur MS. Disease knowledge in patients attending a diabetic foot clinic. *Foot Ankle Int* 2005; **26**: 38–41.

Edmonds ME, Van Acker K, Foster AVM. Education and the diabetic foot. *Diabetic Medicine* 1996; **13**: S61–4.

Lavery LA, Higgins KR, Lanctot DR *et al*. Preventing diabetic foot ulcer recurrence in high-risk patients: use of temperature monitoring as a self-assessment tool. *Diabetes Care* 2007; **30**: 14–20.

Lavery LA, Wunderlich RP, Tredwell JL. Disease management for the diabetic foot: effectiveness of a diabetic foot prevention program to reduce amputations and hospitalizations. *Diabetes Res Clin Pract* 2005; **70**: 31–7.

Mackie S. Developing an education package on diabetic foot disease. *Br J Community Nurs* 2006; **11**: Suppl 6, 8, 10 passim.

Meyers L. Daily foot checks are critical. *Diabetes Forecast* 2005; **58**: 48.

Ooi GS, Rodrigo C, Cheong WK *et al*. An evaluation of the value of group education in recently diagnosed diabetes mellitus. *Int J Low Extrem Wounds* 2007; **6**: 28–33.

Peter-Riesch B, Assal JP. Teaching diabetic foot care effectively. *J Am Podiatr Med Assoc* 1997; **87**: 318–20.

Valk GD, Kriegsman DM, Assendelft WJ. Patient education for preventing diabetic foot ulceration. *Cochrane Database Syst Rev* 2005; **1**: CD001488.

3 Stage 2: the high-risk foot

Many thousands on's
Have the disease, and feel 't not . . ."
(A Winter's Tale, *I, ii*, William Shakespeare)

PRESENTATION AND DIAGNOSIS

People with diabetes and stage 2 feet are at high risk of running into trouble. Their problems are exacerbated by the fact that many patients with feet at stage 2 are unaware that they have any trouble with their feet. The risk factors for ulceration may not be noticed, and once the patient has neuropathy there may be no pain or discomfort to warn him of potential problems.

In *Coriolanus* Act 4 Scene 1 when William Shakespeare writes of:
'Your ignorance – that finds not 'til it feels'.
He could almost have been writing about a diabetic patient with neuropathy who has an ulcer.

The diabetic foot enters stage 2 when it has developed neuropathy or ischaemia, and the further important risk factors for ulceration, namely deformity, swelling and callus, are frequently also present. Deformity, swelling and callus do not commonly lead to ulceration in patients with intact protective pain sensation and a good blood supply, but when they are found in combination with neuropathy or ischaemia they significantly increase the risk of ulceration.

Because these risk factors may not cause symptoms, patients are unlikely to report problems. It is therefore important to screen patients at the annual review, which is an essential part of diabetic foot care. A recent evaluation of a diabetic foot screening programme showed that it could prevent major amputations. A large randomized controlled trial of 2001 diabetic patients compared outcomes in 1001 patients who were screened for risk factors and 1000 in the control group who were not screened. The people at risk of foot ulceration in the screened group were treated with podiatry and education. At the end of

2 years there was only one major amputation in the screened group compared with 12 in the control group, which is a significant difference.

There are other factors that increase risk, including diabetic complications, comorbidities and social problems. Important among these are
- Poor vision
- Old age
- Social isolation—'lack of social connectedness'
- Poverty
- Ignorance
- Intellectual deficit
- Concurrent psychiatric illness
- Obesity.

Every diabetic foot at stage 2 will be classified as neuropathic or neuroischaemic. It is necessary to emphasize that there is a great divide between the neuropathic foot, which lacks protective pain sensation but has a good blood supply, and the neuroischaemic foot with a combination of neuropathy and ischaemia, because the treatment will be different in the two groups and because the neuroischaemic foot offers no leeway for error. The neuroischaemic foot is an unforgiving foot and even well-managed diabetic patients with neuroischaemic feet sometimes come to a major amputation.

When renal impairment develops in the diabetic patient it is accompanied by fluid retention with peripheral oedema, anaemia, reduced microvascular blood flow and increased susceptibility to skin breakdown: thus, the addition of such renal impairment in the patient with a neuropathic or neuroischaemic foot leads to a situation of extreme risk in diabetic patients, and this syndrome is often referred to as the diabetic renal foot and has the worst prognosis of all diabetic feet.

A Practical Manual of Diabetic Foot Care, 2nd edition, Edmonds, Foster and Sanders.
Published 2008 Blackwell Publishing. ISBN 978-1-4051-61473

This chapter considers (under 'Vascular control') two non-ulcerative complications of the neuroischaemic foot:
• Severe chronic ischaemia
• Acute ischaemia.
It also discusses two specific but non-ulcerative complications of the neuropathic foot:
• Painful neuropathy
• Charcot's osteoarthropathy including neuropathic fractures.

MANAGEMENT

Stage 2 feet require multidisciplinary care.

The following components of multidisciplinary care are important at stage 2:
• Mechanical control
• Vascular control
• Metabolic control
• Educational control.
Wound control and microbiological control are not needed as the feet have intact skin.

Mechanical control

To maintain mechanical control, deformity must be accommodated by footwear. Callus, dry skin and fissures are treated. Common non-diabetic foot problems, already described for stage 1, will also occur in stage 2 feet and need management as described in Chapter 2.

Footwear

Deformities in the neuropathic foot may include a raised medial longitudinal arch leading to high pressure points on the sole of the foot, which develops callus and ulceration unless protected by a special insole. The insole will usually need to be accommodated in a bespoke shoe.

The neuroischaemic foot is prone to develop ulcers upon its margins, often over the side of the 1st and 5th metatarsal heads, and 5th metatarsal base. Patients should be advised to wear a sufficiently wide and deep shoe to protect the vulnerable margins of the foot.

The overall approach is to try to accommodate these deformities in properly fitting shoes. The role of prophylactic surgery is discussed in Chapter 8.

The orthotist is a very important member of the diabetic foot team, both in terms of footwear education and provision of shoes and orthotics. Ideally the orthotist should work within the diabetic foot clinic as an integral part of the team, seeing and discussing patients together with his colleagues. The provision of suitable foot care is not a simple matter and very close cooperation is needed between the orthotist and other members of the foot team, whilst the whole process of footwear provision, from prescription to final delivery, is taking place. Some diabetic feet have extreme deformity and several attempts may need to be made before a solution is found. For the multidisciplinary management of deformity, close liaison is necessary between physican, podiatrist and orthotist in the provision of shoes and insoles. Some deformities may be accommodated in high-street footwear. Patients with major deformities whose shoes cause red pressure marks or callus will need either footwear adjustments or special shoes.

An outline of shoes and insoles available is given below, and a further discussion of footwear is given in Chapter 4.

Types of shoe

There are five main categories of shoe.
• Sensible shoes of a correct size and style from the high-street shoe shop. Once patients are high risk they should not wear mail-order shoes unless they can obtain them on a sale or return basis and have them checked by a health-care professional. Athletic shoes (trainers) are a reasonable choice for most patients: one of our patients said he was too old for trainers but agreed to wear golf shoes (Fig. 3.1). Patients, who have neuropathy and don't know it, will be accustomed to the tactile sensation of having shoes on their feet and may progressively buy tighter-fitting shoes to reproduce that sensation. This habit can cause pressure necrosis—patients with neuropathy should be warned to avoid tight shoes, and the implications of sensory loss should be emphasized. High-street shoes are not able to accommodate significant deformity which needs to be housed within stock shoes, modular shoes or bespoke shoes. The heels of

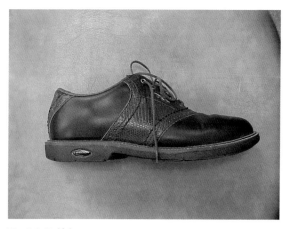

Fig. 3.1 Golf shoes.

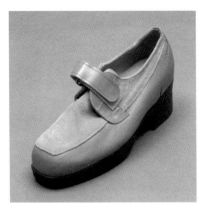

Fig. 3.2 Extra depth stock shoe.

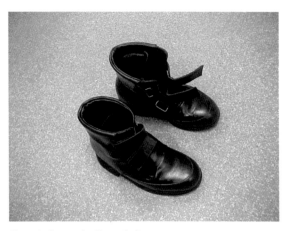

Fig. 3.3 Customized bespoke boot.

shoes should not be more than 2.5 cm high, to avoid throwing weight forward onto the metatarsal heads. Thin-soled shoes render the feet at risk of trauma

- Ready-made, off-the-shelf, stock shoes (Fig. 3.2). These are made with extra depth and width, and without prominent seams. They usually have a low opening, are fully lined and contain a built-in rocker sole and flat-bed insoles made of microcellular rubber. The insoles can be replaced with bespoke insoles. Stretching specific areas, or making 'balloon patches' to accommodate single small deformities may also render off-the-shelf shoes suitable

- Modular shoes, which are the stage between ready-made and bespoke shoes. The orthotist carries out a trial fit using the standard stock shoe and then details a number of fixed modifications to be carried out

- Customized or bespoke shoes. These accommodate the shape of the foot which cannot be fitted within stock or modular shoes. The more abnormal the foot shape the greater the need for bespoke shoes. These may also be necessary if previous ulceration has resulted in scarring, depletion of fibrofatty padding under the metatarsal heads, or bound down plantar tissues leading to high plantar pressures. Bespoke shoes can house moulded insoles which redistribute high plantar pressures in the neuropathic foot. In some cases of ankle deformity, bespoke boots may be necessary (Fig. 3.3)

- Temporary ready-made shoes (for ulcerated feet) that can accommodate dressings. They are usually fitted with flat-bed insoles but a moulded insole can be inserted.

General principles of prescription of stock and bespoke shoes

- The patient's choice of material, colour and style should always be respected as far as possible

- For young patients, shoes made in a trainer style are often acceptable

- Patients need shoes for inside and outside, and may need bespoke shoes or boots for work, sometimes with steel toecaps. Agricultural labourers may develop problems if they wear Wellington boots for long periods in wet climates. In tropical climates agricultural labourers are at risk of deep fungal infections without protective footwear

- Shoe soles should be thick enough to prevent puncture by nails or thorns

- Shoe fastenings should be adjustable to accommodate swelling. Patients should be taught to rest the heel of the shoe on the ground and move the foot well back in the shoe before doing up the laces

- Shoes should be checked at every clinic visit and reassessed frequently for excessive wear and the changing needs of patients

- Patients should have at least two pairs so that they are never without a pair of wearable shoes

- Each pair of shoes should not, if possible, be worn for more than 2 consecutive days at a time

- Patients should wear special shoes at all times except for bed and bathing. They should not 'keep special shoes for best'—they are for everyday use

- Slippers should not be worn round the house: the special shoes are for indoor and outdoor use

- Shoes which become worn down should be brought in for early repair and the orthotist should supervise repair of bespoke shoes

- There is need for regular review of footwear. If foot biomechanics are abnormal there may be uneven

patterns of wear which can rapidly render the shoe likely to cause problems
- New shoes, and repaired shoes, whether bespoke, stock or from high-street stores, should be checked before the patient wears them for the first time. They should never be posted to the patient without a final fitting and check and if new problems develop the patient should be seen without delay. The patient should be asked to bring all his shoes along to the clinic on this visit so that a problem with a specific pair can be detected.

Insoles

Insoles are made from a variety of polyethylene foams, microcellular rubbers and ethyl vinyl acetate foams, and can be flat-bed (usually one layer, provided in stock shoes) or moulded. Moulded insoles are usually made from two or three layers of differing densities.

Insoles are used to reduce or redistribute areas of high pressure, friction and shear in the following ways:
- By loading areas of the sole which are not normally in contact with the ground, such as the medial longitudinal arch, a total contact effect can be achieved, relieving local areas of high pressure
- By extending the insole up the sides of the foot, a cradle effect will reduce friction (so-called cradled insoles)
- Under particularly high-pressure areas, such as prominent metatarsal heads, areas of the insole can be excavated out to form a 'sink'
- Extra cushioning or padding can be used to compensate for reduced fibrofatty padding over the metatarsal heads
- Silicone gel plantar inserts can be used to reduce shear and this material also comes in the form of heel cups, flat-bed insoles and sleeves for individual toes.

All insoles should be regularly checked for 'bottoming-out' or excessive wear.

CASE STUDY
Nail in shoe

A 47-year-old man with type 2 diabetes of 9 years' duration and previous history of neuropathic ulcer, attended the orthotist for review 1 month after receiving new shoes because he was developing new callus in his mid-tarsal area where he had never previously had a problem. When the orthotist removed the ethyl vinyl acetate insole he found that a large nail had punctured the sole of the shoe (Fig. 3.4). Fortunately the insole was thick enough to prevent penetration of the skin, but the increased pressure had led to callus formation.

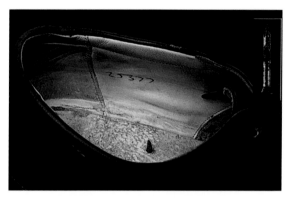

Fig. 3.4 Nail has penetrated the sole of the shoe—the insole has been removed to reveal the nail.

Key points
- Patients who check their feet and report any new problems at an early stage can abort problems
- A thick insole can prevent puncture wounds
- Patients with neuropathy are wise to check the soles of their shoes regularly for penetrating nails.

Persuading patients to wear suitable shoes

There is a need for compromise, flexibility and imagination in footwear provision and education. Young and fashion conscious patients will want to look and dress the same as their peers, and use of trainers and Doc Marten's boots will make them feel less self-conscious. Where bespoke shoes are essential, they can be made in the above styles (Fig. 3.5).

If patients are reluctant to wear special shoes, and do not understand the reason, then taking and showing them in-shoe pressure measurements can demonstrate that

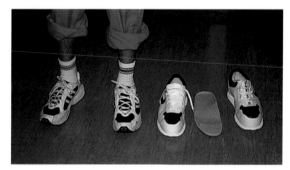

Fig. 3.5 The patient is wearing his favourite trainers on which a pair of bespoke trainers have been modelled, which are deep enough to contain a cradled insole.

areas of the sole are at risk of ulceration because of high pressures.

CASE STUDY
High-tech education

A 25-year-old woman with type 1 diabetes of 10 years' duration and a history of relapsing neuropathic ulceration, was very reluctant to wear bespoke shoes and denied that they would help to prevent ulceration. We explained the association between high plantar pressures, callus and ulceration and then measured plantar pressures when she was wearing her own shoes and when she was wearing trainer-style shoes (Fig. 3.6a,b).

Once she saw the reduction of high pressures in the trainer-style shoes she agreed to wear them and her ulcers healed and remained healed.

Key points
- In-shoe pressure measurement systems are invaluable in demonstrating the reduction of forefoot pressures in special shoes
- When dangerously high pressures are demonstrated to patients they are more likely to agree to change their style of footwear
- When high-tech apparatus is not available, using low-tech educational messages is also effective. An outline of the patient's foot can be traced on paper, cut out and fitted into the patient's shoe: if it will not fit in the shoe, the patient can see clearly that the shoe is too small.

Patients' reasons for refusing to wear special shoes
- Too ugly and unfashionable
- Too heavy
- 'Look like hospital shoes'
- Unacceptable appearance
- High cost
- Excessive time to receive shoes
- Limited colours, styles, materials and durability.

It is better to compromise on design and issue a pair of shoes which are suboptimal but will be worn by the patient rather than issue 'optimal' shoes which stay in the back of the wardrobe.

What to do if patients refuse to wear suitable shoes
- Try to limit the amount of walking patients do in unsuitable shoes
- If patients wear slip-on shoes, the heels should be as low as possible to avoid weight being thrown forward onto the metatarsal heads. If patients are accustomed to

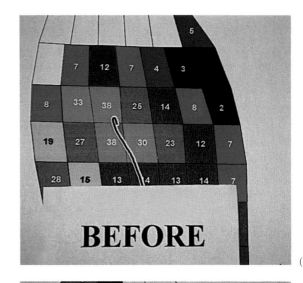

(a)

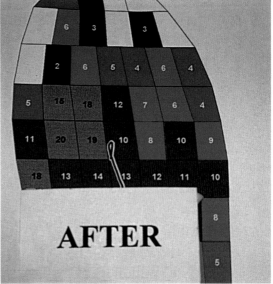

(b)

Fig. 3.6 (a) Forefoot pressure measurements using EMED system reveal red areas of unacceptably high pressure in patient's own shoes. (b) The areas of high pressure are eliminated in a trainer-style shoe.

wearing high heels and agree to adopt a lower style, the heels should be lowered gradually to avoid damage to the Achilles tendon
- If shoes are particularly damaging, try to persuade patients to accept an alternative style
- Ascertain reasons for non-acceptance. Are they spurious or sound?

- Ask another patient who wears special shoes, of similar age, background and lifestyle, to talk to the patient
- Re-educate the patient and explain the importance of special shoes. Try to find a compromise or alternative in every case.

World view of shoes

In many parts of the world people with diabetes do not buy special shoes because they cannot afford them. Sometimes even shop-bought shoes are too expensive. Many wear alternatives which are home-made from pieces of leather or floor covering or old motor tyres. Sandals made from tyres are particularly dangerous when wear exposes a mesh of metal fibres in direct contact with the sole of the foot. In some countries local health-care workers have successfully developed shoes for people with diabetes which are suitable for tropical environments and cost-effective, as in the case of the Singapore sandal, created by the local podiatry team (Fig. 2.4, see Chapter 2). The use of foam sponges, purchased cheaply from kitchen suppliers and incorporated into footwear by workers in India has also been successful.

Management of specific deformities

Deformity and limited joint mobility subject the feet to abnormal mechanical forces which can lead to ulceration unless managed carefully. Some of the most common problems seen in people with diabetes are claw toes, prominent metatarsal heads, fibrofatty padding depletion and displacement, hallux rigidus/limitus, hallux valgus, foot drop and rigid plantar-flexed foot. In patients with continuing or relapsing neuropathic ulcers, hallux rigidus and rigid plantar-flexed foot with limited movement at the ankle joint are common. The latter problem overloads the forefoot as the foot can never achieve an angle of 90 degrees flexion at the ankle joint.

Claw toes

They should be accommodated in shoes with a wide, deep toe box to reduce pressure on the dorsum of the toes. This may be achieved in high-street shoes, but often extra-depth shoes or bespoke shoes are needed. If the deformity is not 'fixed' a silicone rubber device (toe prop) can correct toe position and off-load the apices.

Prominent metatarsal heads

These can be accommodated in an extra-depth stock shoe with a cushioning insole. However, where the medial longitudinal arch is high and the metatarsal heads are extremely prominent, a cradled insole with sinks and bespoke shoes will be needed.

Fibrofatty padding depletion

Where fibrofatty padding is absent or greatly diminished or displaced, a cushioned insole, or felt padding can reduce plantar pressures. Patches of silicone gel can be applied over the metatarsal heads. When it is associated with raised arch and clawed toes, a cradled insole in a bespoke shoe will be needed. Felt padding should not be applied to the diabetic foot long term: removable devices are safer.

Hallux rigidus/limitus

This is a very common cause of neuropathic ulceration in barefoot and sandal-wearing populations. Callus develops under the big toe and if not removed regularly an ulcer develops. A rocker sole can be applied to the sole of a shoe or sandal by an orthotist to reduce pressure at the end of the walking cycle when the toe leaves the ground. This condition may require surgical correction. Callus should be regularly debrided.

Hallux valgus

Extra-width stock shoes or bespoke shoes will be needed to protect the medial prominence.

Foot drop

Foot drop can be accommodated by an ankle–foot orthosis (AFO) which can be of the traditional metal and leather calliper type or the more recent thermoplastic type. Sprung joints to assist dorsiflexion may also be added but will make the AFO heavier.

Rigid plantar-flexed foot

Limitation of dorsiflexion at the ankle joint can be compensated by building up support at the hindfoot: a raise on the other shoe is often needed. Achilles tendon lengthening has been shown to increase ankle dorsiflexion range of motion, decrease forefoot plantar pressure and reduce the rate of ulcer recurrence. Other series have shown that the most important complication of Achilles tendon lengthening is the development of a transfer lesion on the heel. However, such risks of this procedure may be outweighed in patients with recurrent ulcers and reduced dorsiflexion of the ankle joint.

Physiotherapy may help to improve the range of motion at the ankle joint. When plaster casts are made to heal ulcers or manage Charcot's osteoarthropathy in these feet it is necessary to build up the hindfoot area of the cast to compensate for the plantar flexion, and it is nearly always necessary to put a temporary shoe raise on the other side.

Management of corns, callus and fissures

Corns

Corns should be removed by sharp debridement with a scalpel. Interdigital corns may be moist and grasping them with a forceps helps maintain tissue tension. Felt padding may be used short term to deflect pressure but needs to be checked regularly.

- Opaque coverings or padding should be lifted regularly to inspect feet which lack protective pain sensation
- Unequivocal advice should be given to patients to seek help immediately if their feet deteriorate
- For many years we refrained from using adhesive felt padding on high-risk diabetic feet. We now use felt padding as a temporary measure while insoles are awaited, but always advise the patient to lift the padding and check beneath it at regular intervals and review the patient frequently. We prefer to use silicone rubber removable devices or insoles to deflect pressure.

Callus

Plantar callus is a characteristic feature of the neuropathic foot and its potential for causing ulcers should never be underestimated. It is the most important marker of a foot at risk of neuropathic ulceration. Callus concentrates pressure on the plantar aspect and increases the risk of ulceration more than 11-fold. Callus is the most important preulcerative lesion in the stage 2 foot. On the neuropathic foot it is usually hard and dry because of reduced sweating due to autonomic neuropathy. When neglected and allowed to accumulate, it causes pressure necrosis and ulceration of the underlying tissues. Good blood flow is probably necessary for exuberant callus formation.

Callus also develops on the neuroischaemic foot, where it is thin and 'glassy' and rarely causes ulceration. We do not recommend that areas of thin glassy callus on ischaemic feet be debrided unless they develop rough areas which can catch on clothing, are causing pain or develop signs of underlying problems. The practitioner must be aware that the layer of callus may be very thin, that the texture of ischaemic callus is glazed and slippery and that without great care the scalpel blade may slip. Callus in nail sulci should also be cleared with great care when patients are ischaemic. It is very important not to traumatize the ischaemic foot: underoperating should be the rule.

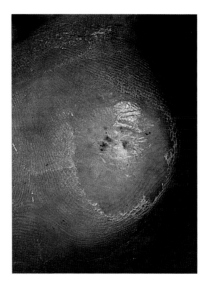

Fig. 3.7 Callus debrided to expose white macerated layer and speckles of blood.

Preulcerative callus

Clear warning signs become apparent when callus becomes too thick and ulceration is imminent. These include:

- Small speckles of blood within callus where individual capillaries are damaged by pressure and begin to leak
- A deeper layer of white, macerated callus within callus (Fig. 3.7) only exposed by sharp debridement of the superficial layers
- An intraepidermal bulla full of clear fluid, but the underlying tissue is intact.

Emergency treatment to remove callus and reduce the excessive mechanical forces by means of footwear adaptations should be undertaken without delay.

CASE STUDY
Preulcerative callus

A 50-year-old man with type 1 diabetes of 30 years' duration underwent amputation of the second ray of his right foot for wet gangrene. At discharge from hospital he was reluctant to wear special shoes. After the foot healed he developed heavy callus over his 1st and 4th metatarsal heads. Speckles of blood within the callus indicated a preulcerative state (Fig. 3.8). He agreed to wear bespoke shoes after the significance of the blood within the callus was explained. The orthotists supplied cradled insoles with poron sinks in bespoke shoes, callus was debrided at monthly intervals, and he did not develop an ulcer.

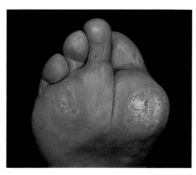

Fig. 3.8 Heavy callus containing speckles of blood indicates a preulcerative state.

Key points

- Speckles of blood within callus indicate that an ulcer is imminent
- Patients with ray amputations should be strongly advised to accept bespoke shoes and taught to return immediately if speckles of blood are observed within their callus
- Regular debridement of callus and bespoke shoes can prevent neuropathic ulcers.

Podiatric removal of callus

Ideally, callus should only be removed by podiatrists who have been trained in the appropriate techniques as follows:

- Callus should be removed with a scalpel held by the operator's dominant hand
- The fingers of the operator's other hand should stretch the tissue being operated on to maintain good skin tension and ensure even removal of callus
- The foot should not be soaked prior to callus removal by scalpel debridement. The operator needs visual and tactile clues to guide him as to the amount of callus that can be safely removed
- Callus contains more moisture in its deeper levels, closer to the epidermodermal junction, and if the skin and callus are macerated by soaking then valuable tactile clues as to the depth the operator has reached are lost
- Patients who develop callus on pressure points need regular treatment and careful follow-up if ulceration is to be prevented
- Speed of regrowth of callus varies and treatment periods must be individually planned
- Formation of callus is a warning that dangerously high mechanical forces are acting on the stage 2 foot, and every effort should be made to achieve effective mechanical control through footwear adaptation and lifestyle changes

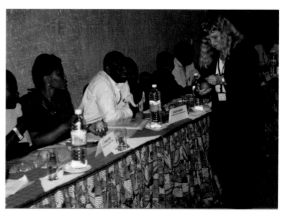

Fig. 3.9 'Step by Step' callus-removal techniques demonstrated by removing peel from sweet limes.

- Patients should be taught the danger signs that callus is becoming preulcerative
- Patients who fail to keep an appointment for callus removal should be recalled.

In countries where there is no tradition of podiatry, nurses and physicians can learn podiatric techniques. To learn precision and gain manual dexterity they should try first to remove the skin from an orange without removing any white pith, and practice paring wax from a candle. The first 'patients' from whom they remove callus should be family or colleagues with low-risk feet, and they can then move on to practising on non-diabetic patients with no risk factors before they treat high-risk patients. In the World Diabetes Foundation funded 'Step by Step' programmes in India, Nepal, Bangladesh, Sri Lanka and Africa, health-care practitioners were trained in callus removal by using scalpels to remove the peel from sweet limes (Fig. 3.9), and pairs of physicians and nurses removed their shoes, performed foot examinations and staging, and cut each other's toe nails.

Removal of callus by patients' carers

Patients should never cut their callus off, or use proprietary corn or callus removers. These contain strong acids and can damage the skin, allowing infection to enter the foot.

For diabetic foot patients who are unable to reach a health-care professional, the following procedure can be undertaken by a carer, family member or friend to reduce the callus.

- Soak the foot in a bowl of warm water containing a handful of salt for 15 minutes

- Rub a pumice stone or a piece of Scotchbrite (nylon kitchen scouring pad) over the area of callus to reduce the thickness
- Tape a piece of clean gauze over the area and keep it covered, and walk as little as possible for 48 hours
- Observe the foot carefully for discharge or tissue breakdown. If these develop the foot should be shown to a health-care professional as soon as possible.

The authors are aware that the above advice is controversial. It is delivered in the belief that preventative foot care delivered by people who have been taught safe techniques and know the importance of not breaking the skin of the high-risk foot is better than no foot care at all.

In addition, correct nail cutting techniques (see Chapter 2) should be taught to stage 2 patients and their families if they live in isolated areas and are unable to obtain sufficiently frequent foot care from professionals. Gentle, regular filing of nails is safer than cutting or paring them with a knife. Regular filing can reduce the nails sufficiently so that they never need cutting. The nails should be filed in one direction only to avoid rocking the nail plate.

Fissures

Fissures are a complication of dry neuropathic skin. Regular application of emollient helps to prevent fissures. The edges of deep fissures should be cleared of callus and the crevice can be held together with Steri-strips to speed healing (Fig. 3.10a–c). Patients who are prone to heel fissures should avoid backless footwear.

Other common foot disorders and their management are described in Chapter 2.

Vascular control

The majority of patients will be asymptomatic and ischaemia will be diagnosed on screening examination. Ischaemia should never be taken lightly. All patients with absent foot pulses should have their pressure index measured to confirm ischaemia and to provide a baseline, so that subsequent deterioration can be detected before the patient presents with irreversible lesions.

Podiatrists should always ascertain their patient's vascular status before they cut the toe nails or remove callus, as any injury to the neuroischaemic foot can result in ulceration.

Furthermore, the detection of peripheral vascular disease provides an extremely important opportunity for management of atherosclerotic risk factors to prevent future vascular events in the coronary and cerebrovascular

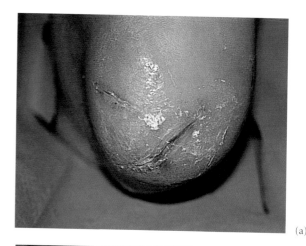

(a)

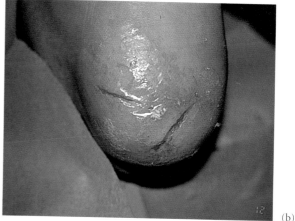

(b)

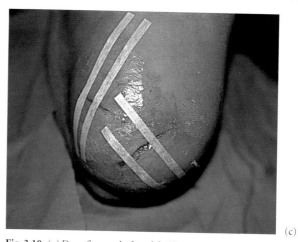

(c)

Fig. 3.10 (a) Deep fissures before debridement. (b) The edges of the fissures have been cleared of callus. (c) The edges of the fissures are held together with Steri-strips.

systems which have a high burden of atherosclerosis in patients with peripheral vascular disease.

Antiplatelet agents significantly reduce myocardial infarction and stroke in high-risk patients. Thus all diabetic patients with evidence of peripheral vascular disease will benefit from antiplatelet agents: 75 mg aspirin daily, or if this cannot be tolerated, clopidogrel 75 mg daily.

Diabetic patients with peripheral vascular disease should also be given statin therapy. The Heart Protection Study has shown that simvastatin reduced the rate of major vascular events in a wide range of high-risk patients including those with peripheral arterial disease or diabetes.

In addition patients should be encouraged to stop smoking and blood pressure should be tightly controlled.

Patients who are above 55 years old and have peripheral vascular disease should also benefit from an angiotensin-converting enzyme (ACE) inhibitor to prevent further vascular episodes (as indicated by the Heart Outcomes Prevention Evaluation [HOPE] and micro-HOPE study). ACE inhibitors protect the vasculature in diabetic patients who have evidence of atherosclerotic disease.

The above recommendations are also discussed in a consensus document which has been produced by the American Diabetes Association on the management of patients with diabetes and peripheral vascular disease.

If symptoms do develop in the foot with ischaemia, there are three main clinical presentations:
- Intermittent claudication
- Severe chronic ischaemia with or without rest pain
- Acute ischaemia.

Intermittent claudication

The classical site of claudication is the calf, although it may occur in the thigh and buttocks in aortoiliac disease. Claudication is less common in diabetic patients compared with non-diabetic patients because of peripheral neuropathy and the very distal site of atherosclerosis in the tibial vessels of the diabetic leg.

However, patients presenting with claudication should be referred for a vascular opinion and undergo Doppler studies for both pressure index and sonograms and also duplex angiography. Patients with claudication rarely have vascular intervention and operative intervention is required in only 1% of diabetic patients per year although it may be indicated when the claudication is severe, i.e. pain comes on within a few yards of walking and the site of the arterial disease is in the iliac arteries. Patients with claudication should enter an exercise programme. Pharmacological treatment with cilostazol can now be

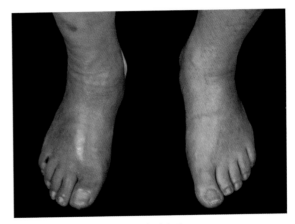

Fig. 3.11 Pink painful ischaemic right foot.

prescribed at a dosage of 100 mg twice daily but it should not be prescribed in patients with heart failure.

Severe chronic ischaemia

With increasing severity of occlusive arterial disease, patients may develop a pink, painful pulseless foot (Fig. 3.11). The colour of the skin is a strikingly bright pink and the foot is cold.

The amount of pain will be related to the severity of the disease and the degree of peripheral neuropathy. When neuropathy is mild, patients will have classical rest pain, which is a constant pain, often worse at night and relieved by hanging the leg down outside the bed at night. It is important not to mistake the pink painful ischaemic foot for an infected cellulitic foot. The pink painful ischaemic foot is usually cool and the infected cellulitic foot is usually hot. If the leg is elevated the pinkness of ischaemia will fade while erythema of cellulitis will remain.

Patients who present with ischemic feet may also have peripheral painful neuropathy, and then it is sometimes difficult to know how much pain is due to ischaemia and how much pain is due to neuropathy. The features of each were described in the Introduction but often there is an overlap. It may be necessary to treat the ischaemia by revascularization with angioplasty if possible, as well as managing the painful neuropathy.

The pink painful ischaemic foot is an indication of severe arterial disease. There is no time to be lost. Urgent vascular investigations will be necessary with a view to vascular intervention. The ankle brachial pressure index will nearly always be less than 0.5, although medial calcification may give an erroneously high value. It is wise to proceed to further investigations including transcutaneous oxygen tension and toe pressure measurements. A level below 30 mmHg confirms severe ischaemia in both tests. Pain control is important. (For further discussion of these investigations, vascular intervention and pain control in the foot with severe ischaemia, see Chapter 4.)

Vascular intervention may not always be possible. If it is possible to control pain, then a trial of conservative treatment may be attempted instead of immediately performing a major amputation.

CASE STUDY
Severe ischaemia

A 57-year-old man with type 2 diabetes of 7 years' duration underwent right femoral popliteal bypass. Eleven years later he flew to Canada. During the return flight he developed pain and numbness in his right foot and leg. He visited his local casualty department. A diagnosis of ischaemia was made but the severity was not appreciated and the patient was sent home. Next day he came to the diabetic foot clinic. The foot and lower leg were bright pink, icy cold and pulseless, with swollen toes and severe pain around the 1st metatarsophalangeal joint. Doppler studies could not detect pulsatile flow in the foot, and transcutaneous oxygen tension was 3 mmHg in the right foot and 50 mmHg in the left foot. He underwent an angiogram which showed that the graft was not patent. Further vascular intervention was not possible.

He developed necrosis on the medial aspect of the 1st metatarsophalangeal joint, and the lateral border of the foot. He also developed severe rest pain which was controlled with morphine sulphate. He refused a major amputation, and elected to undergo conservative treatment of his ischaemic foot in the diabetic foot clinic with aggressive treatment of infection. There was a slow but gradual improvement leading to complete healing of the foot after 4 years. However, during this time he had five further admissions for infections. He had an initial period of 5 months off work but was then able to remain in full-time work.

Fourteen years later he still has two legs.

Key points
- Severely ischaemic feet in the diabetic patient may be difficult to diagnose because rest pain may not be as severe as in non-diabetic patients without neuropathy
- Severely ischaemic feet can sometimes survive without revascularization especially if there is a significant degree of infection at presentation

- Close follow-up care from a multidisciplinary diabetic foot clinic is essential
- Healing can take years.

Acute ischaemia
A sudden occlusion of a major artery, usually popliteal or superficial femoral, will result in a pale, painful cold foot with purplish mottling (Fig. 3.12). Initially the skin is intact, but if treatment is delayed digital necrosis will develop. (Management of necrosis is described in Chapter 6.)

Acute ischaemia is a rare complication of the stage 2 diabetic foot and can present very suddenly in:
- Patients with no previous history of vascular problems
- Patients with a history of steadily deteriorating chronic ischaemia
- Patients who have previously had peripheral arterial bypass which occludes or angioplasty with recurrence of stenosis or occlusion.

Unless the patient is profoundly neuropathic he will complain of sudden onset of pain in the leg and foot. If a hand is run down the leg a 'cut-off' point will be found where the temperature of the skin suddenly decreases.

Symptoms may include:
- Pain
- Numbness
- Paraesthesiae
- Weakness.

Signs are:
- Pallor
- Blueish-grey discolouration with mottling or 'bruised' appearance
- Paralysis.

Acute ischaemia is a clinical emergency associated with severe morbidity and mortality. If the leg is to be saved it is necessary to reperfuse it as a matter of urgency. Immediate vascular intervention is needed.

Metabolic control

Even though neuropathy or ischaemia may now be present, progression may be checked by tight control of blood glucose, blood pressure and blood lipids, and stopping smoking as described for patients with stage 1 feet. All patients with peripheral arterial disease should take aspirin 75 mg daily.

Oedema may complicate both the neuropathic and the neuroischaemic foot and it is an important factor predisposing to ulceration. Its main cause will be impaired cardiac and renal function which should be investigated

STAGE 2

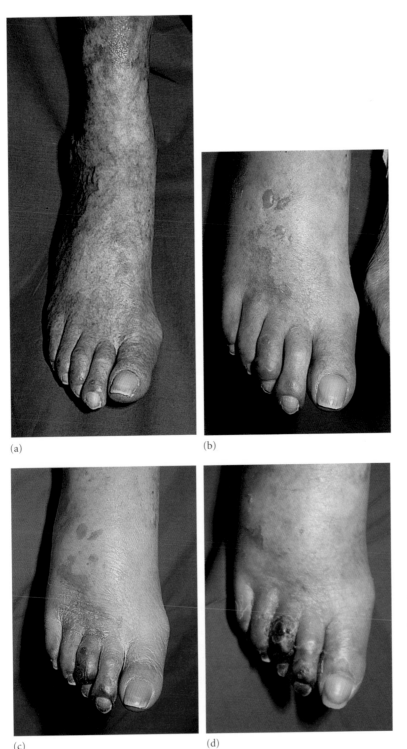

(a)

(b)

(c)

(d)

Fig. 3.12 (a) Acute ischaemia: the foot is grey, pallid and cold and needed distal bypass for limb salvage. (b) Two days after her distal bypass the foot has developed small blisters on the dorsum and the tips of the toes are discoloured. (c) Two weeks later the discoloured areas were necrotic. (d) One month after the discolouration was first noted the necrosis demarcated and stopped extending.

and then treated accordingly. With deteriorating renal function, oedema of the feet becomes a crucial factor leading to the intractable ulceration of end-stage renal failure (see Chapter 6).

When patients go on to haemodialysis the oedema can vary throughout the week according to the time of dialysis and it is important for the footwear to be adjustable, to accommodate fluctuant swelling.

Venous insufficiency can cause swelling of the leg and foot and should be investigated with duplex scanning, treated with support hose and referred for a vascular opinion as to the need for vein surgery.

Neuropathic oedema may respond to ephedrine starting at a dose of 10 mg tds but this may need to be increased up to 30–60 mg tds.

Educational control

General principles

- 'One-to-one' education can be carried out during the routine appointment by the podiatrist while the feet are treated
- 'Little and often' is the rule. When long 'lectures' are delivered, patients 'switch off'!
- Always seize the opportunity to get a point across or to ask a question which might reveal danger. Patients who volunteer that their vision is poor will need help with the foot check
- Changes in the patient's lifestyle (an impending holiday or trip, or a change of occupation) may indicate the need for extra education
- The diabetic foot service should get to know their patients well and be aware of changes going on in their lives which might have adverse effects on their feet
- Education programmes should be flexible, sensitive and individualized
- All patients at stage 2 should be taught the danger signs of actual or impending foot problems and should know what to do and where to go to get rapid help, as described for patients at stage 1, and should know why it is important for them to follow this advice.

Effective education can keep a patient at stage 2 for the rest of his diabetic life. Failure to control the stage 2 foot can lead to a lifetime of disability. Above all, it is important to educate patients at stage 2 in trauma prevention programmes so as to avoid ulceration and entering stage 3.

Psychological factors should also be specifically addressed in patients at stage 2.

Trauma prevention programmes

Trauma is the precursor of many ulcers, fractures and Charcot's osteoarthropathy. A special trauma prevention programme is needed for the successful management of patients at stage 2.

Common causes of trauma

- Wearing of unsuitable footwear which rubs blisters and sores
- Wearing of 'thong' sandals
- Walking barefoot
- Foreign bodies within the footwear (patients should be taught to shake out their shoes before wearing them and to check the inside for rough places or ruckled insoles). One of our patients developed severe ulceration when her small son dropped a Lego brick into her shoe: we found the brick later, deep within an ulcer!
- Nail penetration: one patient travelled from India back to England bringing back a tintack deeply embedded in his foot
- Burns from hot bath and shower water. Patients should check temperature of water with elbow or bath thermometer
- 'Toasting toes' in front of fires or fan heaters
- Falling asleep in front of the fire
- Walking on hot sand
- Spilling boiling water
- Falling asleep on the beach (sunburn)
- Frostbite. One of our patients suffered frostbite after being found lying unconscious in the snow. Another patient with frostbite was a butcher with profound neuropathy who worked within a deep freeze room.

CASE STUDY
Burnt feet

A 52-year-old man with type 2 diabetes of 20 years' duration and profound neuropathy originally attended the diabetic foot clinic with neuropathic ulceration. This healed with regular debridement and special shoes. He was taught to check his feet every day, was careful to avoid trauma and had been ulcer free for 7 years. He attended the diabetic foot clinic at 3-monthly intervals for routine foot care and education.

He went on a business trip to Scotland and stayed in a hotel. During the night he was woken by a strong smell of cooking meat in his bedroom. On investigation he found a hot water pipe running along the wall by his bed, against which his foot had pressed in his sleep. He flew back to London the next morning for an emergency foot clinic appointment. He had a deep burn across the plantar surface of his forefoot which was cellulitic and discharging pus. He was admitted to hospital the same day for intravenous antibiotics. The burn gradually took on the appearance of a neuropathic ulcer, surrounded by heavy callus which needed regular debriding. Even when he was non-weightbearing, callus continued to develop. The foot healed in 17 weeks.

Key points

- No matter how careful patients who lack protective pain sensation are, they will sometimes injure themselves
- Patients in unfamiliar places are particularly vulnerable
- Patients should be specifically warned about the dangers of hot water pipes and radiators on bedroom walls
- Burns are hard to assess in diabetic patients at stage 2 because all burns (and not just third-degree burns) are painless in the neuropathic foot (see Chapter 4).

Traditional remedies and alternative medicine

Some traditional remedies may be hazardous, in particular for feet with neuropathy. We have seen:

- Severe burns following treatment by a traditional Chinese physician who heated eggs in a pan until they were black and charred and slapped them directly onto the foot 'to draw the edges of the ulcer together'
- Maceration and infection following topical papaya ointment application
- 'Animal wool' wrapped around the toes to relieve pressure on interdigital corns, which absorbed perspiration, shrank and constricted the blood supply
- A type 1 patient who was advised to stop taking insulin and rely on herbal remedies instead.

Patients and providers should be wary of unproven therapies.

The internet is full of details of folk remedies and new treatments. We ask patients to discuss the use of these remedies with us first so that we can establish their merits or dangers.

When traditional medicines prevent patients from seeking professional help their use is particularly dangerous.

Proprietary remedies can also be dangerous for the complicated diabetic foot. Many corn and callus removers contain salicylic acid. Many proprietary remedies contain equivocal advice which may be regarded by the patient as an indication that the products are safe. Warnings that patients with diabetes or peripheral vascular disease should not use them are frequently in a very small type which the patient with eye problems may be unable to read.

No matter how careful patients with neuropathy are, problems will sometimes occur. Without protective pain sensation it is extremely difficult to avoid and detect trauma, even if the patient takes great care.

Individualized trauma prevention programmes should take into account personal lifestyle and holiday and occupational activities.

Personal lifestyle

Patients in stage 2 are usually advised to avoid walking barefoot but if this is not possible the following precautions may help:

- Walking barefoot at temple or on pilgrimage to Mecca will be safer at dawn and dusk than in the heat of the day
- Grouting of floor tiles should be smooth
- Patients should clear up spillages immediately so they do not step on spilt uncooked rice or lentils or broken dropped objects.

Holiday foot care

Patients who are in unfamiliar places are at particular risk. We remember a patient whose toes were crushed when a bus driver in Greece unfolded a seat onto his foot trapping his toes, but he was unaware of this until he tried to get up at the end of his 50-mile journey.

Trauma occurrence is particularly common in people on holiday. The reasons include the following:

- Unfamiliar environment exacerbates problems caused by poor vision or unsteady gait
- Lack of easy access to professional help
- Holidays regarded as a carefree time, when one can escape from the usual pressures
- Usual shoes discarded
- Increased alcohol consumption.

Dangers of the beach include:

- Cuts from sharp rocks, sea shells and broken glass
- Abrasions from sharp corals and sand or putting shoes on sandy feet
- Puncture wounds
- Burns from hot sand
- Not drying feet properly, leaving skin soggy and susceptible to trauma
- Insect bites and stings
- Sunburn.

CASE STUDY
Burn on the beach

A 62-year-old woman with type 1 diabetes of 40 years' duration, retinopathy and neuropathy went on holiday to

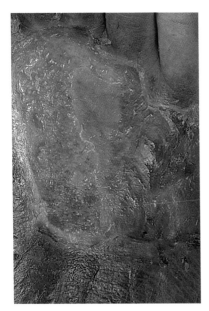

Fig. 3.13 Third-degree burn on the dorsum of the foot.

Blackpool, removed her shoes and socks and sat in a deckchair on the beach for 3 hours. Her head and torso were shaded by an umbrella but her feet and legs were exposed to the sun. She suffered a full-thickness burn on the dorsum of her right foot (Fig. 3.13). She was admitted to hospital for debridement and skin grafting and the foot healed in 6 weeks.

Key points
- Diabetic patients who go on holiday are vulnerable to injury. Thermal injuries are common and patients need to protect themselves from the sun
- Every diabetic foot service should have a special holiday foot care programme.

Dangers of airports
- Carrying heavy luggage which puts extra pressure on feet
- Airport trolleys which may run into or over the feet or lower leg
- Other passengers in a hurry who may step on toes
- Patients losing control of the situation in airports: they cannot limit the distance or speed at which they will need to walk.

Patients who fly should:
- Walk up and down the gangway on the plane to reduce the likelihood of severe oedema or a deep vein thrombosis
- Wear adjustable footwear

- Avoid dehydration: drink plenty of water; avoid tea, coffee, alcohol and fizzy drinks.

We advise patients with a previous history of severe foot problems to organize a wheelchair at each end of the flight, and to allow plenty of time for embarkation and disembarkation.

General safety rules for patients on holiday
- No brand new shoes
- Wear socks
- If skin becomes dry use emollient
- Seek help from a local health-care professional if problems arise
- Telephone home foot care service for advice if necessary
- Always take out health insurance
- Take a first aid kit
- Avoid sunburn
- Wear plastic sandals on the beach and in the sea.

Occupational factors
Neuropathic patients may develop foot problems associated with jobs entailing much walking, and will sometimes need to seek desk jobs. Neuropathic patients whose work entails standing for hours in a factory in front of a machine will need to shift their stance from time to time and can be advised to set their watch beeper to go off at every quarter hour, whereupon they should shift their feet about and take a few steps. (They should probably explain to colleagues why they are doing this!)

Making patients feel safe
It is very frightening for high-risk patients if they sustain a trauma and cannot get immediate help without working their way through bureaucratic barriers and delays.

Many patients say that they only feel safe when they know that if they find a foot problem they can come to the diabetic foot clinic immediately for treatment and advice. The foot clinic should be a safe haven for people with diabetes.

Addressing psychological factors
Educators dealing with diabetic foot patients should be aware of the importance of psychological factors.

Diabetes arouses strong emotions of anger, fear and denial which can be barriers to successful management. Newly diagnosed patients are inundated with advice from health-care professionals and from well-meaning friends. Some advice may be inaccurate or unnecessarily negative. Patients may deny that diabetes or diabetic feet are a problem. On the internet a vast amount of unrefereed information is available which may give patients unrealistic expectations of the future.

In devising education programmes, the clinician should be aware of the psychological importance of the loss of protective pain sensation.

Protective pain sensation keeps behaviour within certain constraints: as we grow up we learn to avoid obvious noxious stimuli because of the unpleasant sensations associated with them. This reinforces safe behaviour, and less obvious stimuli will soon be detected because they give rise to discomfort, but it seems that this pathway needs constant reinforcement. When sensation is lost, behaviour can become reckless and hazardous.

Lack of touch and lack of pain perception have profound effects on the patient's body image and awareness of the physical boundaries of self in the following ways:

- Patients may feel that their neuropathic feet are no longer a part of them, and may ignore them and fail to look after them
- If ulcers or other problems develop, the patient is also likely to neglect them because they are not painful (and we have all been brought up to believe that if there is no pain the problem is not serious)
- Patients may therefore not perceive themselves to be at risk.

Psychological factors can worsen outcomes because they:

- Prevent a patient from understanding his foot problems
- Make him underestimate the risks he faces
- Make him refuse treatment or neglect to follow advice. Work with paraplegic patients has indicated that patients who do not perceive themselves to be at risk are more likely to neglect themselves and are more likely to develop foot problems. It is essential that patients at stage 2 are made aware that they are at risk.

Management of patients with psychological problems
The health-care professional should always:

- Tell the truth to patients
- Avoid deliberately frightening patients unless there is an urgent need to change their behaviour, for example when a very sick patient wishes to discharge himself from hospital or refuses a life-saving operation
- Issue realistic advice. It is well worth taking time to explain to patients that they lack protective pain sensation, so that they understand the practical implications of their inability to feel a 10-g monofilament. In theory, lack of protective pain sensation can be compensated for if patients are made aware that they will not feel pain, and taught trauma prevention and the need for regular foot inspections.

There are some patients who, despite regular and frequent education, appear to be unable to care for themselves or to take responsibility for their feet. They are labelled 'difficult patients'. They often have associated problems including:

- Old age
- Concurrent medical conditions
- Poverty
- Intellectual deficit.

Once such patients are identified it may be necessary to provide:

- Frequent treatment
- Home contact (telephone calls and postcard reminders) between appointments to ensure that all is well
- 'Conspiracy' with the community nurses or other carers to organize regular foot checks at home.

Some patients learn a sharp lesson the first time they develop a serious problem and never let it happen again, but others seem to be incapable of learning from previous experiences.

Diabetes coupled with renal disease may make patients even more reckless. There is a singularly high incidence of trauma in renal transplant patients. The reasons for this are not entirely clear. Patients with long-term chronic diseases who are subjected to lengthy treatments and frequent advice and are never free of hospital appointments may be less likely to follow instructions from health-care practitioners, including advice on the need to avoid trauma to their feet. Alternatively it may be that the tissues of renal patients are more fragile so that an insult which might be unperceived in a normal patient can lead to frank tissue damage in a renal patient.

SPECIFIC COMPLICATIONS OF NEUROPATHY

Painful neuropathy

The most common presentation is that of a bilateral painful peripheral neuropathy. However, pain can also be unilateral, when it is usually secondary to a focal neuropathy or mononeuritis.

Peripheral painful neuropathy
Presentation
This is a singularly disagreeable complication of diabetes. Patients in severe pain who cannot sleep become profoundly disturbed, confused, depressed and unwell. Relentless, burning pain and contact dysaesthesia make patients extremely miserable. It is particularly difficult to

bear because apart from the pain there are often no signs which make it obvious that something is wrong. Some patients have described severe painful neuropathy after a period of rapid glycaemic control, usually after starting insulin. This has been called insulin neuritis, but the symptoms gradually improve if tight control is maintained.

Some health-care practitioners are unsympathetic because of the absence of signs.

The pain may be sharp, shooting, stabbing or burning. There may be paraesthesiae or deep muscular aching pain, restless legs, cramps and/or sensation of cold. Painful neuropathy is worse in bed at night, when the feet and legs are in contact with clothes, including bedclothes and when the feet are warm.

Distribution of pain is usually in both feet extending into the lower legs in a stocking distribution. One limb may be slightly worse than the other. However, unilateral pain suggests either a diabetic mononeuropathy, such as femoral neuropathy, or nerve root pain due to compression such as in a prolapsed intervertebral disc.

Some patients with painful neuropathy lose weight. Often the first sign that they are entering the recovery phase is that they begin to gain weight again.

Examination

On examination the feet and legs may be normal, although some patients may show a stocking distribution of loss of sensation. There may be an increased sensation to a normal stimulus such as light touch and this is termed allodynia or contact hypersensitivity. When there is increased sensation to normal painful stimuli such as pinprick, this is referred to as hyperalgesia.

When the pain is unilateral it is important to look for focal signs of root or nerve pathology, for example focal muscular weakness or unilateral loss of reflexes.

It is important to attempt to distinguish painful neuropathy from ischaemic rest pain. Rest pain is relieved by dependency but painful neuropathy is not affected by position change. In limbs with painful neuropathy, pulses are usually present. However, in the limb with rest pain there are definite signs of ischaemia, with absent pulses.

Investigations

Patients suspected of having peripheral painful neuropathy should have:

- Full blood count
- Urea/creatinine/electrolytes
- Liver function tests
- Protein electrophoresis
- Serum B_{12} levels.

Thus, other causes of painful neuropathy include B_{12} deficiency, renal failure, alcoholic neuropathy associated with liver dysfunction and myeloma and these should be excluded, before confirming a diagnosis of diabetic painful neuropathy. When the pain is predominantly unilateral it is important to investigate for the presence of root compression. This is best done with magnetic resonance imaging (MRI) of the lumbosacral spine.

Vascular investigations should be carried out to rule out an ischaemic cause of the pain. In patients with painful neuropathy, transcutaneous oxygen tension is usually greater than 30 mmHg but in the ischaemic limb, transcutaneous oxygen tension is usually less than 30 mmHg. However, both painful neuropathy and ischaemia may coexist and it is sometimes difficult to be sure whether neuropathy or ischaemia is the cause of lower limb pain. Although certain features suggest a neuropathic aetiology, such as burning and contact discomfort, both neuropathic and ischaemic pain are worse at night.

CASE STUDY
Ischaemic or neuropathic pain

A 68-year-old man with type 2 diabetes of 9 years' duration complained of pain in both legs for the previous 3 months. This pain was worse at night. He got relief by hanging the legs over the side of the bed. He was a heavy smoker. On examination he had a stocking distribution symmetrical neuropathy. However, his foot pulses were absent and his transcutaneous oxygen was 28 mmHg on the right and 25 mmHg on the left. Duplex angiography showed bilateral iliac disease. He underwent iliac angioplasty and his pain was partially resolved but not eradicated. Therefore, he was also treated for painful neuropathy.

Key points

- Pain in the lower limb in the diabetic patient may be due to neuropathy or ischaemia or a combination of both
- When ischaemia is present and is thought to contribute to the pain it should be treated by revascularization (angioplasty where possible)
- The clinical problem arises when angioplasty is not technically possible and bypass is the only option. The risk of bypass then has to be measured against the estimated gain of bypass in relieving what is considered to be predominantly ischaemic pain
- If in doubt as to the cause of the pain, treat both neuropathy and ischaemia.

Management

The first important step is to reassure the patient that he will get better. Painful neuropathy nearly always resolves within 2 years although the pain may be replaced by numbness. The patient with painful neuropathy alone and palpable pulses should be told that there is no danger of amputation.

The next step is to explore the many treatment options and try to find something to tide the patient over the next months before the pain resolves. If one treatment does not work there will be others to be tried. Reassurance, sympathy and tender loving care alone will help considerably: the knowledge that the pain will not last forever and that every attempt will be made to relieve it is also helpful. Frequent appointments should be made for review and assessment so that patients do not feel abandoned. This role has been taken on by the multidisciplinary diabetic foot clinic.

Simple measures may help. Pain may be relieved by cold: a basin of cool water may be kept beside the bed. One of our patients purchased a small refrigerator, kept it at the end of the bed, and inserted his feet when woken by pain! One patient wore a pair of his wife's tights under his trousers: another patient wore silk pyjamas underneath his city suit. A bed cradle can be used to prevent the bedclothes from touching the lower limb. If the patient can be helped to sleep he will feel better.

Treatment can be divided into four modalities:
- Topical therapy
- Glycaemic control
- Drug therapy
- Physical treatment.

Topical therapy

OpSite film stuck directly onto the skin and OpSite spray may help to relieve burning pain and contact dysaesthesia.

Capsaicin is applied as a cream, and depletes peripheral pain fibres of substance P thereby blocking transmission of painful signals from the periphery to central neurones. It should be applied sparingly in a thin layer four times daily to the affected area. It should only be used on intact skin. Burning or tingling may occur in the first 2 weeks but the patient should be encouraged to persist. Patients should wash their hands immediately after use. The analgesic effect may take 6 weeks to develop.

Isosorbide dinitrate spray and glyceryl trinitrate patches have been shown to be useful in small double-blind studies and lidocaine patches have been shown to relieve pain in open-label studies.

Glycaemic control

Hyperglycaemia is known to lower the threshold to pain and in general diabetic control is usually poor in patients with painful neuropathy. It is important to improve control and aim for a glycated haemoglobin $< 7\%$. In patients with type 2 diabetes, oral hypoglycaemic therapy should be optimized, but if this fails then insulin therapy should be started.

Drug therapy

This consists of simple analgesics, anticonvulsants, antidepressants, opiates and hypnotics.

Analgesics. Initial therapy should be simple analgesics such as aspirin or paracetamol. If necessary, stronger analgesics may be given, such as co-dydramol.

Anticonvulsants. Gabapentin and pregabalin have become the predominantly used anticonvulsants and we use them for first-line therapy. The starting dose for gabapentin is 300 mg on the first day, 600 mg on the second and 900 mg on the third day. Thereafter the dose may be eventually increased to 1800 mg daily. It is usually well tolerated and initial drowsiness resolves. Similarly, pregabalin is started at 75 mg bd and is then increased at intervals through 150 mg bd to 300 mg bd. It is also well tolerated. The dose of both gabapentin and pregabalin should be reduced if the patient is in renal failure. If pain is not fully controlled by such anticonvulsants, then a tricyclic antidepressant or the opioid-like drug tramadol can be added.

Carbamezapine, sodium valproate, phenytoin, lamotrigine and topiramate can also be used. Carbamezapine can be started at 100 mg once or twice daily and increased up to the maximum tolerated dosage (usually 800–1000 mg daily). Sodium valproate (100–1500 mg daily) and phenytoin (100–800 mg daily) have been used with variable results. Newer generation anticonvulsants such as lamotrigine (200–400 mg daily) and topiramate (100–400 mg daily) may be helpful.

Antidepressants. Imipramine or amitriptyline as tricyclic antidepressants may relieve burning pain. It is best to commence at a low dosage at night to avoid the side-effect of postural hypotension. The dose of amitriptyline should be 25 mg initially and this should be increased to 150 mg over a period of 16–20 weeks as long as serious side-effects do not occur. Mild side-effects include drowsiness, constipation, blurred vision, dry mouth and sweating. However, these symptoms should not persist on continuing therapy. If they do, the dose should be reduced. If the patient has difficulty in passing urine or becomes confused or develops palpitations then the medication should be stopped immediately by the patient, who should be reviewed urgently.

Two serotonin-noradrenaline re-uptake inhibitors have been shown to be useful in painful neuropathy: venlafaxine extended release at a dosage of 150–250 mg/day and duloxitene at 60–120 mg daily. In general, selective serotonin re-uptake inhibitors have not been successful in painful neuropathy.

Opiates. In severe pain, opiates may be necessary. These drugs should only be prescribed when anticonvulsants and antidepressants have been tried. Tramadol is an opioid-like, non-narcotic analgesic with a dosage of 50–400 mg daily. It is useful either alone or with anticonvulsant therapy when it is used for breakthrough pain. If there is no response to tramadol or it cannot be tolerated, then sustained release opioids can be used. Controlled release oxycodone 10–60 mg daily has been effective in randomized, double-blind, placebo-controlled studies. Anecdotally, patients have reported that cannabis helps although a recent controlled study of cannabis was negative.

Hypnotics. Hypnotics are extremely helpful as loss of sleep makes the patient more sensitive to pain and induces depression.

Physical treatment
Transcutaneous electrical nerve stimulation (TENS) can be used to block the pain. Electrodes are placed on either side of the painful area. Acupuncture has anecdotally been reported as useful. In very severe cases, spinal cord stimulation with implanted spinal electrodes has been beneficial.

Focal neuropathy
When lower limb pain is unilateral, a focal neuropathy may be the cause. The commonest focal neuropathy is femoral neuropathy, otherwise known as proximal motor neuropathy, diabetic amyotrophy, or plexopathy.

Femoral neuropathy can present with:
• Pain in thigh
• Weakness of quadriceps
• Difficulty in walking
• Weight loss.
It usually resolves in 18 months.

Focal neuropathy can also present as a truncal radiculopathy on the thorax or abdomen. It is associated with unilateral sensory loss, muscle weakness, which leads to a laxity and bulging of the abdominal muscles, and weight loss. Patients are often thought to have a malignancy because of the weight loss and the impression of an abdominal mass. Pain usually resolves within 9–12 months.

Charcot's osteoarthropathy

This is an acute osteoarthropathy, with bone and joint destruction, that occurs in the neuropathic foot. It commonly presents in the mid-foot but also occurs in the forefoot and hindfoot. The prognosis for the hindfoot is much more serious with the high risk of instability of the ankle and the necessity for a major amputation.

It is extremely important to have a high index of suspicion and to encourage early presentation of the patient. This should be followed by a rapid diagnosis and early intervention, and with such a modern approach many Charcot feet can now be healed and deformity prevented. There may be a history of minor trauma such as tripping, twisting the ankle or walking over rough surfaces such as cobbles. About 30% of patients complain of pain or discomfort. Rarely, pain may be very severe. Charcot's osteoarthropathy may follow injudicious mobilization after surgery, a period of bedrest or casting.

Patients who develop Charcot's osteoarthropathy usually have evidence of a peripheral neuropathy, autonomic neuropathy and a good blood supply to the lower limb. Patients may have symptoms of autonomic neuropathy such as gastroparesis, diabetic diarrhoea, gustatory sweating or postural hypotension. Diabetic patients with renal transplants have an increased risk of Charcot's osteoarthropathy. Rarely, in diabetes, the knee can also be affected by Charcot's osteoarthropathy. Patients with type 1 diabetes have reduced bone density which renders them susceptible to fractures and then to Charcot's osteoarthropathy. Patients with type 2 diabetes have normal bone density and Charcot's osteoarthropathy is more frequently associated with subluxation and fracture-dislocation.

Charcot's osteoarthropathy can be divided into two phases:
• Acute active phase
• Chronic stable inactive phase.

Acute active Charcot's osteoarthropathy
The acute active phase is characterized by unilateral erythema and oedema (Fig. 3.14). The foot is at least 2°C hotter than the contralateral foot and the difference may be as great as 10°C. This may be measured with an infrared skin thermometer. Patients may present early in

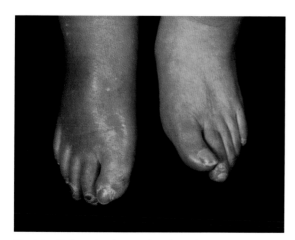

Fig. 3.14 Unilateral oedema and erythema in acute onset Charcot's osteoarthropathy.

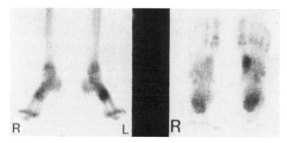

Fig. 3.15 MDP bone scan showing increased uptake at the base of the 1st metatarsal of the left foot, indicating early bony damage despite normal X-ray.

the acute active phase when the X-ray is normal, or later when there may be already existing deformity and radiological changes of Charcot's osteoarthropathy.

Presentation in the acute active phase with normal X-ray

If the X-ray is normal, we then proceed to two investigations. Initially a technetium methylene diphosphonate (MDP) bone scan, which will detect early evidence of bone damage (Fig. 3.15). If the result of the bone scan is positive, we would proceed to an MRI which will describe in more detail the nature of the bony damage. The other advantage of carrying out the bone scan is that it locates the site of the damage and therefore it allows the MRI to be focused in detail on that particular part of the foot.

Patients awaiting bone scan should be treated as if the diagnosis has been confirmed. Although patients with an early injury may appear to be developing Charcot's osteoarthropathy, it is not possible yet to differentiate

between those who have a soft tissue injury only and those who will develop extensive bony destruction. For this reason, all patients in stage 2 with a history of trauma, redness, warmth and oedema should be treated with a cast, and all aspects of casting are described in full in Chapter 4. If the problem is not a Charcot's osteoarthropathy, but a simple sprain, it will resolve rapidly.

CASE STUDY
Differential diagnosis of acute Charcot's osteoarthropathy

A 65-year-old man with type 2 diabetes of 21 years' duration developed a hot, red, swollen left foot, after tripping in the street. On examination the foot was hot and swollen, particularly over the lateral aspect of the ankle. However, pulses were not palpable and the pressure index was 0.6. X-ray was normal. The differential diagnosis was an acute Charcot's osteoarthropathy or a soft tissue injury. Charcot's osteoarthropathy was thought to be less likely in view of the moderate ischaemia; however, it could not be excluded. The foot was put in a cast until an MDP bone scan was performed. This showed a diffuse uptake around the left ankle but no focal bony change, indicating a soft tissue injury (Fig. 3.16a,b). The patient was mobilized without a cast and the swelling gradually resolved.

Key points
- Patients presenting with a hot, swollen foot should be regarded as having a Charcot's osteoarthropathy until proved otherwise
- Until an MDP bone scan can be performed, the foot should be casted
- The MDP bone scan can differentiate between soft tissue and bony damage.

However, we recently saw a rare case of Charcot's osteoarthropathy in a neuroischaemic foot.

CASE STUDY
Acute Charcot's osteoarthropathy in a neuroischaemic foot

A 71-year-old man with type 1 diabetes of 45 years' duration and a previous history of neuropathic ulceration attended the diabetic foot clinic for a routine appointment. We noticed that his left foot was very red and oedematous with a medial convexity and sent him by wheelchair for an X-ray which confirmed a Lisfranc's fracture-dislocation. He denied any trauma to the foot

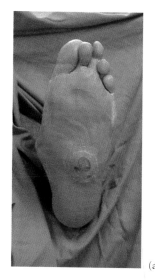

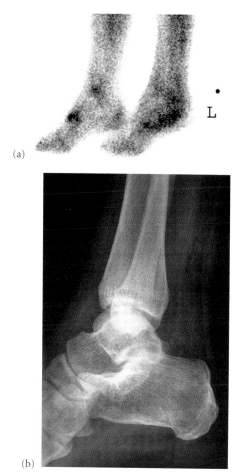

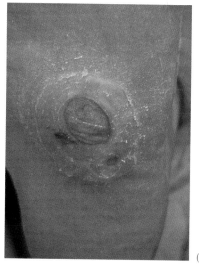

Fig. 3.16 (a) MDP bone scan showing diffuse uptake around the left ankle. (b) Normal X-ray of left ankle.

but said that the previous day he had performed his duties as a guide at St. Paul's Cathedral, London, which entailed him staying on his feet for many hours, during which he had worn his hospital shoes. At the time the Charcot foot developed his pedal pulses were absent and his ankle brachial pressure index was 0.8.

Within a few hours the area of skin overlying the medial prominence was blue and became necrotic leading to ulceration, which was treated in a total-contact cast. Duplex angiography revealed peroneal artery stenoses which were angioplastied. The ulcer healed but he subsequently developed a rocker-bottom deformity and a plantar ulcer (Fig. 3.17a,b). This ulcer was also treated in a total-contact cast and healed. This is very unusual in cases of acute Charcot's osteoarthropathy, although it should be noted that the ischaemia was mild.

Fig. 3.17 (a) Plantar ulcer has developed over this rocker-bottom deformity in a rare case of Charcot's osteoarthropathy associated with ischaemia. (b) Close-up view of the plantar ulcer which subsequently healed in a total-contact cast.

Key points
- Although Charcot's osteoarthropathy is very rare in the neuroischaemic foot it is not unheard of. However, the ischaemia is usually mild. The Charcot foot can also develop in patients who have undergone a successful vascular procedure
- Sudden development of a bony prominence can jeopardize the integrity of overlying soft tissue
- Total-contact casting is the gold standard treatment.

Differential diagnosis of acute onset Charcot's osteoarthropathy

It is important to differentiate between the red, hot, swollen appearance of Charcot's osteoarthropathy and the red, hot, swollen cellulitic foot. Cellulitis is more likely in the presence of an ulcer which may show typical signs of infection. Infection severe enough to cause generalized redness, warmth and swelling will usually cause local signs such as discolouration of the bed of the wound, and discharge from the ulcer. The swelling of Charcot's osteoarthropathy responds more rapidly to elevation than does that of the infected foot. In a recent series of 25 Charcot feet with acute presentation, C-reactive protein was normal in 47% of the cases and only moderately elevated in the remainder. However, infection and Charcot's osteoarthropathy can sometimes be present concurrently in the same foot. If in doubt, treat for both.

Gout and deep vein thrombosis may also masquerade as Charcot's osteoarthropathy but can be excluded by measurement of serum uric acid (which is usually raised in gout, although not always) and duplex vein angiography.

CASE STUDY
Acute Charcot foot with normal X-ray but microfracture on MRI

A 55-year-old woman with type 1 diabetes of 35 years' duration presented with a hot, painful, swollen foot after minimal trauma. X-ray was normal (Fig. 3.18a). An MDP bone scan showed increased uptake in the mid-foot (Fig. 3.18b). An MRI demonstrated changes as shown in Fig. 3.18c,d,e. The patient was fitted with a total-contact cast and this was continued for 5 months until the skin temperature of the affected side was less than 2°C hotter than the opposite side. Repeat MRI showed healing of the microfracture (Fig. 3.18f,g,h) and the X-ray remained normal (Fig. 3.18i). The patient was rehabilitated in a bivalved cast and then bespoke footwear.

Key points
- Early diagnosis is essential and can be confirmed with MDP bone scan and MRI
- MRI can show the initial bony lesion of Charcot which is often a microfracture, especially in type 1 patients

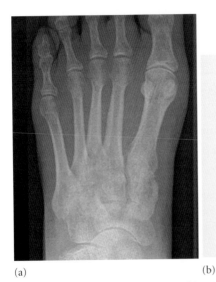
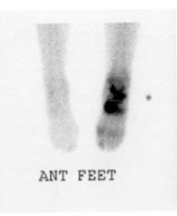
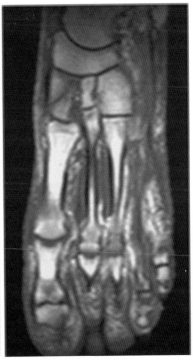

(a)　　　　　　　　(b)　　　　　　　　(c)

Fig. 3.18 (a) Normal X-ray of mid-foot. (b) MDP bone scan showing increased uptake in the mid-foot. (c) MRI scan: T1 sequence shows a fracture of the medial cuneiform with reduced fat signal.

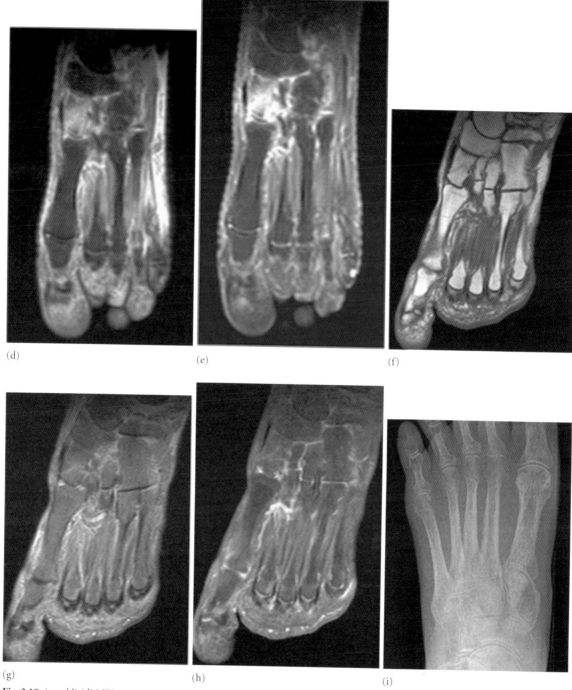

(d) (e) (f)

(g) (h) (i)

Fig. 3.18 (*cont'd*) (d) MRI scan: STIR sequence shows increased signal indicating oedema in the medial cuneiform. (e) MRI scan: gadolinium sequence shows increased signal in the medial cuneiform indicating inflammation. (f) MRI scan: T1 sequence now shows healing of the fracture and return of the fat signal.

(g) MRI scan: STIR sequence shows reduction in the oedema in the medial cuneiform. (h) MRI scan: gadolinium sequence shows reduction in the oedema of the medial cuneiform. (i) Follow-up X-ray remains normal.

- Early treatment of these fractures can achieve healing with the prevention of deformity.

Presentation in the acute active phase with existing bony changes

If treatment is not given early in the acute Charcot foot or the patient presents late, then extensive bone damage is incurred leading to joint subluxation and dislocation with subsequent deformity. These changes can develop very rapidly and lead to extensive fragmentation and dislocation within a few weeks.

A specific forerunner to the development of joint disruption in the acute Charcot foot is fracture. This can occur painlessly in the neuropathic foot and may be an isolated episode. However, neuropathic fractures may precipitate Charcot's osteoarthropathy and it is impossible at the outset to predict those fractures which will or will not develop this complication. Therefore, all fractures in the neuropathic foot must be treated promptly with the utmost care in conjunction with orthopaedic surgeons. There has often been a delay in diagnosis and management of fractures that do lead to Charcot's osteoarthropathy. Fractures should be treated with non-weightbearing and plaster immobilization, supported by crutches and/or wheelchair. Fractures in diabetic neuropathic patients do not heal at the same rate as in non-diabetic patients and plaster casts should therefore be continued until healing is confirmed by X-ray. In our experience, fractures in patients with neuropathy take two or three times as long to heal as they do in low-risk or normal feet. Many healthcare professionals appear to be unaware of this. Many neuropathic patients with type 1 diabetes have osteopaenic bones and are prone to fracture bones after minimal trauma. Because of the lack of symptoms, fractures are frequently only detected after a routine X-ray.

In the late presentation of the acute active phase, deformity can present in the forefoot, mid-foot and hindfoot and ankle. This is still accompanied by swelling, warmth, and a temperature 2°C greater than the contralateral foot. Advanced changes show fragmentation of bone, new bone formation, subluxation and dislocation. These changes often develop very rapidly, within a few weeks of the onset, and sometimes within a few days.

CASE STUDY
Acute Charcot's osteoarthropathy with rapid onset of bony destruction and deformity

A 46-year-old man with type 1 diabetes of 33 years' duration, end-stage renal failure treated by renal

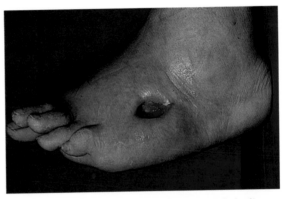

Fig. 3.19 The Charcot foot with dorsal swelling and a healing surgical wound where infection was drained.

transplantation and severe neuropathy, received regular foot checks under a renal foot study protocol. Three days before he went on holiday to the Channel Islands his feet were routinely checked and nothing abnormal was discerned. Two weeks later he came to the clinic on his return from holiday to report that his foot was 'a little swollen'. He reported no trauma to the foot, but had been walking more than usual on cobbled pavements. The foot was red, 5°C hotter than the contralateral foot and very swollen. X-ray revealed a Lisfranc's fracture-dislocation and he developed a rocker-bottom foot. He was treated in a total-contact plaster cast for 6 months following which he wore bespoke boots to accommodate his deformity. The foot remained ulcer free apart from one episode of sepsis which was precipitated by dropping a heavy object on the foot. This led to a break in the skin with resulting infection on the dorsum of the foot which needed surgical drainage (Fig. 3.19).

Key points
- Charcot's osteoarthropathy can develop with great rapidity
- Severe injuries normally associated with gross trauma can develop in high-risk patients simply through walking or unperceived trauma
- Renal transplant patients have a very high risk of Charcot's osteoarthropathy
- Deformed feet can be successfully accommodated in footwear.

Bone and joint destruction can occur in any part of the foot or ankle, but the common presentations can be divided into forefoot, mid-foot and hindfoot. The forefoot involves the metatarsophalangeal and interphalangeal joints. The mid-foot involves the tarsometatarsal joints and the hindfoot includes the ankle and subtalar joints.

Each region of the foot has specific clinical presentations of bone and joint destruction or deformity.

Forefoot
This presents with generalized swelling of the forefoot and osteonecrosis of the metatarsal heads. It is rare for a significant structural deformity to develop in forefoot Charcot's osteoarthropathy. The resorption of the distal metatarsal bones giving 'sucked candy' appearances is in our experience usually associated with chronic ulceration and infection. Rarely, Charcot's osteoarthropathy may present as a red, hot, swollen toe, usually the first toe.

CASE STUDY
Acute Charcot's osteoarthropathy of the forefoot

A 21-year-old woman with type 1 diabetes of 15 years' duration developed painless swelling of both forefeet (Fig. 3.20a). There was no evidence of ulceration. X-ray revealed fragmentation and lucency of the 2nd, 3rd and 4th metatarsal heads of both feet (Fig. 3.20b). The patient was supplied with a wheelchair and underwent strict non-weightbearing for 4 weeks. The oedema gradually resolved.

Deformity did not develop and the radiological changes stabilized.

Key points
- The radiological changes of osteonecrosis are typical of forefoot osteoarthropathy in the absence of foot ulceration and sepsis when sucked sugar candy appearances may be noted
- Charcot's osteoarthropathy may present spontaneously with no history of trauma
- Young type 1 diabetic women are known to have osteopaenia and are susceptible to fractures, including foot fractures.

CASE STUDY
Charcot toe

A 45-year-old woman with type 2 diabetes of 10 years' duration presented with a red, hot, painful and swollen first toe. X-ray showed a fracture line in the subchondral area adjacent to the interphalangeal joint with erosions (Fig. 3.21). There was no history of trauma. She was on haemodialysis. Serum urate was raised but it is likely that this was associated with her impaired renal function. The

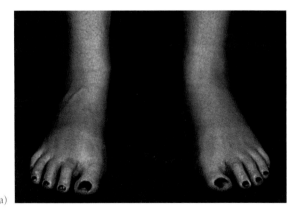

(a)

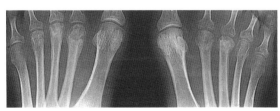

(b)

Fig. 3.20 (a) Swelling of the forefeet. (b) X-ray of both feet showing fragmentation and lucency of the 2nd, 3rd and 4th metatarsal heads.

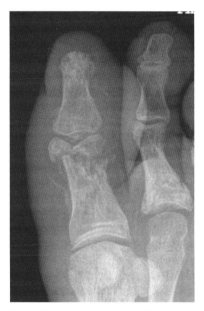

Fig. 3.21 X-ray of the toe shows a fracture line in the subchondral area adjacent to the interphalangeal joint with erosions.

patient was treated in a cast and the swelling and discomfort resolved over the subsequent 3 months.

Key points
- A red, hot, swollen toe may be due to Charcot's osteoarthropathy although infection and gout must be considered in the differential diagnosis
- The Charcot toe can be successfully treated with casting.

Mid-foot
This is the commonest site of presentation of Charcot's osteoarthropathy and it is recognized clinically by the rocker-bottom deformity and the medial convexity.

The medial convexity is associated with the classical Lisfranc's tarsometatarsal fracture-dislocation (Fig. 3.22). A clinical presentation is shown in Fig. 3.23.

The rocker-bottom deformity develops when there is disintegration and displacement of the cuneiforms or the proximal tarsal bones, resulting in collapse of the mid-foot. Rocker-bottom deformity is frequently associated with plantar ulceration (Fig. 3.24).

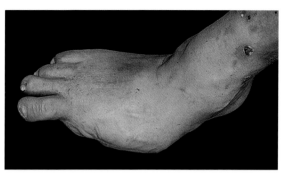

Fig. 3.23 Medial convexity of mid-foot developing after amputation of first toe.

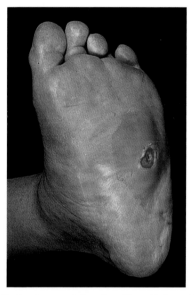

Fig. 3.24 Rocker-bottom deformity of the mid-foot with early breakdown.

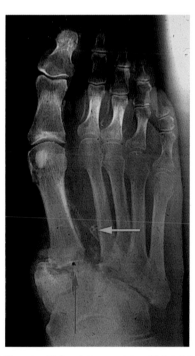

Fig. 3.22 There is a Lisfranc's tarsometatarsal joint dislocation (red arrow) with metatarsal bases shifted laterally. Yellow arrow shows vascular calcification.

Fractures of the base of the first metatarsal may precipitate Charcot's osteoarthropathy in the mid-foot (Fig. 3.25a,b).

Hindfoot
The early presentation is of a swollen ankle. Later, there is severe structural deformity and instability of the ankle joint (Fig. 3.26). This can lead to a flail ankle on which it is impossible to walk. Ulceration can often develop over the malleoli.

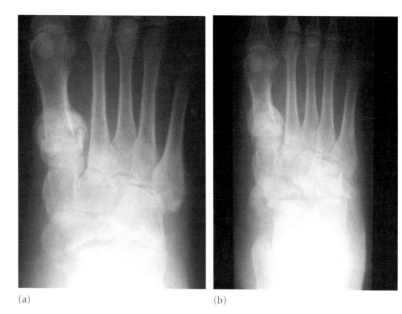

Fig. 3.25 (a) Fractured base of first metatarsal. (b) The development of a Charcot foot with disorganization of the tarsus and fragmented navicular and cuboid.

(a)   (b)

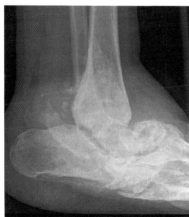

Fig. 3.26 Severe disorganization and disruption of the hindfoot and ankle joint leading to instability.

CASE STUDY
Neuropathic fracture of the tibia with Charcot's osteoarthropathy of the ankle

A 50-year-old woman with type 1 diabetes of 35 years' duration attempted to board a bus and missed her step and fell to the ground. She sustained a spiral fracture of the tibia and was treated conservatively with a below-knee plaster cast (Fig. 3.27a). However she developed Charcot changes at the ankle joint (Fig. 3.27b).

Key points
- Diabetic patients with type 1 diabetes have osteopaenia and are susceptible to fractures
- Fractures can precipitate Charcot's osteoarthropathy.

Treatment of the acute active phase of Charcot's osteoarthropathy with normal X-ray

Initially the foot is immobilized in a non-weightbearing plaster cast. The cast is checked after 1 week, and replaced if it has become loose due to reduction of oedema, then regularly checked and replaced as necessary. The patient should use crutches and be encouraged to avoid weightbearing on the affected side. However, we recognize that in many cases it is difficult to be completely non-weightbearing because the patient has multiple comorbidities including loss of proprioception, postural hypotension, high body mass index and, in some cases, neuropathy of the upper limbs, all of which can make it difficult for patients to use crutches. Furthermore, a wheelchair existence is impractical in many home environments. In addition, total immobility has disadvantages in itself with loss of muscle tone, reduction in bone density and loss of body fitness. The casting is continued until the swelling has resolved and the temperature of the affected foot is within 2°C of the contralateral foot.

An alternative treatment is a prefabricated walking cast, such as the Aircast, described in Chapter 4. A moulded insole should replace the standard insole provided with the cast by the manufacturer. The hindfoot Charcot is probably best treated in a total-contact cast.

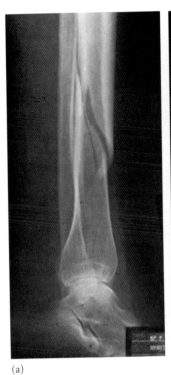
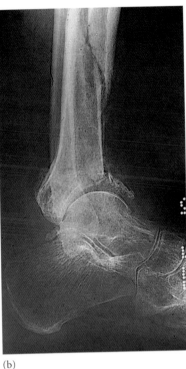

(a)   (b)

Fig. 3.27 (a) Spiral fracture of the tibia. (b) Charcot changes at the ankle joint following spiral fracture of the tibia.

Patients at this stage may receive further treatment with bisphosphonates. A randomized controlled study of a single 90 mg pamidronate infusion has shown a significant reduction of the markers of bone turnover and skin temperature in treated subjects compared with controls, although the fall in skin temperature was similar in both groups. There was a similar finding in a recent study with alendronate. Calcitonin has also been used in the acute stage of Charcot's osteoarthropathy and it was found that there was a more rapid transition to the stable chronic phase in the treated group compared with controls.

If treatment is given early in acute Charcot's osteoarthropathy, when the X-ray is normal, as described above, it should be possible to prevent bony destruction and deformity.

Treatment of the acute active phase of Charcot's osteoarthropathy with bone/joint destruction and deformity

The aim of treatment is immobilization in a plaster cast (see Chapter 4) until there is no longer evidence on X-ray of continuing bone or joint destruction, and the foot temperature (which can be measured with an infrared thermometer) is within 2°C of the contralateral foot.

When this is achieved, the foot will have reached a chronic inactive stage.

Deformity in Charcot's osteoarthropathy can predispose to ulceration, particularly on the plantar surface of the rocker-bottom deformity. It may also occur on the medial convexity. These ulcers may become infected and lead to osteomyelitis. This may be difficult to distinguish from neuropathic bone and joint changes, as on X-ray, nuclear bone scan or MRI, the appearance is similar.

Treatment of specific fractures

Toe fractures
The toe is strapped to its neighbour for a splinting effect.

Metatarsal fractures
The patient is put into a total-contact cast until X-rays confirm healing, which may take up to 6 months. In some cases full union is not attained. However, at this stage the initial swelling has usually resolved and patients are mobilized slowly out of the cast.

Calcaneal fractures
The limb should be immobilized in a plaster cast until radiological healing has occurred.

Tibial and fibular fractures

These fractures can be treated either by open reduction and internal fixation or by cast immobilization.

Chronic stable inactive Charcot's osteoarthropathy

The foot is no longer warm and red. There may still be oedema but the difference in skin temperature between the feet is usually less than 2°C. The X-ray shows fracture healing, sclerosis and bone remodelling. The average amount of time spent in a cast by diabetic patients before reaching the chronic stage is 6 months but some patients may need a cast for over a year. This is a crucial stage in the treatment. The patient must now be rehabilitated and gradually moved from cast treatment to suitable footwear. The patient needs close observation to detect any relapse which will be evident from further swelling and heat in the foot.

Careful rehabilitation is always necessary after a long period in a cast.

Forefoot

This usually stabilizes without bony deformity but patients may need moulded insoles in bespoke shoes.

Mid-foot

When the mid-foot has stabilized, the patient can progress from a total-contact cast to a bivalved cast or Aircast or other cast walker (see Chapter 4) fitted with a cradled moulded insole. When the patient comes out of the cast there will be wasting of the calf muscles and joint stiffness. The physiotherapist must be aware of the dangers of re-activating the bony destruction phase by excessively rapid mobilization or protracted weightbearing in the early stages of rehabilitation.

Too rapid mobilization can be disastrous, resulting in further bone and joint damage. Extremely careful rehabilitation should be the rule, beginning with just a few short steps in the new footwear. The patient rests for the remainder of the day and monitors the foot. If there is no increase in warmth, swelling and redness then he can walk a few more steps the next day, and very carefully build up to a reasonable amount of walking.

Finally, the patient may progress to bespoke footwear with moulded insoles. The rocker-bottom foot with plantar bony prominence is a site of very high pressure. Regular reduction of callus can prevent ulceration. If ulceration does occur, an ostectomy (see Chapter 8) may be needed. If stabilization cannot be achieved by conservative means then it is possible to carry out operative procedures in the mid-foot.

Hindfoot

Hindfoot Charcot's osteoarthropathy may be difficult to stabilize. An attempt may be made with total-contact casting. The cast may have been used during the acute phases, to reduce oedema and halt progressive bony changes and deformity. Continued use of the cast will help to achieve stability of the hindfoot. Alternatively, a Charcot restraint orthotic walker (CROW) may be used, followed by an ankle–foot orthosis (AFO) with bespoke footwear.

The CROW

This is a bespoke bivalved total-contact device which externally fixates the ankle (Fig. 3.28a,b). Extra internal padding has been added to cushion the vulnerable medial malleolar area. The yellow corrugations contain ethyl vinyl acetate (EVA) to strengthen the device without increasing the bulk. All internal metal rivets have extra padding. The rigid, durable outer shell is constructed out of polypropylene and is lined with EVA. There is a bespoke moulded insole to accommodate any existing deformity and to redistribute plantar pressures. A rocker-bottom, crepe sole is attached to facilitate roll-off during walking. It is used after swelling is controlled and progressive destruction halted by total-contact casting.

AFO

The AFO is a device used to stabilize the foot and ankle. There are two main forms of AFO, the traditional conventional metal and leather calliper and the newer thermoplastic types which are more cosmetic.

CASE STUDY
Conservative management of Charcot's osteoarthropathy of the hindfoot

A 46-year-old male with type 1 diabetes of 40 years' duration presented with bilateral Charcot's osteoarthropathy. He was referred from a clinic 80 miles away and had been advised to have a right below-knee amputation. The left foot had stable mid-foot Charcot's osteoarthropathy with rocker-bottom deformity: the right foot was hot with unstable hindfoot Charcot's osteoarthropathy with lateral talotibiofibular displacement. The Charcot's osteoarthropathy was diagnosed 3 years previously following a first ray amputation (Fig. 3.29a). In view of the considerable distance he had to travel it was decided that casting him would be unwise. As an alternative, the treatment plan was to try to achieve stability by providing a CROW. After 5 weeks in the CROW, swelling had improved and the

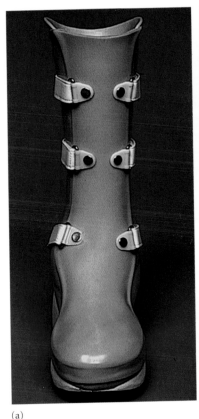 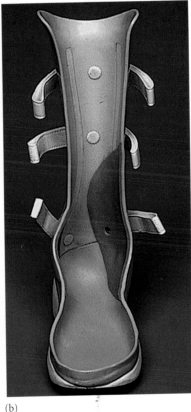

(a)   (b)

Fig. 3.28 (a) Anterior view of the CROW (with front piece). (b) Anterior view of the CROW with removal of the front piece to show interior. Extra internal padding (blue) has been added to cushion the vulnerable medial malleolar area.

skin temperature difference between the two feet was less than 2°C. An AFO was manufactured containing a moulded EVA insole (Fig. 3.29b,c). The patient was advised to take 5–10 steps daily for the first week and then at each week to double the steps taken. At 10 months he was taking up to 50 steps daily and the temperature difference was still less than 2°C. At this stage there was clinical and radiological evidence that the hindfoot had stabilized. He remained in the AFO for his long-term orthotic prescription. There was no relapse and he has remained ulcer free.

Key points
- Charcot's osteoarthropathy can develop after a first ray amputation or other surgical procedure
- Casting should not be undertaken if patients cannot return to the casting clinic quickly when problems arise
- Unstable hindfoot Charcot's osteoarthropathy can be stabilized, in some cases, by conservative means using a CROW, and maintained long term in an AFO and bespoke footwear.

If conservative care is unsuccessful, and the patient has a 'flail ankle', which is often associated with intractable ulceration over the malleoli, then internal stabilization may be necessary, and this is discussed in Chapter 8.

Following reconstructive ankle surgery, the lower limb is usually managed in a cast for several months and then a CROW is supplied to maintain the stability of the hindfoot. When all is stabilized, temperatures have stayed down and patient is fully ambulant, an AFO provides long-term stability.

CASE STUDY
Surgical reconstruction of Charcot's osteoarthropathy of the hindfoot

A 61-year-old woman with type 1 diabetes of 40 years' duration developed a hot, red, swollen foot and ankle, and Charcot's osteoarthropathy was diagnosed. She was unwilling to wear a total-contact cast, but agreed to wear an Aircast. One month later she attended a wedding and discarded the Aircast for 1 day. She returned to the foot

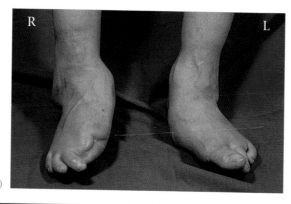

(a)

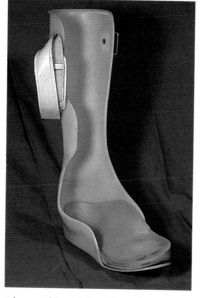

(b)

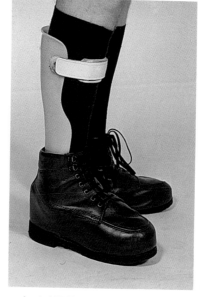

(c)

Fig. 3.29 (a) Left foot shows stable mid-foot Charcot's osteoarthropathy; right foot shows unstable hindfoot Charcot's osteoarthropathy and first ray amputation. (b) Ankle–foot orthosis (AFO) containing a moulded ethyl vinyl acetate insole. (c) Patient wearing AFO in bespoke boot.

clinic the following week with an unstable flail ankle. She underwent surgical reconstruction (Fig. 3.30) and returned to the foot clinic in a non-weightbearing plaster cast which she wore for 4 months, using a knee scooter to off-load the foot. A CROW was made and she began to remobilize. She developed a swelling on the front of her ankle where a screw from her internal fixation metal plate had worked loose, and the screw was surgically removed. The joint remained stable and an AFO was made for her long-term management with bespoke footwear and insoles. She did not relapse and remained ulcer free.

Key points
- Reconstructive surgery can solve the problem of unstable Charcot's osteoarthropathy of the ankle
- In the rehabilitation phase a CROW achieves stability and an AFO maintains stability
- The problem with removable casts during the phase of bony destruction is that some patients may remove them.

Recent advances in the management of the Charcot foot include the application of a Taylor Spatial Frame to the deformed foot. This is applied at operation and secured

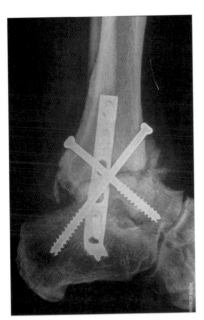

Fig. 3.30 X-ray of reconstructed Charcot hindfoot and ankle (courtesy of Dr M. Myerson).

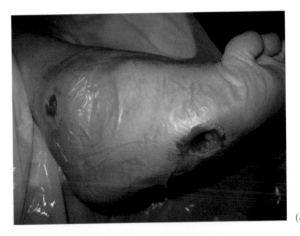

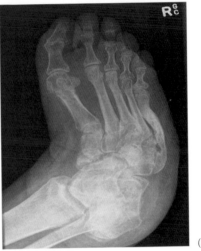

(a)

(b)

Fig. 3.31 (a) Charcot foot with rocker-bottom and hindfoot deformity and ulceration. (b) X-ray showing disorganization of mid- and hindfoot.

by pins through the bones of the foot. The wires within the frame are adjusted daily via a computer program to gradually change the shape of the foot, particularly the soft tissues. When this has been achieved, the patient then undergoes internal stabilization.

CASE STUDY
Use of Taylor Spatial Frame in Charcot's osteoarthropathy

A 43-year-old woman with type 1 diabetes of 30 years' duration developed a Charcot foot with rocker-bottom and hindfoot deformity leading to persistent ulceration which did not respond to casting treatment. Fig. 3.31a shows the presenting foot deformity complicated by ulceration with X-ray demonstrating mid- and hindfoot disorganization (Fig. 3.31b). She was treated with a dynamic Taylor Spatial Frame which was adjusted through a computer-based system to distract and reduce joint subluxation (Fig. 3.31c). She then underwent internal stabilization (Fig. 3.31d) and this restored the foot to a plantigrade position (Fig 3.31e) with healing of the ulceration (Fig. 3.31f) and successful accommodation in bespoke footwear.

Key points
- The dynamic Taylor Spatial Frame can help to correct deformity in Charcot's osteoarthropathy

- It can be used to restore rearfoot-to-leg and forefoot-to-rearfoot relationships
- Internal fixation can then stabilize the foot and ankle.

Follow-up of patients with Charcot's osteoarthropathy

We believe that patients with a history of Charcot's osteoarthropathy are among the most high risk of all and that they should never be discharged from the care of the multidisciplinary foot clinic.

Occasionally there may be a relapse in an already established but stabilized foot with Charcot's osteoarthropathy. This will present with erythema, swelling and warmth. The patient should be treated as if he was again in the acute phase.

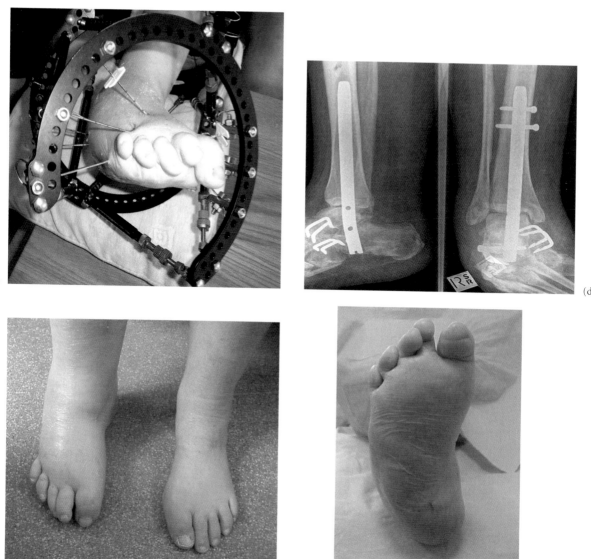

(c)

(d)

(e)

(f)

Fig. 3.31 (*cont'd*) (c) Taylor Spatial Frame applied to lower limb. (d) Internal operative stabilization. (e) Foot restored to a plantigrade position. (f) Healing of the ulcer. (Courtesy of Mr M. Phillips)

Many patients will eventually develop Charcot's osteoarthropathy in both feet. All patients with Charcot's osteoarthropathy should therefore be taught to check their feet and ankles regularly for hot spots and danger signs.

Charcot's osteoarthropathy of the knee is rarely seen in diabetic patients; however, the authors have seen four cases in the knee and all patients previously had Charcot's osteoarthropathy of the foot.

Education for patients with Charcot's osteoarthropathy

Patients should be warned of the dangers of unprotected walking during the acute phase. Even one step without cast or brace can injure the foot irrevocably. They should be told always to wear the cast or walker, even in bed at night, otherwise the temptation to go to the lavatory in the middle of the night without bothering to wear it may be too great. Patients should walk as little as possible and always use crutches: the more the foot is rested and elevated the sooner it will recover. Patients should be advised to borrow or hire a folding wheelchair so that they can get out without overloading the foot. The foot should be elevated whenever possible, so the wheelchair should be fitted with an extending plank on which to support the leg.

The clinician should never underestimate how difficult a diagnosis of acute Charcot's osteoarthropathy is for patients. Following advice and keeping off the foot is certain to have profound effects on their daily life, at home and at work, socially and emotionally.

During the rehabilitation period the patient will be under particularly great stress, when he knows the foot is recovering and the urge to get back to a normal life will become very strong. This is a dangerous period as failure to rehabilitate slowly and gently can trigger the destructive phase into action again.

PRACTICE POINTS

- The majority of deformities in stage 2 can be accommodated in special footwear
- Callus is an important precursor of ulceration and should be treated aggressively, especially in the neuropathic foot
- The cold, pink, painful foot is an indication of severe ischaemia and requires urgent vascular intervention
- Patients must understand the implications of lack of protective pain sensation
- Education in trauma prevention is important
- Patients with painful neuropathy will need therapy of various modalities which can be delivered in a supportive environment in the diabetic foot clinic
- Early diagnosis, immediate cast immobilization and careful rehabilitation are important for successful management of Charcot's osteoarthropathy.

FURTHER READING

Presentation and diagnosis

McCabe CJ, Stevenson RC, Dolan AM. Evaluation of a diabetic foot screening and protection programme. *Diabetic Medicine* 1998; **15**: 80–4.

Mayfield JA, Reiber GE, Sanders LJ *et al.* American Diabetes Association. Preventive foot care in diabetes. *Diabetes Care* 2004; **27** Suppl 1: S63–4.

Murray HJ, Young MJ, Hollis S *et al.* The association between callus formation, high pressures and neuropathy in diabetic foot ulceration. *Diabetic Medicine* 1996; **13**: 979–82.

Orendurff MS, Rohr ES, Sangeorzan BJ *et al.* An equinus deformity of the ankle accounts for only a small amount of the increased forefoot plantar pressure in patients with diabetes. *J Bone Joint Surg Br* 2006; **88**: 65–8.

Pinzur M, Freeland R, Juknelis D. The association between body mass index and foot disorders in diabetic patients. *Foot Ankle Int* 2005; **26**: 375–7.

Smith DG, Assal M, Reiber GE *et al.* Minor environmental trauma and lower extremity amputation in high-risk patients with diabetes: incidence, pivotal events, etiology, and amputation level in a prospectively followed cohort. *Foot Ankle Int* 2003; **24**: 690–5.

Mechanical control

Abouaesha F, Van Schie CH, Griffiths GD *et al.* Plantar tissue thickness is related to peak plantar pressure in the high risk diabetic foot. *Diabetes Care* 2001; **24**: 1270–4.

Boffeli TJ, Bean JK, Natwick JR. Biomechanical abnormalities and ulcers of the great toe in patients with diabetes. *J Foot Ankle Surg* 2002; **41**: 359–64.

Brand PW. Repetitive stress in the development of diabetic foot ulcers. In Levin ME, O'Neal LW (eds). *The Diabetic Foot.* Mosby, St Louis, USA, 1988, pp. 83–90.

Bus SA, Maas M, Cavanagh PR *et al.* Plantar fat-pad displacement in neuropathic diabetic patients with toe deformity: a magnetic resonance imaging study. *Diabetes Care* 2004; **27**: 2376–81.

Bus SA, Maas M, de Lange A *et al.* Elevated plantar pressures in neuropathic diabetic patients with claw/hammer toe deformity. *J Biomech* 2005; **38**: 1918–25.

Cavanagh PR, Ulbrecht JS. What the practising physician should know about diabetic foot biomechanics. In Boulton AJM, Cavanagh PR, Rayman G (eds). *The Foot in Diabetes*, 4th edn. John Wiley & Sons, Chichester, UK, 2006, pp. 68–91.

Kastenbauer T, Sokol G, Auinger M *et al.* Running shoes for relief of plantar pressure in diabetic patients. *Diabetic Medicine* 1998; **15**: 518–22.

Ledroux WR, Shofer JB, Smith DG *et al.* Relationship between foot type, foot deformity, and ulcer occurrence in the high risk diabetic foot. *J Rehabil Res Dev* 2005; **42**: 665–72.

Macfarlane DJ, Jensen JL. Factors in diabetic footwear compliance. *J Am Podiatr Med Assoc* 2003; **93**: 485–91.

Maciejewski ML, Reiber GE, Smith DG *et al.* Effectiveness of diabetic therapeutic footwear in preventing reulceration. *Diabetes Care* 2004; **27**: 1774–82.

Nube VL, Molyneaux L, Yue DK. Biomechanical risk factors associated with neuropathic ulceration of the hallux in people with diabetes mellitus. *J Am Podiatr Med Assoc* 2006; **96**: 189–97.

Pataky Z, Golay A, Faravel L *et al.* The impact of callosities on the magnitude and duration of plantar pressure in patients with diabetes mellitus. A callus may cause 18,600 kilograms of excess plantar pressure per day. *Diabetes Metab* 2002; **28**: 356–61.

Tovey FI. The manufacture of diabetic footwear. *Diabetic Medicine* 1984; **1**: 69–71.

Uccioli L, Faglia E, Monticone G *et al*. Manufactured shoes in the prevention of diabetic foot ulcers. *Diabetes Care* 1995; **18**: 1376–7.

Van Schie, CHM, Boulton AJM. Biomechanics of the diabetic foot. In Veves A, Giurini JM, LoGerfo FW (eds) *The Diabetic Foot*, 2nd edn. Humana Press, New Jersey, USA, 2006, pp. 185–200.

Young MJ, Cavanagh PR, Thomas G *et al*. The effect of callus removal of dynamic plantar foot pressures in diabetic patients. *Diabetic Medicine* 1992; **9**: 55–7.

Zimny S, Schatz H, Pfohl M. The role of limited joint mobility in diabetic patients with an at-risk foot. *Diabetes Care* 2004; **27**: 942–6.

Vascular control

American Diabetes Association. Peripheral arterial disease in people with diabetes. *Diabetes Care* 2003; **26**: 3333–41.

Heart Outcomes Prevention Evaluation Study investigators. The effects of ramipril on cardiovascular and microvascular outcomes in people with diabetes mellitus: results of the HOPE study and MICRO-HOPE sub study. *Lancet* 2000; **355**: 253–9.

Heart Protection Study Collaborative Group. MRC/BHF Heart Protection Study of cholesterol lowering with simvastatin in 20,536 high-risk individuals: a randomised placebo controlled trial. *Lancet* 2002; **360**: 7–22.

Kansal N, Hamdan A. Clinical features and diagnosis of macrovascular disease. In Veves A, Giurini JM, LoGerfo FW (eds). *The Diabetic Foot*, 2nd edn. Humana Press, New Jersey, USA, 2006, pp. 147–62.

Tooke JE (ed). *Diabetic Angiopathy*. Arnold, London, UK, 1999.

TransAtlantic Inter-Society Consensus (TASC). Management of peripheral arterial disease (PAD). *J Vasc Surg* 2000; **31** (Suppl): S1–S296.

Metabolic control

Chaturvedi N, Stephenson JM, Fuller JH, The EURODIAB IDDM Complications Study Group. The relationship between smoking and microvascular complications in the EURODIAM IDDM Complications Study. *Diabetes Care* 1995; **18**: 785–92.

Educational control

Assal JP, Albeanu A, Peter-Riesch B *et al*. The cost of training a diabetes mellitus patient. Effects on prevention of amputation. *Diabetes Metab* 1993; **19**: 491–5.

Brand P. *Insensitive Feet*. The Leprosy Mission, London, UK, 1981.

Valk GD, Kriegsman DM, Assendelft WJ. Patient education for preventing diabetic foot ulceration. A systematic review. *Endocrinol Metab Clin North Am* 2002; **31**: 633–58.

Painful neuropathy

Spruce MC, Potter J, Coppini DV. The pathogenesis and management of painful diabetic neuropathy: a review. *Diabet Med* 2003; **20**: 88–98.

Benbow SJ, Daousi C, MacFarlane IA. Painful diabetic neuropathy. In Barnett AH (ed). *Diabetes Best Practice and Research Compendium*. Elsevier, Oxford, UK, 2006, pp. 127–36.

Tesfaye S. Diabetic polyneuropathy. In Veves A, Giurini JM, LoGerfo FW (eds). *The Diabetic Foot*, 2nd edn. Humana Press, New Jersey, USA, 2006, pp. 105–30.

Watson CP, Moulin D, Watt-Watson J *et al*. Controlled-release oxycodone relieves neuropathic pain: a randomized controlled trial in painful diabetic neuropathy. *Pain* 2003; **105**: 71–8.

Charcot's osteoarthropathy

Berendt AR, Lipsky B. Is this bone infected or not? Differentiating neuro-osteoarthropathy from osteomyelitis in the diabetic foot. *Curr Diab Rep* 2004; **4**: 424–9.

Bem R, Jirkovska A, Fejfarova V *et al*. Intranasal calcitonin in the treatment of acute Charcot neuroosteoarthropathy: a randomized controlled trial. *Diabetes Care* 2006; **29**: 1392–4.

Chantelau E, Poll LW. Evaluation of the diabetic Charcot foot by MR imaging or plain radiography – an observational study. *J Am Podiatr Med Assoc* 2003; **93**: 485–91.

Chantelau E. The perils of procrastination: effects of early vs. delayed detection and treatment of incipient Charcot fracture. *Diabet Med* 2005; **22**: 1707–12.

Connolly JF, Csencsitz TA. Limb threatening neuropathic complications from ankle fractures in patients with diabetes. *Clin Orthop* 1998; **348**: 212–9.

Fabrin J, Larsen K, Holstein PE. Long-term follow-up in diabetic Charcot feet with spontaneous onset. *Diabetes Care* 2000; **23**: 796–800.

Giurato L, Uccioli L. The diabetic foot: Charcot joint and osteomyelitis. *Nucl Med Commun* 2006; **27**: 745–9.

Jude EB, Selby PL, Burgess J *et al*. Bisphosphonates in the treatment of Charcot neuroarthropathy: a double-blind randomised controlled trial. *Diabetologia* 2001; **44**: 2032–7.

McGill M, Molyneaux L, Bolton T *et al*. Response of Charcot's arthropathy to contact casting: assessment by quantitative techniques. *Diabetologia* 2000; **43**: 481–4.

Mehta JA, Brown C, Sargeant N. Charcot restraint orthotic walker. *Foot Ankle Int* 1998; **19**: 619–23.

Myerson MS, Alvarez RG, Lam PW. Tibiocalcaneal arthrodesis for the management of severe ankle and hindfoot deformities. *Foot Ankle Int* 2000; **21**: 643–50.

Pitocco D, Ruotolo V, Caputo S *et al*. Six-month treatment with alendronate in acute Charcot neuroarthropathy: a randomized controlled trial. *Diabetes Care* 2005; **28**: 1214–5.

Petrova NL, Foster AV, Edmonds ME. Calcaneal bone mineral density in patients with Charcot neuropathic osteoarthropathy: differences between Type 1 and Type 2 diabetes. *Diabet Med* 2005; **22**: 756–61.

Petrova NL, Foster AV, Edmonds ME. Difference in presentation of Charcot osteoarthropathy in type 1 compared with type 2 diabetes. *Diabetes Care* 2004; **27**: 1235–6.

Petrova NL, Moniz C, Elias DA *et al.* Is there a systemic inflammatory response in the acute Charcot foot? *Diabetes Care* 2007; **30**: 997–8.

Rajbhandari SM, Jenkins RC, Davies C, Tesfaye S. Charcot neuroarthropathy in diabetes mellitus. *Diabetologia* 2002; **45**: 1085–96.

Roukis TS, Zgonis T. The management of acute Charcot fracture-dislocations with the Taylor's spatial external fixation system. *Clin Podiatr Med Surg* 2006; **23**: 467–83,viii.

Sanders LJ, Frykberg RG. The Charcot Foot (Pied de Charcot). In Bowker J, Pfeifer MA (eds). *Levin and O'Neal's* The Diabetic Foot, Seventh Edition. Elsevier Inc., September 2007.

Smith DG, Barnes BC, Sands AK *et al.* Prevalence of radiographic foot abnormalities in patients with diabetes. *Foot Ankle Int* 1997; **18**: 342–6.

Tan PL, Teh J. MRI of the diabetic foot: differentiation of infection from neuropathic change. *Br J Radiol* 2006; May 10.[Epub ahead of print.]

4 Stage 3: the ulcerated foot

O, he's a limb that has but a disease,
Mortal, to cut it off, to cure it easy.
(Coriolanus, III, i, William Shakespeare)

PRESENTATION AND DIAGNOSIS

The ulcer is a pivotal event in the natural history of the diabetic foot. Once patients develop skin breakdown and ulceration they enter stage 3. For too many people with diabetes, stage 3 is the point of no return along the road to amputation. Neuroischaemic feet are the most likely to come to major amputation, but neuropathic patients with ulcers are also at risk of amputation if their feet are mismanaged; all ulcers, both neuropathic and ischaemic, need very rapid and active management.

The aim is always to close the ulcer as quickly as possible, thus minimizing the incidence of secondary infection and changes to the architecture of the foot. If ulcers heal quickly, while they are still small and shallow, then scarring and destruction of fibrofatty padding and bone infection will be minimized, and the risk of relapse reduced. Neglected ulcers may eventually heal, but their residual effects may include bone and joint damage, fibrofatty padding depletion, and a lifetime of foot problems.

Throughout their lifetime 15% of diabetic patients will develop ulceration; 85% of amputations result from non-healing ulcers. Every break in the skin of the diabetic foot is a portal of entry for bacteria and has the potential for disaster. It is dangerous ever to assume that an ulcer on a diabetic foot is small, or trivial or unimportant. As Malvolio said in Romeo and Juliet, 'A scratch . . . tis enough . . . t'will serve'.

Furthermore, the development of an ulcer is a marker of multi-organ disease in the diabetic patient which must be actively assessed and treated. When the diagnosis of ischaemia is made in the diabetic foot, it presents the opportunity to protect the rest of the vasculature from ischaemic episodes by intensive atherosclerotic risk factor management. Patients with diabetic foot problems do not usually die directly from foot complications but from cardiovascular disease.

CLASSIFICATION

We have already emphasized the importance of differentiating between ulcers in neuropathic feet and ulcers in neuroischaemic feet because their treatment will differ. The basis of this classification is the presence or absence of ischaemia in the common background of neuropathy. The majority of ischaemic feet in diabetes will also have neuropathy and therefore we describe the ischaemic foot as neuroischaemic. However, there may be some ischaemic feet with minimal or no neuropathy and the ulcers in these feet are perhaps more accurately called ischaemic. For simplicity, we shall refer to them as neuroischaemic ulcers because the simple staging system is a treatment-based system and ischaemic and neuroischaemic ulcers need the same treatment.

The simple staging system does not classify ulcers according to depth. It is difficult to assess the depth of an ulcer accurately, except where it is clear that it probes to bone, suggesting possible infection, which already has its own separate stage within the system. Describing ulcers as superficial can lead to false reassurance, as any ulcer, even a small shallow one, can deteriorate and become very serious in a short space of time. It is dangerous for diabetic patients or their carers ever to regard small superficial lesions as trivial because the destructive potential of a break in the skin cannot be accurately assessed by measuring its depth.

A Practical Manual of Diabetic Foot Care, 2nd edition, Edmonds, Foster and Sanders.
Published 2008 Blackwell Publishing. ISBN 978-1-4051-61473

Although ulceration can present in many different ways, we believe the most relevant classification of ulcers is the simple division of ulcers in neuropathic feet or ulcers in neuroischaemic feet, as such a division has the most relevant and important implications for treatment. However, it is also important to recognize specific categories of ulcer within this simple classification.

Specific categories of ulcer

These include:
- Decubitus heel ulcers caused by unrelieved pressure
- Ulcers of Charcot's osteoarthropathy associated with rocker-bottom deformity, medial convexity and hindfoot deformity
- Ulcers over the Achilles tendon
- Puncture wounds caused by standing on sharp objects
- Traumatic wounds, including burns
- Artefactual (factitial) ulcers caused deliberately by the patient
- Malignant ulcers.

The main part of this chapter will concentrate on the presentation and management of neuropathic and neuroischaemic ulcers, describing the multidisciplinary approach, with mechanical, wound, vascular, microbiological, metabolic and educational control. The chapter will finish with a discussion of the presentation and management of the specific categories of ulcers described above.

Neuropathic ulcer

Neuropathic ulcers are commonly found at the apices of the toes and on the plantar aspect of prominent metatarsal heads. Callus forms in these areas in response to high vertical pressures or shearing forces. This leads to inflammation, further callus formation, increased pressure and tissue breakdown. Failure to remove callus regularly leads to ulceration. Developing and established neuropathic ulcers are usually painless. Pain associated with neuropathic ulceration may be the first symptom of infection.

Neuroischaemic ulcer

Ulceration in the neuroischaemic foot usually occurs on the margins of the foot. The first sign of ulceration is a red mark which blisters and then develops into a shallow ulcer with a base of sparse pale granulations or yellowish closely adherent slough. In ischaemia, there is often a halo of erythema around the ulcer where local blood vessels have dilated in an attempt to improve perfusion of the area (Fig. 4.1).

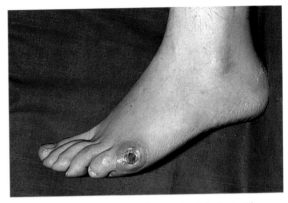

Fig. 4.1 An ischaemic ulcer on the margin of the foot with a halo of erythema.

Pain associated with a neuroischaemic ulcer may be due to the ischaemia itself or to infection. The degree of pain will depend on the severity of concomitant neuropathy.

It is now necessary to classify the ulcer as neuropathic or neuroischaemic. This is achieved by:
- Taking a history
- Examination of the foot and the ulcer
- Investigations, including assessing the neurological and vascular status.

Taking a history
A short history of the ulcer should be taken to ascertain its cause, duration and previous treatment.

Examination
Foot examination should be carried out as described in the Introduction (Chapter 1). The ulcer should then be examined noting:
- Site
- Size
- Appearance of the ulcer and surrounding tissues
- Discharge
- Oedema
- Tenderness
- Smell
- 'Probe-ability'.

The implications of these are discussed below.

Site
Ulcers on the plantar surface are usually neuropathic and ulcers on the margins of the foot are usually neuroischaemic. However, ulcers can appear in other sites.

Interdigital ulcers can be caused by the toes being squeezed together in tight, ill-fitting shoes in both neuropathic and neuroischaemic feet.

Ulceration on the dorsal aspect of the toes is often associated with pressure from tight shoes in either class of foot.

Ulcers on the plantar aspect of the heel are usually caused by acute trauma, particularly treading on foreign bodies. Indeed, trauma can cause ulceration at any site in either class of foot.

Size
Any break in the skin, however small, can lead to disaster. However, larger ulcers usually take longer to heal.

Appearance of the ulcer and surrounding tissues
The colour of the base of the ulcer is important. A pink, clean, glistening ulcer bed is healthy. Variation in the colour of the ulcer bed may be significant: for example, a wound bed which is largely pink but has an area of grey discolouration often overlies a sinus. Many poorly perfused ischaemic wound beds are grey or yellow and sloughy. Moist green or yellow slough indicates infection and patients should be managed as described in Chapter 5.

Black tissue indicates necrosis and the foot should be regarded as at stage 5 and managed accordingly.

Neuropathic ulcers are usually surrounded by callus, which is often white and rubbery because it is macerated by discharge from the ulcer. The neuropathic ulcer may be almost completely covered over by callus.

Neuroischaemic ulcers may be surrounded by a small halo of thin, glassy callus.

Diffuse redness of the surrounding tissues may indicate infection in both neuropathic and neuroischaemic feet, especially if this is associated with swelling and purulent discharge. A purplish colour indicates reduced oxygen supply to the tissues, which may result from ischaemia or severe infection or both: it is a clinical emergency.

Healing ulcers are surrounded by an area of shiny new pink and white epithelium (Fig. 4.2).

Discharge
Purulent discharge is indicative of infection. Clear or yellow-tinged viscous bubbly discharge from an ulcer which probes to bone may be synovial fluid, indicating involvement of the joint. Increased amounts of clear discharge may be an early indication of infection.

Oedema
Oedema around an ulcer is usually suggestive of infection but may be related to ischaemia.

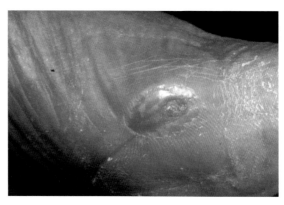

Fig. 4.2 This healing ulcer is surrounded by an area of shiny new pink and white epithelium.

Tenderness
This should be elicited by gentle palpation and may be due either to infection or to ischaemia.

Smell
Any smell associated with an ulcer is suggestive of infection.

Probe-ability of the ulcer
The depth and dimensions of the ulcer are determined by probing, which is an important part of the examination. Probing reveals the presence of:
- Undermined edges where the probe can be passed from the ulcer under surrounding intact skin (Fig. 4.3a,b)
- Sinuses when the probe can be inserted deeper than in other areas of the ulcer bed and may reach tendon or bone. A sinus may not be immediately apparent, but may be sometimes disclosed by probing suspicious areas of the ulcer, which are a different colour to the remainder of the ulcer bed. These areas may also be less firm and resilient.

Some ulcers appear to pout, or stand proud of the surrounding epithelium. If such an ulcer is producing copious amounts of discharge there will often be a sinus present. The aperture of the sinus may be slit-shaped rather than round (Fig. 4.4).

When probing the practitioner should determine the following:
- The depth and breadth of the ulcer
- The depth and direction of any sinus
- Does the probe reach bone? If so, this suggests osteomyelitis and the foot is at stage 4. Previously it was thought that probing to bone was an accurate indicator of osteomyelitis, particularly in patients who actually

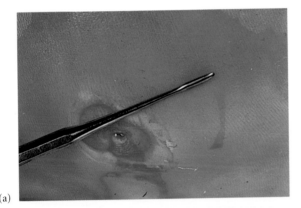

(a)

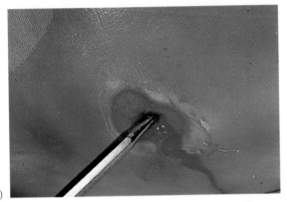

(b)

Fig. 4.3 (a) Ulcer with a probe placed over the skin to indicate position of sinus. (b) Probe inserted into sinus of same ulcer.

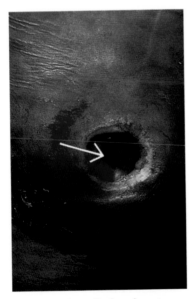

Fig. 4.4 This deep sinus has a slit-shaped aperture.

Table 4.1 Clinical features of neuropathic and neuroischaemic feet

Neuropathic foot	Neuroischaemic foot
Ulcer on plantar surface	Ulcer on margins
Heavy callus	Thin glassy callus or no callus
Warm foot	Cold foot
Pulses present	Pulses absent
TcPo$_2$ above 30 mmHg	TcPo$_2$ below 30 mmHg

present with significant soft tissue limb-threatening infection. However, in a recent study of a population of outpatient diabetic patients, in whom osteomyelitis was found in only 12% of diabetic foot wounds, probing to bone had a low positive predictive value of 0.57 but it was concluded that a negative test could exclude the diagnosis of osteomyelitis.

Investigations

These should include neurological, vascular, laboratory and radiological investigations as described in Chapter 1.

While it is not necessary to X-ray every stage 3 foot with a presenting ulcer, it may be advisable to do so in the following circumstances:
- When the history suggests that the patient may have trodden on a foreign body
- When the ulcer probes to bone, possibly suggesting osteomyelitis
- If there are clinical signs of infection
- When there is unexplained pain or swelling which may be related to neuropathic fracture or Charcot's osteoarthropathy
- When the ulcer has been present for longer than 1 month.

Having completed the history, examination and investigations, it is possible to make a firm diagnosis of ulceration either in the neuropathic foot or the neuroischaemic foot. The characteristic features are described in Table 4.1.

Follow-up of ulcerated feet

In the short term, the ulcer will need close review at each visit. Signs of progress or deterioration should be looked for.

Signs that an ulcer is healing
- Ulcer bed becomes pink
- Ulcer bed becomes shiny with glistening granulations

- Dimensions of ulcer decrease with new epithelium around the edges
- Ulcer bed becomes drier with less discharge
- Swelling diminishes
- Ulcer becomes less painful
- Malodour ceases
- There is no undermining
- Sinus depth reduces
- No surrounding cellulitis.

Signs of deterioration
- Colour of ulcer bed changes
- Matt surface develops over ulcer bed
- Dimensions of ulcer become static or increase
- Ulcer becomes moist with increased discharge
- Local swelling develops or increases
- Foot becomes painful
- Malodour develops
- Ulcer becomes undermined
- Cellulitis develops in surrounding tissues.

These warning signs should never be ignored.

In the long term, it should be remembered that patients with neuropathic feet may eventually develop ischaemia, and the classification should be repeated at every annual review.

MANAGEMENT

All of these components of multidisciplinary management are important in stage 3:
- Mechanical control
- Wound control
- Microbiological control
- Vascular control
- Metabolic control
- Educational control.

The aim is to heal ulcers within the first 6 weeks of their development. This is the time for aggressive management and is a window of opportunity that should be taken seriously. All diabetic foot ulcers should be referred for multidisciplinary care without delay so that the opportunity of early healing is not wasted. The ulcer is a pivotal event on the road to amputation, and the diabetic patient with an ulcer on the foot is at great risk of infection, gangrene and loss of the leg.

Because it is difficult to predict which ulcers will do well and which will do catastrophically, it is essential to organize optimal care for all ulcers. When ulcers are healed, the foot is treated as stage 2 to prevent recurrence. Neuroischaemic ulcers may be painful and thus pain control will also be considered.

Mechanical control

Ideally, ulcers must be managed with rest and avoidance of all pressure. Surgery such as exostectomies to remove bony prominences and Achilles tendon lengthening to reduce pressure on the plantar forefoot may help to achieve successful mechanical control. However, surgery is not without risks and the main way to achieve mechanical control is to use casting in order to redistribute pressure on the plantar aspect of the foot. Total off-loading will heal ulcers; however, total non-weightbearing is rarely practical and is difficult to achieve. For these reasons, ambulatory methods of achieving mechanical control are best; however, the patient should always be advised to walk as little as possible.

In the neuropathic foot, the overall aim is to redistribute plantar pressures evenly, thus avoiding areas of high pressure that will prevent or delay healing.

In the neuroischaemic foot, the aim is to protect the vulnerable margins of the foot.

Thus, mechanical control will be considered separately in the neuropathic and the neuroischaemic foot.

Neuropathic foot
The most efficient way to redistribute plantar pressure is by the immediate application of some form of cast: the total-contact cast is usually best. If casting techniques are not available, temporary ready-made shoes with a cushioning insole can be supplied to off-load the site of ulceration. Alternatively, weight-relief shoes can be supplied, and felt padding can also be used. Additional off-loading measures are crutches, wheelchairs and Zimmer frames.

Moulded insoles in bespoke shoes are sometimes used to treat ulcers. However, shoes with insoles are not an efficient way to off-load diabetic foot ulcers. Their main function is to prevent recurrence.

Casts
Various casts are available and their use is governed by local experience and expertise. Techniques include:
- Total-contact cast
- Scotchcast boot
- Aircast (walking brace) and other removable cast walkers.

Total-contact cast
The total-contact cast (Fig. 4.5a) is an extremely efficient method of redistributing pressure from the plantar surface of the foot. However, it is not without its complications, and should be reserved for patients whose ulcers

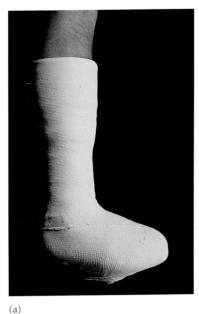

(a)

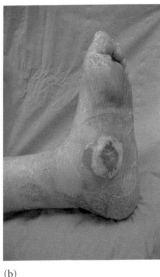

(b)

Fig. 4.5 (a) The total-contact cast: an extremely efficient method of redistributing pressure. (b) Indolent ulcer on a Charcot foot before treatment by total-contact casting.

have not responded to other treatments. It is a close fitting cast, applied over minimal padding. The casting procedure is described below.

Materials needed for each total-contact cast are as follows:

- A foam pyramid or roll of towels to elevate the leg
- Stockinette: a length double the distance from the tips of the toes to the knee. The size of stockinette used will depend on the diameter of the patient's leg
- 5 mm adhesive felt: two circles, each with a diameter of 5 cm, which cover the malleoli, and a strip 3 cm wide and long enough to reach from the tibial crest to the ankle. If there are additional bony prominences more pieces of felt will be needed to protect them
- Cast padding: usually three rolls, 7 cm wide, per cast
- Casting tape: usually three rolls, 7 cm wide, per cast, but if the patient is very heavy more rolls will be needed. Wet casting tape should not come into contact with chairs, clothes, trolley top or bare skin
- A pair of gloves for each operator
- Plastic sheeting to protect the chair
- A bucket of warm water in which to dip the casting tape. The water can be cold, in which case the casting tape takes longer to set
- Written advice for the patient
- A vibrating cast saw for adaptation or removal of the cast.

Fig. 4.5b shows an ulcer on a Charcot foot before treatment by total-contact casting. Fig. 4.5c shows a close-up view of the ulcer.

- When patients attend the casting clinic, they wear shorts or tracksuit bottoms otherwise they will need to unpick trouser seams to remove the cast
- The health-care professionals applying the cast must wear protective gloves. Total-contact casting is a job for two people, one of whom will hold the foot and leg in position while the other applies the cast
- A layer of stockinette is applied to the patient's foot and lower leg. The stockinette will line and cover the cast. The length of the stockinette needed is twice the distance from knee to tips of toes (two-and-a-half times if the leg is plump) and the excess should be gathered up over the knee (Fig. 4.5d). When the cast is finished the excess stockinette is brought down to cover the cast and protect the contralateral leg from rubs
- The foot is held in a plantigrade position and any excessive creases in the stockinette around the ankle area are cut out and taped flat
- A strip of 5 mm felt padding is applied over the tibial crest and circles of felt are applied over each malleolus and any other bony prominences (including, in this case, a circle of felt around the ulcer). Small pieces of cast padding are inserted between the toes to keep them apart and absorb perspiration (Fig. 4.5e)

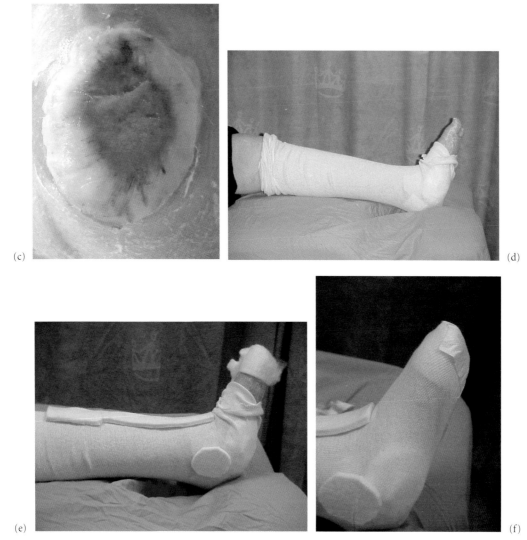

(c)

(d)

(e)

(f)

Fig. 4.5 (*cont'd*) (c) Close-up view of the same ulcer. (d) A layer of stockinette is applied to the patient's foot and lower leg and the excess is gathered up over the knee. The extra stockinette will cover the cast later. (e) Felt padding is applied over the tibial crest, over each malleolus and any other bony prominences (including, in this case, a circle of felt around the ulcer). Small pieces of cast padding are inserted between the toes. (f) The distal end of the stockinette is taped together to enclose the toes.

- The distal end of the stockinette is taped together to enclose the toes (Fig. 4.5f)
- A double layer of cast padding is applied to the entire lower limb (Fig. 4.5g) with three extra layers at the proximal end of the cast and three extra layers over the toes where the padding is fanned across to provide extra cushioning
- Fibreglass casting tape (Fig. 4.5h) is applied to form a supporting layer. The tape hardens in contact with air

and is therefore only removed from its foil packaging when the operators are ready to apply the tape. It is removed from its foil packaging, dipped into the bucket of water, submerged until bubbles of air stop rising and then removed from the water and gently squeezed to remove excess water. Speed of hardening of the tape will increase proportionally to the heat of the water used; therefore, experienced operators may want to use hot water, and beginners start with cold water. The tape is

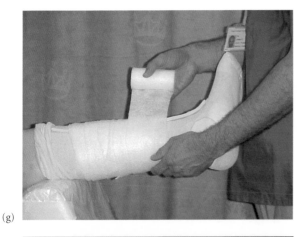

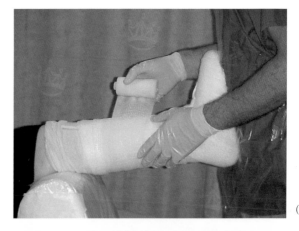

(g)

(h)

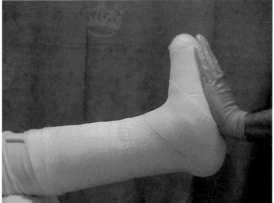

(i)

(j)

Fig. 4.5 (*cont'd*) (g) Cast padding is applied to the entire lower limb. (h) Fibreglass casting tape is applied. (i) The foot is maintained in a plantigrade position throughout the application of the cast. (j) The excess stockinette which was gathered up over the knee when casting commenced is rolled down to cover the outer fibreglass layer.

applied around the foot and leg, starting at the top of the leg, 3 cm below the cast padding, and below the tibial tuberosity. It is wound around the leg three times at the proximal end and then descending down the leg overlapping the previous section of tape by two-thirds with each circumnavigation. When all the tape has been applied the layers of tape are rubbed gently to accommodate the contours of the foot and leg and to ensure that the layers of tape adhere to each other. The finished cast should be at least three layers of tape thick and for heavy patients more will be needed. Very heavy patients will need up to six layers. Patients should be told not to touch the wet fibreglass which can cause skin irritation. The foot is maintained in a plantigrade position throughout the application of the cast (Fig. 4.5i)

- The excess stockinette which was gathered up over the knee when casting commenced is rolled down to cover

the outer fibreglass layer (Fig. 4.5j). Rubbing the stockinette provides a smooth finish (Fig. 4.5k). A cast walker fastened with velcro straps is provided (Fig. 4.5l)
- Casts should be checked after 1 week and replaced if reduction of oedema renders them loose
- The maximum period a cast should be left on without renewing is 1 month. This patient was healed when the cast was removed after 1 month (Fig. 4.5m).

The original total-contact cast adopted by Brand and colleagues in the management of complications of leprosy did not use cast padding but a layer of foam padding at the proximal and distal ends of the cast. Brand's cast also incorporated a strengthening plywood platform. However, we have found a reduced incidence of iatrogenic lesions in casts with additional padding, and rarely incorporate a platform as this increases leg length disparity. The original total-contact cast used plaster of Paris bandage and took

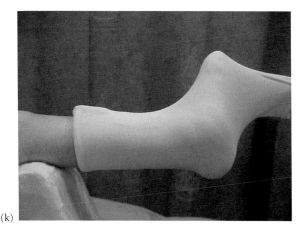

(k)

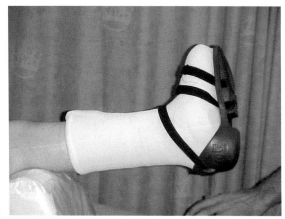

(l)

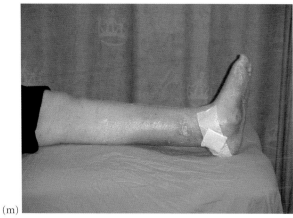

(m)

Fig. 4.5 (*cont'd*) (k) Rubbing the stockinette has provided a smooth finish. (l) A cast walker fastened with velcro straps is provided. (m) The foot was healed when the cast was removed after 1 month.

2 days to set, during which time the patient could not walk and we found that some patients walked too early and dented their casts.

When undertaking total-contact casting it is essential for practitioners to try to avoid problems.

An emergency cast removal service should be available for patients if they develop problems with the cast. The most common mistakes made when applying casts are:

- The cast comes too high up the leg, so that when the knee is bent the cast presses on the back of the thigh
- The cast is wrapped too tightly around the toes and border of the forefoot, causing pressure lesions
- The rough fibreglass outside layer is not covered with stockinette and rubs occur on the contralateral limb
- The cast is too lightweight for heavier patients and collapses
- Fibreglass is dented by pressure from finger tips—the cast should be handled with the flat of the hands
- The foot is insufficiently dorsiflexed. If the cast is applied to a rigid plantar flexed foot there should be compensatory building up of the heel area of the cast.

Advantages of the cast include:

- Redistributes pressure very evenly over the sole; 30% of pressure is transferred further up the leg in a 'coning' effect
- Enforces compliance—the patient cannot remove it
- 'Ball and chain'—patients walk less in a heavy cast
- Reduces oedema
- Ulcers heal very quickly—mean healing time of 6 weeks.

Disadvantages of the cast include:

- Cannot be removed so ulcer progress cannot be checked daily
- Heavy and reduces mobility
- Patient may not drive a car in a cast unless fitted with suitable controls and with permission from insurers
- A few patients develop 'cast phobia' and will not wear them. One of our patients borrowed her neighbour's electric saw and removed her cast (but fortunately not her leg). Another used a claw hammer to bash the cast off and sustained trauma to her leg
- Iatrogenic lesions (rubs, pressure sores, infections) may be undetected
- Leg may develop 'cast disease' from prolonged immobilization, e.g. muscle wasting, weakness and osteopaenia
- Leg length disparity may cause discomfort and problems with knee, hip and spine (this can be prevented with a shoe raise on the contralateral side; however, providing a shoe raise may be regarded as tacitly encouraging the patient to walk more)

- Danger of fracture and the development of a Charcot foot when the cast is discontinued without careful rehabilitation
- Frail patients may suffer falls
- Casts are unsuitable for patients with ulcers or skin eruptions on the leg
- Problems may also arise if patients fail to care for the cast or miss appointments for review.

CASE STUDY
Problems with total-contact cast

A 63-year-old woman with type 1 diabetes mellitus of 20 years' duration, developed an acute Charcot's osteo-arthropathy which was treated in a total-contact cast. She was a very successful milliner who was currently making hats for Royal Ascot Races, and was working from a studio at home with a team of assistants. She failed to attend for her 1-week cast check. We telephoned her and she said that the cast was fine but she was frantically busy making hats and really did not want to come in. We persuaded her to attend. When she came the following day she looked tired and unwell, and the cast was in poor condition with dehiscence of the lamina. Before the cast was removed she volunteered that she 'might have dropped some pins down it'. On cast removal she had a deep necrotic ulcer on the plantar surface of the foot caused by a pin which had penetrated the inner layers of the cast (Fig. 4.6a,b) and punctured her foot. She was admitted to hospital the same day (she booked a private room and continued to direct her team preparing for Ascot over the telephone). She underwent surgical debridement and the foot healed in 2 months.

Key points
- Regular cast inspections are essential
- A patient's report on the condition of the cast may be unreliable
- A patient's occupation may be hazardous without special precautions.

Rarely, a total-contact cast causes an eczematous eruption.

CASE STUDY
Eczematous eruption within cast

A 42-year-old neuropathic man with type 1 diabetes of 40 years' duration was given a total-contact cast for acute Charcot's osteoarthropathy. After 3 weeks he developed an eczematous eruption of the whole area covered by the cast and some areas on the other leg and arms.

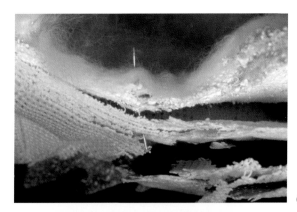

(a)

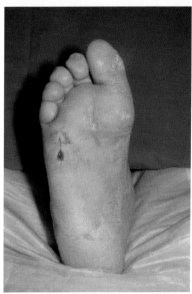

(b)

Fig. 4.6 (a) Cast in poor condition with pin protruding. (b) Site of ulcer on plantar surface of 5th ray indicating area where pin penetrated the foot.

He underwent patch testing by the dermatology clinic including testing to epoxy resins (the most likely culprit among the components of the casting tape). These tests were all entirely negative, making a contact eczema rather unlikely, although it is possible that he was allergic to another component of his plaster.

Our solution was to enclose the cast, inside and out, with three layers of stockinette to reduce any possibility of direct contact of the patient's skin with any other component of the cast, and his skin condition improved.

Key points
- Eruptions beneath the cast may be due to allergy to cast components
- A cast with extra protective layers of stockinette may be useful when patients develop eruptions under the cast
- Patch testing may be helpful.

Rehabilitation programme. Once the ulcer is healed, the patient should be assessed for moulded insoles and bespoke shoes.

He should remain in the cast until the new shoes are ready.

It is helpful if the orthotist attends the casting clinic so that footwear preparations can be under way during the last weeks of healing and unnecessary delays are avoided.

When the patient has been healed for 1 month, the rehabilitation programme can commence as follows:
- The cast should be bivalved and made removable by cutting out the front, padding the raw edges of both pieces with Elastoplast, and holding the two pieces in place with Velcro strapping or bandage. The padding should be incorporated into the cast
- The patient may walk for five steps without the cast on the first day of rehabilitation, wearing his new shoes and walking within the house. He should then replace the cast
- The foot should be checked for red marks on the following day. If all is well, the patient can walk for 10 steps without the cast
- Very gradually he can build up the amount of walking he does, within the house at first and then outside, but always wearing the special shoes and checking the foot every day for problems
- If blistering or ulceration occurs he should return to the diabetic foot clinic at once
- Patients may require physiotherapy to build up wasted muscles.

Courses in the UK in the manufacture of total-contact casts are available for health-care professionals at King's College Hospital.

Education for patients in casts. It is dangerous to enclose an insensitive leg and foot in a closed cast without careful education of the patient as follows:
- Keep your cast clean and dry. Walk as little as possible. If you go out in wet weather cover the cast with a plastic bag or cling film, but remove these as soon as you are under cover again
- You can obtain a plastic cast protector from the Chemist (Pharmacy) for bathing and showering
- Check your cast every morning and evening for:

  Cracks
  Soft areas
  Dirty areas
  Stained areas (where blood or pus has come through the cast from the inside)
  Wet areas
  Bad-smelling areas
  If any of these occur, please telephone the diabetic foot clinic immediately and come in for a cast check
- Check your temperature with a clinical thermometer every morning and evening. If it rises above 37.5°C, ring the clinic and come in for a check
- Check your blood glucose every morning and evening. If it rises above 15 mmol/L (270 mg/dL) please ring the clinic and come in for a check
- If you feel unwell, tired, hot, achy, shivery or have flu-like symptoms, please ring the clinic and come in for a check
- Never poke or pour anything down your cast
- Never try to remove the cast yourself
- Do not go a long distance from home
- Do not fly as there is increased danger of deep vein thrombosis.

Scotchcast boot

Not every patient is suitable for total-contact casting, and the Scotchcast boot is a useful alternative (Fig. 4.7a). It can also be used for patients with neuroischaemic foot or cast phobia.

It is a simple removable or non-removable boot made of stockinette, cast padding, felt and fibreglass tape. Originally the fibreglass tape used was of the Scotchcast brand name: other fibreglass casting tape can, however, also be used. The boot is effective in reducing pressure on the plantar surface and the margins of the foot. It is made as follows:
- A layer of stockinette is applied to the lower limb from mid-calf to 10 cm distal to the toes
- One piece of 7 mm felt is applied to the sole of the foot extending to the tips of the toes, 5 cm up the back of the heel and 2.5 cm up each side of the foot. Lateral borders should not be higher than the top of the foot. Triangles are cut out of the felt so that it sits snugly around the heel
- Cast padding is wrapped loosely around the foot over the felt (Fig. 4.7b)
- Three strips of fibreglass tape are cut and overlapped longitudinally so that they cover the sole of the foot. More fibreglass tape is then wrapped around the foot over the strips, keeping well within the area covered by cast padding (Fig. 4.7c)

- The fibreglass is trimmed away below the malleoli, round the back of the heel and along the sides of the foot below the level of the felt (Fig. 4.7d). The fibreglass covering the dorsum of the foot is lifted away (Fig. 4.7e), leaving behind as much cast padding as possible. Any sharp corners of fibreglass are rounded off
- The stockinette is folded back over the foot from each end
- The entire boot is wrapped round with Elastoplast tape. At this stage the boot cannot be removed by the patient. If a removable boot is wanted, the procedure is as follows:
- The dorsal area of the boot is cut open from toes to ankle (Fig. 4.7f) through all the layers of cast padding and stockinette, and the boot is removed

- The raw edges where the cut was made are sealed with Elastoplast (Fig. 4.7g)
- A tongue is made as extra protection to the dorsum of the foot to avoid rubbing by the straps (Fig. 4.7h). This can be made out of a thick padded dressing or a piece of felt.
- Ready-made straps or Velcro fastenings over the midfoot and high on the foot should be adjustable to accommodate oedema (Fig. 4.7i)
- A large sock worn over the cast offers extra protection to the toes. The boot can be worn inside a cast sandal.

Courses in the UK for the manufacture of the total-contact cast and Scotchcast boots are available at King's College Hospital and the Blackburn diabetic foot clinic have run a course on Scotchcast boot manufacture.

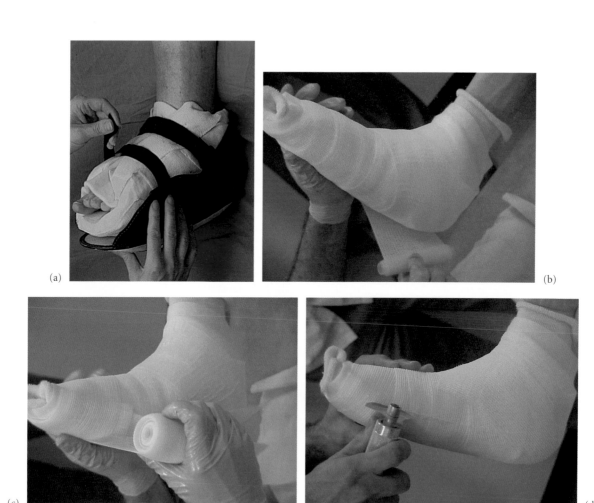

(a)

(b)

(c)

(d)

Fig. 4.7 (a) The Scotchcast boot is a useful bespoke fibre glass boot, and is effective at reducing pressure on the plantar surface and the margins of the foot. (b) Cast padding is wrapped loosely around the foot over felt. (c) Fibreglass tape is wrapped around the foot. (d) The excess fibreglass is trimmed away.

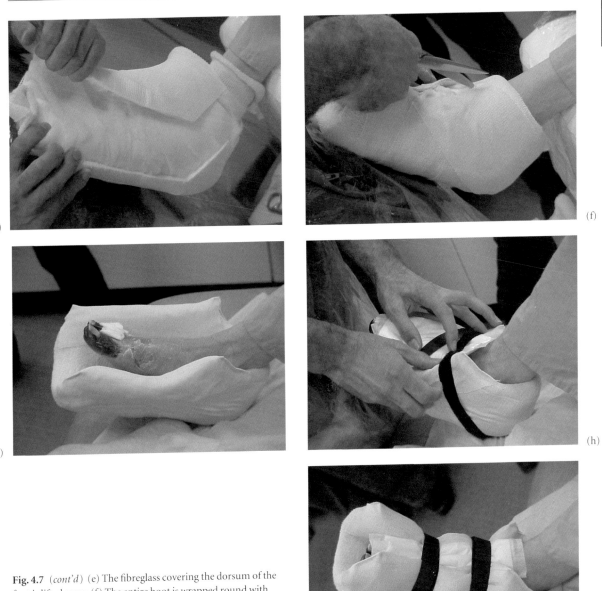

(e)

(f)

(g)

(h)

(i)

Fig. 4.7 (*cont'd*) (e) The fibreglass covering the dorsum of the foot is lifted away. (f) The entire boot is wrapped round with Elastoplast tape and the dorsal area of the boot is cut open from toes to ankle. (g) The raw edges where the cut was made are sealed with Elastoplast tape. (h) A tongue is made as extra protection to the dorsum of the foot to avoid rubbing by the straps. (i) Adjustable ready-made straps or Velcro fastenings are applied to hold the boot in place and to accommodate oedema.

Removable cast walkers

There are several models of removable cast walker. We have first-hand experience with the prefabricated pneumatic walking brace called Aircast (Fig. 4.8).

The Aircast is a bivalved device and the two halves are joined together with strapping. The cast is lined with four air chambers which are inflated with a hand pump to ensure a snug fit. Care must be taken that the cast does not impinge upon the margins of the foot. The Aircast has a rocker sole.

Flat-bed insoles are supplied with the Aircast although they can be replaced by bespoke moulded insoles.

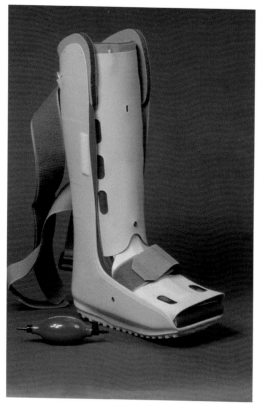

Fig. 4.8 Aircast, a prefabricated pneumatic walking brace, provides an immediate off-loading device.

Advantages of the Aircast include:
- Practitioners can view the wound and inspect the foot. This is important for practitioners who fear iatrogenic lesions or undetected infections
- It avoids the labour-intensive programme required for plaster casting
- It provides an immediate off-loading device
- It fits either foot and can be retained for future problems after one episode of ulceration is healed.

Disadvantages of the Aircast include:
- It will not accommodate severe deformity
- The cast is easily removable which renders it unsuitable for some patients who may use it only intermittently
- Aircasts should not be issued to very frail and unsteady patients who might fall and injure themselves.

Many other removable ready-made casts and walkers are available. These can be useful but often they do not accommodate deformity adequately. These devices can, if wished, be made non-removable by wrapping bands of fibreglass tape around the cast after it has been fitted, thus enforcing compliance. This technique produces a similar healing rate to that of the total-contact cast, whose efficacy may be largely due to the patient being unable to remove it.

Temporary ready-made shoes

When it is not possible to provide a cast, ready-made temporary shoes with cushioning insoles that can accommodate dressings, or weight-relief shoes are helpful.

Dressing shoes

The Darco shoe provides closed toe protection and accommodates bulky dressings. It can also be fitted with a Plastazote or bespoke moulded insole.

Weight-relief shoes

- Orthowedge: this shoe off-loads pressure from the metatarsal head and toes using a rocker-bottom wedge design
- Forefoot relief shoe: this transfers weight from forefoot to hindfoot with 10 degrees of dorsiflexion built into the shoe. A semi-rigid heel counter provides stability
- Heel relief shoe: this eliminates weightbearing on the posterior end of the foot, which is put into a plantar flex mode to facilitate off-loading of the heel area. Weight is transferred from heel to mid-foot and forefoot
- Half shoe: the front area of the sole is 'cut away' to relieve pressure on the forefoot for forefoot ulceration and the posterior area of the sole is 'cut away' to relieve hindfoot pressure if the ulcer is on the heel. They are available off-the-shelf but can be customized.

Felt padding and felted foam

Felt padding or felted foam may be used to divert pressure from ulcers but can prevent complications from being detected if the padding covers a large area.

Felt padding should be lifted regularly and should not be used as a substitute for good footwear and insoles (Fig. 4.9). The felt used is made of sheep's wool with a hypoallergenic adhesive backing, and is similar to the adhesive felt used within total-contact casts and Scotchcast boots.

Crutches

Young and active patients with neuropathic ulcers may do well with crutches as an adjunct to other pressure-relieving techniques. However, patients with impaired joint position sense or postural hypotension may be unsteady on crutches. Many patients with diabetes of long standing, especially the elderly, do very poorly with crutches and are prone to falls. It is important to check

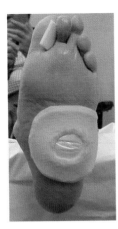

Fig. 4.9 Felt padding can be used temporarily to divert pressure but should not be regarded as a permanent solution.

for Romberg's sign, before dispensing crutches. When asked to stand with a narrow base of support and then to close their eyes, neuropathic patients may lose their sense of balance. If this is so, then the test is positive and the patient should not be given crutches. Patients with neuropathy of the hands or Dupuytren's contracture may find hand-held crutches difficult to manage. Untrained patients can risk falls especially on stairs, so crutches should always be fitted by a health-care professional. Care should be taken to avoid nerve compression injuries to the arms, to which diabetic patients may be particularly susceptible.

Patellar tendon weight-relieving orthosis
In some patients a total non-weightbearing patellar tibial brace allows patients a moderate degree of mobility while still allowing non-weightbearing status to the limb.

Pressure relief ankle–foot orthosis (PRAFO)
This is a custom-fitted ankle–foot orthosis suitable for the treatment of decubitus heel ulcers. It is discussed fully under the section on special ulcers.

Ankle–foot orthosis (AFO)
The AFO is a device used to stabilize the foot and ankle. There are two main forms of AFO, the traditional conventional metal and leather calliper and the newer thermoplastic types which are more cosmetic. This bespoke device is moulded to a plaster cast of the limb.

Walking stick
These must be the correct length and should have a non-slip cover on the end.

Wheelchair
A wheelchair which is used constantly is the best off-loading device of all. Self-drive models are better than chairs which can only be pushed. An extending platform can be attached to elevate the foot. A lightweight folding wheelchair can be of great help in achieving maximum off-loading while still enabling the patient to carry on with social activities. However, many patients become depressed at the idea of having a wheelchair and feel there is a stigma attached to their use.

Zimmer frame
These are exceedingly useful stability and off-loading aids: unfortunately they are associated with elderly and frail patients and some young patients will not use them. However, many patients who cannot cope with crutches find that a Zimmer frame is more helpful, being lightweight and providing more stability.

Electric carts and buggies
Small electrically powered carts and buggies with rechargeable batteries can be used by diabetic foot patients with great success (Fig. 4.10).

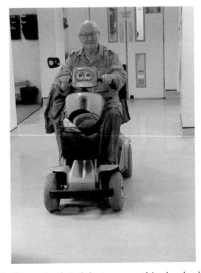

Fig. 4.10 This patient's indolent neuropathic ulcer healed very quickly after he acquired an electric cart.

Moulded insoles

These are mainly used to prevent recurrence of ulcers. They are designed to redistribute weightbearing away from vulnerable pressure areas and at the same time provide a suitable cushioning and total contact with the sole. These insoles may occupy too much space for them to be accommodated in anything but bespoke shoes, although an extra-depth stock shoe can sometimes accommodate the insole if the foot itself has a reasonably normal shape.

A plaster cast is taken of the foot to represent the overall contours including the sole. The cast is filled with a foam to make a last, over which the insoles are moulded and shoes constructed.

A variety of polyethylene foams, microcellular rubbers and ethyl vinyl acetate (EVA) foams are used to construct moulded insoles which are usually made of two or three layers of different densities, with the most compressible at the foot–insole interface.

Materials

Closed cell polyethylene foam, e.g. Plastazote:
- Easily mouldable
- Cushions
- Bottoms out.

Open cell polyurethane, microcellular rubber, e.g. Poron, or closed cell, rubber-like polymers, e.g. Neoprene:
- Not mouldable
- Excellent shock absorption
- Good long-term resilience and will not bottom out.

EVAs, e.g. Nora or Evalon range of different densities of EVAs:
- Mouldable
- Resilient
- Elastic.

Design

Various designs of moulded insoles are in use, including a design that forms a cradle by extending the insole up the sides of the foot.

Recently, EVA insoles have been used. These insoles have a top layer of low-density EVA for cushioning, followed by two to four layers of medium-density EVA and a base layer of high-density EVA, with the most dense and rigid layer acting as a cradle. Under particularly high-pressure areas, areas of the insole can be excavated out to form a 'sink' which is filled in with pressure-relieving material (Fig. 4.11).

Alternatively, the Tovey insole uses a high-density Plastazote material for the cradle. Pressure areas are marked on this and these areas are cut away to be filled in

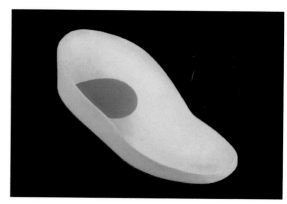

Fig. 4.11 Cradled insole with excavated sink filled with Neoprene over the mid-foot to accommodate plantar deformity.

with Neoprene cushioning. The whole cradle is covered with an upper layer of Neoprene cushioning.

Composite moulded insoles can also be made, with an upper layer of low-density Plastazote and a lower layer of polyurethane rubber.

Moulded insoles may also incorporate other modifications such as metatarsal pads or metatarsal bars which are placed behind the metatarsal heads to relieve focal pressure and to transfer load more proximally.

Bespoke shoe and boots

This footwear is custom-made for the patient (Fig. 4.12) and involves the production of a last which is specific to that individual's foot. Bespoke shoes can house cradled insoles.

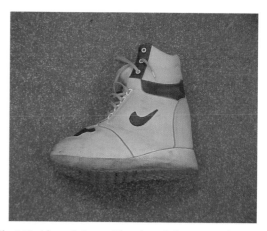

Fig. 4.12 A bespoke boot with rocker sole incorporated to off-load a hallux rigidus with previous ulceration in a young patient who wanted to wear trainers.

The shoes may be adapted to redistribute pressures further. Examples of this are the rigid rocker sole in which the shoe rocks forward to allow walking without extension of the metatarsal-phalangeal joints and to reduce plantar pressures in this area.

When these shoes are first issued they will need to be worn for short periods only. Their main role is prevention of recurrence.

CASE STUDY
Footwear-related blisters

A 72-year-old woman with type 2 diabetes of 10 years' duration, with a rocker-bottom Charcot foot treated in a total-contact cast, was issued with a new pair of special shoes. She was instructed to wear them for only 5 minutes a day at first, but went shopping and wore them for 2 hours. She developed blisters on the side of her foot with a halo of erythema (Fig. 4.13a). The blisters were opened and drained in the diabetic foot clinic. Sterile dressings were applied and lifted every day to check for deterioration. The blisters were dry and healing well within 2 weeks (Fig. 4.13b) and fully healed within 2 months.

(a)
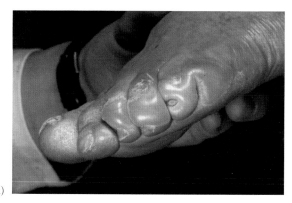

(b)
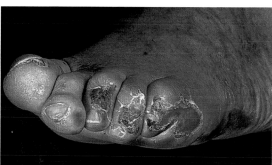

Fig. 4.13 (a) Bullae over lesser toes caused by footwear. (b) The bullae are dry and healing well after 2 weeks.

Key points
- Patients should receive very careful education about the timescale for rehabilitation
- New shoes should only be worn for periods of a few minutes per day, building up gradually to full-time use.

Neuroischaemic foot
Ulcers in neuroischaemic feet usually develop around the margins of the foot. Revascularization is the definitive treatment, although it is still important to off-load the ulcer. A high-street shoe that is sufficiently long, broad and deep, and fastens with a lace or strap high on the foot, may be all that is needed to protect the vulnerable margins of the foot and allow healing (Fig. 4.14). Neuroischaemic ulcers may be prevented from healing because the patient wears tight shoes or slip-on styles.

It may be necessary to provide special footwear. In the first instance, a temporary shoe such as a Darco may be used if dressings are bulky. Alternatively, a ready-made stock shoe which is wide fitting may be suitable. The Scotchcast boot may also be used, when ulcers are large, for postsurgical feet or for feet which fail to respond to treatment in footwear. Crutches and Zimmer frames may be useful for the neuroischaemic patient as described above for the neuropathic patient.

Wound control

Wound control of the neuropathic and neuroischaemic ulcer is based upon:
- Sharp debridement of the ulcer
- Dressings
- Advanced wound healing products
- Supplementary wound healing techniques
- Topical therapy.

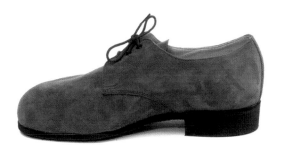

Fig. 4.14 A high-street shoe suitable for an undeformed neuroischaemic foot.

Sharp debridement of the ulcer

We prefer sharp debridement as the ideal method. We do not favour autolytic, enzymatic, whirlpool or chemical debriding techniques for the diabetic foot.

Debridement of the neuropathic ulcer

Debridement is the most important part of wound control. It is not possible to assess a neuropathic ulcer properly without debriding away all associated callus. Sometimes the presence of the ulcer will only be determined following removal of callus which exposes a hitherto unsuspected lesion (Fig. 4.15a–c).

If an ulcer is suspected the patient should always be warned before the overlying callus is removed because he may otherwise feel that it was the callus removal that caused the ulcer.

Rationale

- Removes callus, thus lowering plantar pressures
- Enables the true dimensions of the ulcer to be seen
- Stimulates ulcer healing
- Removes any physical barrier to growth of new epithelium across the ulcer from the margin
- Prevents callus from sealing off an ulcer, which would prevent drainage and promote infection
- Enables drainage of exudate and removal of dead tissue (this renders infection less likely by reducing bacterial load and removing material which is a suitable growth medium for bacteria)
- Enables a deep swab or deep tissue to be taken for microscopy and culture
- Encourages healing by converting a chronic ulcer into an acute ulcer.

The debridement procedure

- Ensure that patient has not developed ischaemia by checking the pedal pulses. Only continue if they are present: otherwise follow procedure for neuroischaemic patients below
- Remove all callus surrounding the ulcer with a sterile scalpel (Fig. 4.15d,e)
- When debriding the ulcer bed, work from the middle outwards: this carries debris and bacteria away from the ulcer bed
- Cut away all slough and non-viable tissue. It is helpful to grip the material that is to be cut away with a pair of forceps and to apply gentle traction so that the material to be cut is under tension. If the slough is slimy and difficult to grasp with the forceps, dry gauze can be applied to it. This will remove moisture so that it can then be grasped more easily with the forceps to apply

traction. It is difficult to remove macerated callus or slough evenly and precisely, unless tension is applied
- The forceps are additionally useful as one arm can be used as a probe to explore the dimensions of the ulcer
- Probe ulcer. If the probe reaches bone this is suggestive of osteomyelitis and the foot should be regarded as a stage 4 foot
- Clean ulcer with sterile normal saline
- Take deep swab/tissue samples (see Chapter 5 for details) and send for culture without delay
- Apply sterile dressing held in place with light bandage, which should not be wrapped too tightly or encircle the toe
- Review at regular intervals (ideally weekly) and repeat the procedure
- Always ensure the patient is reminded that if problems develop he should return to the clinic immediately.

Control of bleeding

Neuropathic feet can bleed with considerable exuberance. Have gauze swabs and calcium alginate to hand. Most bleeding will stop with pressure. Apply pressure over a swab damped with saline, as when the swab is removed it will be less likely to dislodge the clot if it is damp. When debriding around an ulcer apply digital pressure locally to a bleeding point while still continuing to debride with the other hand, or apply a damp swab under pressure from bandage or tape to free both hands for further debridement.

When patients go home after bleeding is stopped, they can be given extra gauze and plaster to apply on top of the clinic dressing if bleeding strikes through.

If patients are prone to bleeding after debridement they should rest and elevate the foot at home for the next 24 hours.

Before debriding the neuropathic foot, ask the patient whether he is on warfarin or heparin or haemodialysis or has any bleeding disorder, in which case debridement should be cautious.

CASE STUDY
Bleeding after debridement

An 89-year-old man with type 2 diabetes of 29 years' duration was taking warfarin. He had dry necrosis of the apex of his right hallux and regularly underwent gentle debridement in the diabetic foot clinic. On one occasion, on the day following debridement, his family noticed that blood was seeping through the dressings on his hallux. Despite rest and elevation the foot continued to bleed and the patient attended Casualty. The bleeding was stopped by applying a calcium alginate dressing with digital pressure and elevation of the limb.

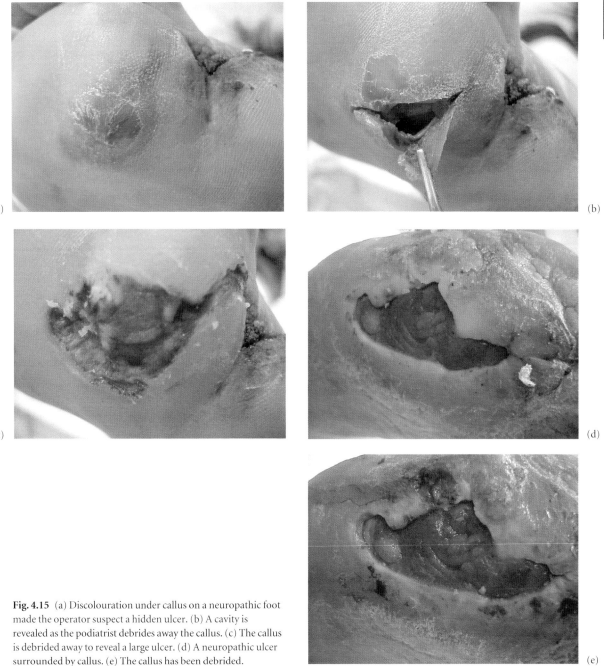

Fig. 4.15 (a) Discolouration under callus on a neuropathic foot made the operator suspect a hidden ulcer. (b) A cavity is revealed as the podiatrist debrides away the callus. (c) The callus is debrided away to reveal a large ulcer. (d) A neuropathic ulcer surrounded by callus. (e) The callus has been debrided.

Key points
- Some feet bleed with alarming rapidity when debrided
- Application of topical calcium alginate dressing assists clotting
- In severe bleeding the limb should be elevated and a pressure pack bandaged on
- No patient should be sent home until bleeding is under control
- Patients should be warned that if the foot starts to bleed again when they arrive home after a debridement, they should not remove the clinic dressings but should elevate the foot, bandage additional dressing material over

existing dressings, and seek medical help if the bleeding does not stop.

One of our patients developed severe bleeding at home after walking barefooted to the bathroom at night unprotected except for his ulcer dressing, and needed hospital treatment. Some neuropathic patients develop calcification of veins and arteries in the lower limb, and the pressures of walking unprotected had fractured a small calcified vein in his foot.

Renal patients on dialysis may be prone to bleeding if debrided during or soon after dialysis because of anticoagulants administered as part of the dialysis process. Extra care should be taken if debridement is performed on these patients.

Debridement of the neuroischaemic ulcer
Rationale
- Enables the true dimensions of the ulcer to be seen (Fig. 4.16a,b)
- Drainage of exudate and removal of dead tissue renders infection less likely
- Enables a deep swab to be taken for culture
- Removal of the surrounding halo of glassy callus (if present) prevents it from catching on the dressing and causing tissue trauma.

The debridement procedure
- Vascular status should be quantified by measuring the pressure index before debridement because only very cautious debridement should be performed if the pressure index is below 0.5
- Some neuroischaemic ulcers develop a halo of thin glassy callus which dries out, becomes hard and curls up. Exudate may also form hard crusts. It is necessary to smooth off these rough areas with the scalpel as they can both catch on dressings and cause trauma to underlying tissues (Fig. 4.16c–e)
- If a subungual ulcer beneath a thickened toe nail is suspected (revealed by pain, discolouration or maceration of the nail plate or exudate escaping from the periungual tissues), the nail should be very gently cut back, or layers of nail can be pared away with a scalpel to expose or drain the ulcer
- If the foot is very sensitive it may be necessary to anchor the area of tissue being debrided with forceps so that tissue can be cut away without pulling on the wound bed. This also avoids painful dragging of the scalpel blade through slack tissues. It is very important to reassure the patient that the operator will stop if debridement is painful
- It is very unwise to inject local anaesthetic into an ischaemic foot

- If a neuroischaemic ulcer bed is proud of the surrounding tissues and surrounded by thin, tightly bound down glassy callus which you want to remove, you are less likely to cut the patient if you work outwards from the centre of the ulcer towards its margin.

Recently, a high powered water jet hydrosurgery system which combines lavage with debridement by the water jet, the Versajet has been described.

Dressings
Diabetic foot ulcers are chronic wounds and we believe that they should be kept dry. The value of moist wound healing has only been demonstrated on acute wounds. Sterile, non-adherent dressings should cover all open diabetic foot lesions at all times except when they are inspected and debrided.

The rationale for keeping ulcers covered is to:
- Protect the wound from noxious stimuli
- Prevent infestation with insects
- Keep the wound warm
- Protect the wound from mechanical traumas
- Reduce the likelihood of infection.

There is no robust evidence from sufficiently large controlled studies that any one dressing is better for the diabetic foot than any other. However, the following properties are useful:
- Easy to lift
- Able to accommodate pressures of walking without disintegrating
- Absorbent.

Dressings should be lifted every day for wound inspection if possible, because when patients lack protective pain sensation the only signs of infection may be visual. For this reason, dressings which need to be left on a wound for several days to achieve their best effect may be inappropriate for diabetic feet.

In our diabetic foot clinic we frequently see the dire results of failure to detect wound deterioration early because the signs were masked by a dressing in a patient who lacked protective pain sensation. Where it is not possible to inspect the wound, any exposed adjoining areas of the foot and leg should be checked for:
- Colour change
- Swelling
- Change in temperature.

These can be signs either of uncontrolled infection or of worsening ischaemia which need urgent action.

Fever or hyperglycaemia should also be looked for.

Types of dressings used in diabetic foot patients and their relevant features
Films
- Clear, so wound inspection can be achieved without disturbing the wound

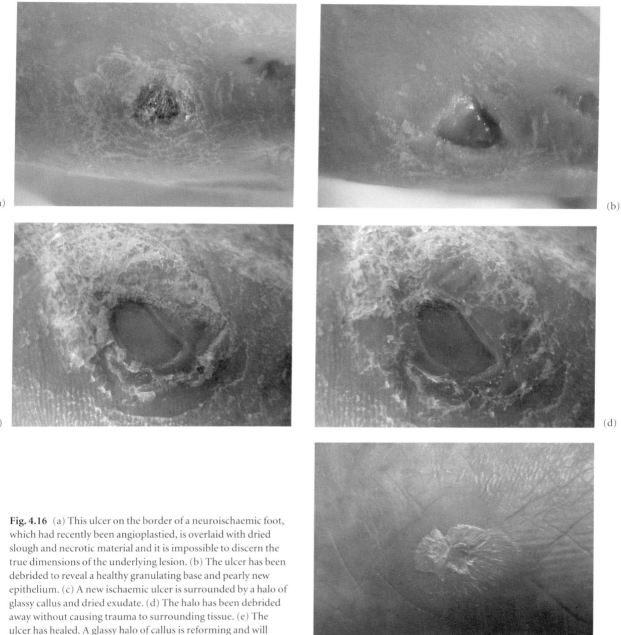

Fig. 4.16 (a) This ulcer on the border of a neuroischaemic foot, which had recently been angioplastied, is overlaid with dried slough and necrotic material and it is impossible to discern the true dimensions of the underlying lesion. (b) The ulcer has been debrided to reveal a healthy granulating base and pearly new epithelium. (c) A new ischaemic ulcer is surrounded by a halo of glassy callus and dried exudate. (d) The halo has been debrided away without causing trauma to surrounding tissue. (e) The ulcer has healed. A glassy halo of callus is reforming and will need to be removed.

- Cannot absorb exudate which will collect under the film and form a blister and may irritate underlying tissue. Therefore contraindicated in exuding wounds
- Should never be used on infected or necrotic wounds. When used on dry necrosis will cause maceration and possibly promote infection

- Rarely appropriate for diabetic feet.

Foams
- Very absorbent
- Cushioning effect
- Bulky—may need specially roomy shoe to accommodate

- Widely used for diabetic feet
- May be preformed, for application to particularly tricky areas, such as the heel cup.

Hydrocolloids
- Can be used only in patients with protective pain sensation
- Patient can bathe and shower
- Designed to be left on for several days. Daily changing prevents dressing from acting optimally.

Alginates
- Only to be used on moist exuding wounds
- Daily removal is time consuming
- Drying out of dressing may prevent wound drainage
- Calcium alginate is a good haemostatic agent
- Do not use on infected or necrotic wounds.

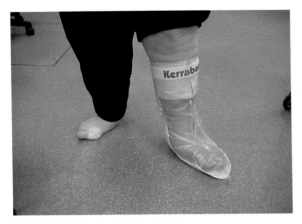

Fig. 4.17 Kerraboot.

Hydrogels
- Promote autolysis and therefore promote debridement by apparently rehydrating the wound
- As we do not favour moist wound healing in the diabetic foot we see no strong indication for hydrogel therapy.

Hydro fibre dressings
- Non-woven pad or ribbon made of hydrocolloid (carboxymethycellulose) fibres absorbs wound fluid and forms a gel
- Used on light-moderately exuding wounds.

Other dressings
Simple non-adherent dressings may be useful. Saline-soaked gauze is widely used throughout the world.

Kerraboot is a transparent boot which allows easy inspection of the lower limb and the free drainage of exudate from a wound (Fig. 4.17).

Fastening dressings
Hypoallergenic tape and tubular bandages are useful. Conventional bandaging may cause excessive tightness. Only small amounts of tape should be applied to the skin. Encircling the entire toe with tape should be avoided in case the toe swells. It is important to issue precise requests to patients and nurses about techniques for holding dressings in place.

Advanced wound healing products
There may be intrinsic defects in ulcer healing in the diabetic patient. There is impairment of fibroblast function, deficiency in growth factors and abnormalities of the extracellular matrix. Initially it is important to try to achieve healing by standard techniques such as casting and debridement and in the case of ischaemic ulcers by revascularization. However, an ulcer that does not heal is a risk for infection in the diabetic patient and advanced wound healing products should be considered.

Skin substitutes
Skin substitutes can be divided into cell-containing matrices and cell-free matrices.

Cell-containing matrices
Cell-containing matrices include living cells such as keratinocytes or fibroblasts within a matrix.

Dermagraft.
- Dermagraft is bioengineered living human dermis manufactured by seeding dermal fibroblasts onto a three-dimensional bioabsorbable scaffold
- A randomized, controlled multicentre study demonstrated that 50.8% of the Dermagraft group experienced complete wound closure which was significantly greater than in the controls, of whom 31.7% had complete closure. In a further 12-week randomized study, incidence of complete wound closure of neuropathic foot ulcers was 30% in the active group and 18% in the control group
- It must be stored at −80°C. Prior to application it is thawed, warmed and rinsed with sterile saline.

Apligraf.
- Apligraf is a bioengineered bilayered skin substitute consisting of human fibroblasts embedded in type 1 bovine collagen and covered by human keratinocytes
- A randomized, controlled study demonstrated a healing rate of 56% for those who were treated by application of Apligraf and standard wound care; this was significantly greater than 39% healing rate for patients who received only standard wound care
- It is delivered in a ready-to-use form on nutrient agarose in a sealed plastic bag in a disposable, battery-powered incubator.

Bilayered cellular matrix.
- Porous collagen sponge containing co-cultured allogeneic keratinocytes and fibroblasts harvested from human neonatal foreskin
- It has shown promising use in initial studies with diabetic neuropathic ulcers.

Cell-free matrices
Cell-free matrices interact with the wound bed, releasing growth factors that stimulate wound healing and angiogenesis. Several cell-free matrices have been evaluated in the treatment of diabetic foot ulcer. These include GraftJacket, Oasis and Integra.

GraftJacket. GraftJacket is an allogeneic acellular matrix, made from donated skin. It initially undergoes a process that removes the epidermis and dermis cells and thus does not trigger an immune response. It serves as a repair matrix that is rapidly converted to the patient's own tissue by quickly renewing blood, cellular and nutrient activity throughout the matrix. Initial experience has been gathered with the use of this allogeneic acellular matrix therapy in the treatment of diabetic wounds. Seventeen patients received surgical debridement and were placed on therapy consisting of a single application of an acellular matrix graft with dressing changes taking place weekly. This led to healing of 82.4% of wounds measuring a mean 4.6 ± 3.2 cm^2 in the 20-week evaluation period.

Oasis Wound Matrix. Oasis Wound Matrix is derived from the pig small intestine submucosa. It consists of a natural collagenous, three-dimensional extracellular matrix which acts as a framework for cytokines and cell adhesion molecules for tissue growth. In contrast to allografts and other bioengineered regeneration materials, Oasis does not contain any cells that trigger rejection. A recent study has compared the healing rates at 12 weeks

for full-thickness diabetic foot ulcers treated with Oasis Wound Matrix versus Regranex Gel. This study reported that complete wound closure after 12 weeks of treatment was observed in 49% of the Oasis-treated patients (n = 18), compared with 28% of the Regranex-treated group (n = 10), p = 0.055.

Integra. Integra consists of a bilayer, biodegradable matrix that provides a scaffold for dermal regeneration and organization and provides protection for the treated wound. The dermal replacement layer is made of a porous matrix of fibres of cross-linked bovine tendon collagen and a glycosaminoglycan (chondroitin-6-sulphate) that is manufactured with a controlled porosity and degradation rate. The temporary epidermal substitute layer is made of synthetic polysiloxane polymer (silicone) and acts to control moisture loss from the wound. As healing progresses an endogenous collagen matrix is deposited by fibroblasts. When the dermal layer is adequately revascularized, the temporary silicone layer is removed and a thin, meshed layer of the person's own skin (epidermal autograft) is placed over the 'neodermis'. Integra Dermal Regeneration Template was approved in 1996 to treat full-thickness and some partial-thickness burns and has been used to treat complex diabetic wounds.

Growth factors
Regranex
- This is platelet-derived growth factor which stimulates chemotaxis and mitogenesis of neutrophils, fibroblasts and monocytes
- A pivotal study in 382 patients demonstrated that Regranex gel 100 µg/g healed 50% of chronic diabetic ulcers which was significantly greater than 35% healed with placebo gel
- It presents as a tube of gel which is stored in a domestic refrigerator and applied every day.

Recombinant human epidermal growth factor
- This has had a positive effect on healing in three randomized, controlled trials.

Platelets and platelet-derived products
Several studies of these products have shown a reduction in ulcer area when compared with placebo.

Protease inhibitors
Promogran
- Promogran consists of oxidized regenerated cellulose and collagen

- It inhibits proteases in the wound and protects endogenous growth factors
- In a 12-week study of 184 patients, 37% of Pomogran-treated patients healed compared with 28% of saline gauze-treated patients but this did not reach a significant difference.

Extracellular matrix proteins
Hyaff
- Hyaff is a fibrous ester of hyaluronic acid which is a polysaccharide that is integral to the extracellular matrix and controls extracellular matrix hydration and osmoregulation
- When Hyaff is applied to the wound, hyaluronic acid is released
- Pilot studies in diabetic patients have shown promising results in the treatment of neuropathic foot ulcers, especially with sinuses. Hyaff-based autologous grafts have also been used to treat plantar ulcers and post-operative wounds on the dorsum of the foot. There was no difference in the rate of healing in patients with plantar ulcers compared with controls but in the dorsal ulcers the Hyaff-based graft showed an increased rate of ulcer healing at 67% vs. 31% (p = 0.049) .

Collagen
The lyophilized form of extracted Type I collagen increases granulation of damaged tissue and stimulates local haemostasis. This can accelerate wound healing by encouraging platelet adhesion and aggregation. One study has indicated that it accelerates wound healing as a therapy for diabetic foot ulcers.

The place of advanced wound healing products in the management of diabetic foot ulcers is not fully worked out. The clinical evidence is limited and many of the products listed below are so expensive that the cost will be prohibitive for many practitioners. Most clinics concentrate on the basics of debridement, off-loading and revacularization.

Supplementary wound healing techniques
Several supplementary wound healing techniques have been used in diabetic foot ulcers including the following.

Skin grafts
- To speed healing of large, clean ulcers with a granulating wound bed, a split-skin graft may be harvested from the patient and applied to the ulcer
- If the donor site is chosen from an area within the distribution of the neuropathy, local anaesthetic infiltration

of the donor site with a spinal needle will provide sufficient analgesia
- A general anaesthetic can thus be avoided and a donor site from within the distribution of the neuropathy will be less painful
- Careful follow-up of plantar skin grafts will be needed as they often develop callus and if this is allowed to accumulate it will result in neuropathic ulceration.

CASE STUDY
Skin graft

A 54-year-old woman with type 2 diabetes of 7 years' duration developed a plantar corn over her 1st metatarsal head, and applied a proprietary corn cure containing salicylic acid, purchased over the counter from her local pharmacy. She presented at Casualty 1 week later with an infected acid burn causing a large tissue defect. She was given intravenous antibiotics and underwent surgical debridement. Two weeks later when the wound had a good bed of granulations and was ready to be closed, the surgeon infiltrated an area on the calf of her leg with local anaesthetic using a long spinal needle, and harvested a split-thickness skin graft. This was applied to the wound and healed in 1 month (Fig. 4.18). The patient had no postoperative pain from the donor site which was within

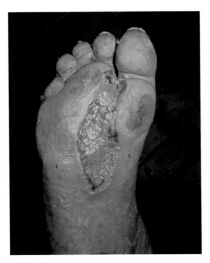

Fig. 4.18 Healed plantar skin graft with callus formation which needed regular debridement.

the distribution of her neuropathy. She had regular debridement of callus and special shoes to prevent the graft from breaking down. A recent study has shown similar healing rates of split-skin grafts compared with meshed skin grafts.

Key points
- Corn cures can cause severe ulceration
- When repairing plantar defects, split-thickness grafts harvested from within the area affected by neuropathy reduce postoperative donor site pain
- Plantar skin grafts on weightbearing areas are prone to develop callus and patients should see a podiatrist.

Vacuum-assisted closure (VAC)
This is topical negative pressure therapy and can be used to achieve closure of diabetic foot wounds.

The pump applies subatmospheric pressure, through a tube and foam sponge applied to the wound over a dressing and sealed in place with a plastic film. The dressing is replaced every 2–3 days (Fig. 4.19a–f).
- Negative pressure improves the dermal blood supply, and stimulates granulation which can form over bone and tendon. It reduces bacterial colonization and diminishes oedema and interstitial fluid
- The technique is useful in healing large postoperative wounds in the diabetic foot, particularly in ischaemic feet and also in patients with renal impairment.

In a recent study 162 patients with postoperative wounds, following partial foot amputation, were enrolled in a 16-week, 18-centre, randomized clinical trial in the USA. More patients were healed in the VAC pump group than in the control group (56% vs. 39%; p = 0.040). The rate of wound healing, based on the time to complete closure, was faster in the VAC pump group than in controls (p = 0.005). A recent consensus statement on negative pressure wound therapy (VAC therapy) for the management of diabetic foot wounds has been published and summarizes current clinical evidence.

Larva therapy (maggots)
- The larvae of the green bottle fly *Lucilia sericata* are used to debride ulcers, especially in the neuroischaemic foot
- This results in relatively rapid atraumatic physical removal of necrotic material
- Larvae also produce secretions that have antimicrobial activity against Gram-positive cocci including methicillin-resistant *Staphylococcus aureus* (MRSA), and a recent study showed success in eliminating MRSA from diabetic foot ulcers.

CASE STUDY
Maggot therapy

A 75-year-old man with type 2 diabetes of 10 years' duration with neuropathy and peripheral vascular disease underwent distal bypass followed by amputation of four toes which had become necrotic following late presentation with an infected foot. After surgery he had palpable foot pulses and a pressure index of 0.72, but the foot wound became very sloughy and he complained of severe pain when the podiatrist attempted to debride it. Maggots were obtained from a medical maggot farm and placed within the wound. Fig. 4.20a shows the wound 2 days after the maggots had been applied: the maggots were wriggling very vigorously. Fig. 4.20b shows some feeding maggots with their heads down and their blunt ends exposed: in this position they look like cells in honeycomb. In Fig. 4.20c a jet of saline squeezed from a litre bag is being used to swill the maggots out of the wound. In Fig. 4.20d, post maggot therapy, the wound is clean and the sloughy tissue has been painlessly removed. The foot went on to heal in 9 weeks.

Key points
- Maggot therapy is useful in debriding the painful neuro-ischaemic foot ulcer
- Maggots destroy necrotic tissue and bacteria but leave viable tissue
- Maggot therapy is usually painless.

Hyperbaric oxygen
- Studies involving relatively small groups of patients have shown that adjunctive hyperbaric oxygen accelerates the healing of ischaemic diabetic foot ulcers. A recent Cochrane review concluded that hyperbaric oxygen significantly reduced the risk of major amputation and may improve the chance of healing of foot ulcers at 1 year. However, this should be regarded cautiously because of the modest number of patients and methodological shortcomings in previous studies
- It is reasonable to use hyperbaric oxygen as an adjunctive treatment in severe or life-threatening wounds which have not responded to other treatments.

Topical therapy
This consists of cleansing agents and antimicrobials.

Cleansing agents
- Saline: we use saline as a wound cleansing agent. It does not interfere with microbiological samples and is not damaging to granulating tissue

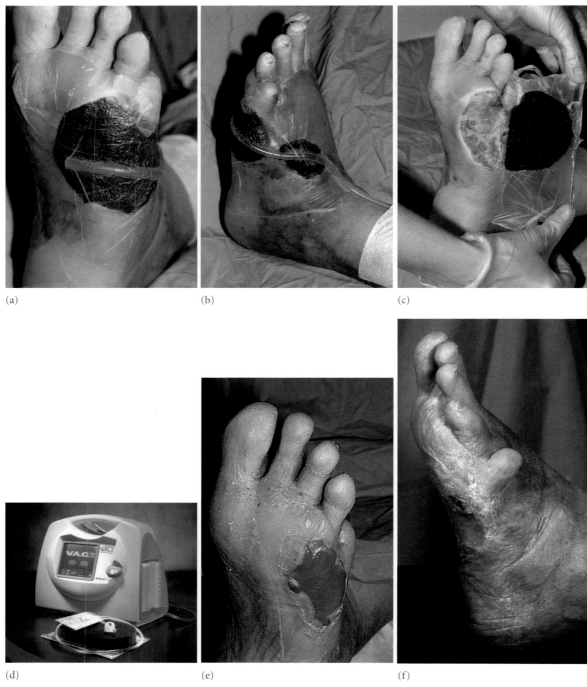

(a)

(b)

(c)

(d)

(e)

(f)

Fig. 4.19 (a) VAC pump sponge attached to plantar aspect of foot. (b) VAC pump sponge also attached to dorsolateral aspect of foot. (c) Pump sponge being removed from foot. (d) The VAC pump and drainage tube, canister and sponges. (e) Ulcer healing after 10 days of VAC therapy. (f) Ulcer healed after 8 weeks.

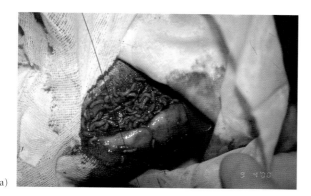
(a)

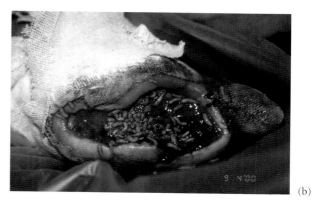
(b)

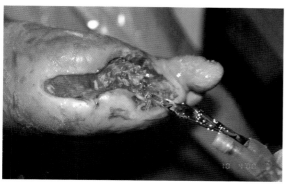
(c)

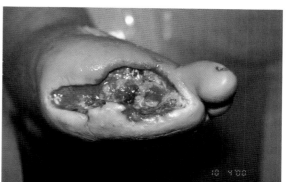
(d)

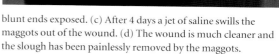

Fig. 4.20 (a) Two days after application the maggots are wriggling very vigorously and have not settled down to feed. (b) Some feeding maggots are seen with their heads down and their blunt ends exposed. (c) After 4 days a jet of saline swills the maggots out of the wound. (d) The wound is much cleaner and the slough has been painlessly removed by the maggots.

- Cetrimide-based cleansing agents are not recommended because of their cytotoxic action which impedes wound healing.

Antimicrobials

- Iodine is effective against a wide spectrum of organisms and comes in a variety of formulations including solutions, alcoholic tinctures, powder sprays and impregnated dressings. At high concentrations it can be toxic to human cells but bacteria are more sensitive to these effects than human cells such as fibroblasts, and thus it is believed that iodine may be useful for antisepsis without impairing wound healing. At present two types of iodine are available, povidone-iodine and cadexomer-iodine. Povidone-iodine is effective in antibacterial prophylaxis in burn patients but the evidence of its efficacy in other wound types is awaited. Cadexomer-iodine consists of microspheres formed from a three-dimensional lattice of cross-linked starch chains (cadexomers) and has been used with success in the diabetic foot ulcer

- Hypochlorite is most useful in sloughy wounds which are infected and therefore is more appropriate for ulcers in stage 4

- Silver compounds: ionic silver has broad-spectrum antimicrobial action against Gram-negative and Gram-positive organisms. *In vitro*, it is effective in killing *Staphylococcus aureus*, including MRSA, and *Pseudomonas* species. Silver has been impregnated into dressings and may be useful in diabetic foot ulcers. In a recent study of sustained silver-releasing dressings in the treatment of diabetic foot ulcers, there was good exudate management and good wound progress of clinically un-infected diabetic foot ulcers with only two infections occurring in 27 ulcers. Although a recent Cochrane review of silver-based wound dressings and topical agents for treating diabetic foot ulcers found no suitable randomized trials or controlled clinical trials to evaluate their clinical effectiveness, a recent prospective, randomized controlled study of non-ischaemic diabetic foot ulcers compared Hydrofiber dressings containing ionic silver with calcium alginate dressings. Subjects who received silver experienced more overall ulcer improvement (p = 0.06), which was most marked on patients taking antibiotic (p = 0.02). Ulcers treated with silver reduced in depth nearly twice as much as did alginate-treated ulcers (2.5 mm vs. 1.3 mm; p = 0.04). Thus silver compounds may have a role in treating the early stages of, or preventing infection in, the diabetic foot ulcer.

- Mupirocin is active against Gram-positive infections including MRSA. To avoid the development of resistance, mupirocin should not be used for longer than 10 days and should not be regarded as a prophylactic
- We have recently returned to the use of potassium permanganate solution, in which the patients immerse their feet. It is an oxidizing agent liberating nascent oxygen and thereby acts as a moderately potent antiseptic, effective against bacteria and fungi.
- Recently honey has been used as a topical antibacterial agent. There is a risk of introducing microorganisms into the wound with honey but this can be avoided by sterilization to produce medical grade Manuka honey.

Microbiological control

Now that the skin is broken, the stage 3 patient is at great risk of infection because there is now a clear portal of entry for invading bacteria to enter the foot. Additionally, in the presence of neuropathy and ischaemia, the inflammatory response is impaired. The patient lacks protective pain sensation which would otherwise automatically force him to detect the problem and rest the foot.

Bacterial growth in ulcers impedes the wound healing rate. Quantitative microbiology has shown that with increased bacterial load, wound healing slows. There is a complex host–bacteria relationship. Many wounds are colonized with a stable bacterial population. If the bacterial burden increases there will be bacterial imbalance which may show itself as increased exudate before frank infection develops. The crucial problem is when to intervene with antibiotics.

Uniform agreed practice on the role of antibiotics in the clinically uninfected stage 3 diabetic foot, where no signs or symptoms of infection are present, has not been established. Over many years of experience managing the diabetic foot, we have established the following plan for neuropathic and neuroischaemic ulcers, which has achieved significant reductions in amputations.

Our approach is also based on the results of a study of 64 diabetic patients with clean foot ulcers who were randomized into two groups: 32 patients receiving oral antibiotics and 32 patients who did not. In the non-antibiotic group 15 patients developed clinical infection compared with none in the antibiotic group, which was a highly significant difference. In the 32 patients who did not receive antibiotics there were 12 with neuroischaemic ulcers and 20 with neuropathic ulcers: 8/12 neuroischaemic ulcers developed infection which was significantly greater than 7/20 neuropathic ulcers. This indicated that neuroischaemic ulcers were more likely to develop clinical infection. Furthermore, 11 of the 15 patients who developed clinical infection had positive ulcer swabs taken at their last clinic visit compared with only one positive swab taken at the prior visit in the 17 patients who did not develop clinical infection. This indicated that properly taken ulcer swabs can be a useful indicator of impending infection.

From this study we concluded that patients with diabetes and clean ulcers associated with peripheral vascular disease and positive ulcer swabs should be considered for early antibiotic treatment. We therefore pay close attention to the results of properly taken ulcer swabs, taken at the first clinic visit and at subsequent visits. Some authors question the value of performing swab cultures in the absence of signs or symptoms of infection, or of ever prescribing antibiotics based on positive wound cultures alone in the absence of signs or symptoms of infection. In non-diabetic patients this approach is probably reasonable.

However, we feel that in dealing with high-risk diabetic feet, failure to take swabs deprives the clinician of advance warning that infection may be imminent. Infection is alarmingly common in high-risk diabetic feet, and signs and symptoms of infection are frequently absent or greatly reduced. We believe that properly taken swabs are useful.

All swabs taken from diabetic foot ulcers should be deep swabs taken after debridement has been carried out. We accept that curettings and tissue from the base of the ulcer may be a more acceptable microbiological sample compared with the deep ulcer swab and we do send such samples instead of an ulcer swab where possible. However, in many cases, particularly in the neuroischaemic foot, it is not possible to safely and painlessly obtain such samples and the deep wound swab is then the only alternative.

Neuropathic ulcers
Our microbiological approach to neuropathic ulcers is as follows.

At the first visit, if there is no cellulitis, discharge or probing to bone, the foot is deemed to be at stage 3. Debridement, cleansing with saline, application of dressings and daily inspection will suffice. The patient is reviewed at, preferably, 1 week or less, together with the result of the deep ulcer swab or tissue culture. If the neuropathic ulcer shows no sign of infection and the swab is negative, treatment is continued without antibiotics. If the ulcer has a positive swab, the patient is treated with the appropriate antibiotic, according to antibiotic sensitivities until the repeat swab, taken at weekly intervals, is negative. It is accepted that some organisms isolated from the swab may be commensals; however, if there are Gram-positive organisms or anaerobes or a pure growth of Gram-negative organisms we regard this as a significant result and microbiological evidence of infection. It was shown in a study of the bacterial population of chronic crural ulcers that a swab should be obtained routinely from patients with diabetic ulcers as 70% of diabetic ulcers with a positive swab developed clinical infection. Recently the persistence of microorganisms in an ulcer has been shown to reduce the rate of healing.

Neuroischaemic ulcers

We prescribe antibiotics more readily for the neuroischaemic foot because untreated infections in neuroischaemic feet lead rapidly to extensive necrosis, destruction of the foot and major amputation.

- At the first visit, if the ulcer is superficial, we prescribe oral amoxicillin 500 mg tds and flucloxacillin 500 mg qds. (If the patient is penicillin allergic, we prescribe clarithromycin 500 mg bd.) If the ulcer is deep, extending to subcutaneous tissues, we add ciprofloxacin 500 mg bd or trimethoprim 200 mg bd, and metronidazole 400 mg tds to cover Gram-negative and anaerobic organisms that may be present in the deep tissues. If, on review, the neuroischaemic ulcer shows no signs of infection and the swab is negative, antibiotics may be stopped. However, in cases of severe ischaemia (pressure index < 0.5) we may continue antibiotics until the ulcer is healed. If the neuroischaemic ulcer has a positive swab, the patient is treated with the appropriate antibiotic, according to antibiotic sensitivities until the repeat swab, taken at weekly intervals, is negative
- At every patient visit, examination for local signs of infection, cellulitis or osteomyelitis is performed. If these are found, action, including antibiotic therapy, is taken as described in Chapter 5.

Vascular control

In the neuroischaemic foot the reduction of perfusion contributes to the predisposition to ulceration and also the delay in healing. Therefore, it is necessary to be very active in assessing the circulation in such patients and proceeding with revascularization, preferably with angioplasty, if the ulcer does not immediately respond to conservative measures described above. Atherosclerotic lesions commonly occur in the tibial arteries but also occur in the popliteal and femoral arteries, with the iliacs rarely involved. A careful non-invasive vascular assessment is necessary, to determine the degree of ischaemia and to decide when to proceed with invasive investigations with a view to revascularization.

The modern management of the ischaemic foot is underpinned by principles that we have stressed throughout this book—to encourage early presentation leading to rapid diagnosis and intervention. In practical terms, to make this feasible, a fast-track service to receive patients with ischaemic ulcers and quickly assess them with modern non-invasive investigations should now be a feature of modern diabetic foot care. This is best carried out in a diabetic foot clinic which can see the neuroischaemic patient without delay. Initially the ankle brachial pressure index should be measured, supplemented by assessment of the Doppler waveform. Further tests such as measurement of transcutaneous oxygen tension and toe pressure may be helpful in deciding whether to pursue a duplex arteriography with a view to vascular intervention. Such decisions are made when the patient is seen in a joint diabetic/vascular surgical clinic within the diabetic foot clinic.

Pressure index

The pressure index is widely criticized because, when the arteries are calcified, it may be artificially raised. However, we feel that it is very relevant to the investigation of the diabetic foot as long as the potential difficulties of its interpretation are understood.

If the pressure index is 0.5 then it is truly low, and indicates severe ischaemia whether the arteries are calcified or not. Indeed, if the artery is calcified the true pressure index may be even lower and even more urgent action is required.

Difficulty comes at pressure indices of 0.5 and above, when one should always pay attention to the Doppler waveform, either in audible or visible form. The normal waveform is pulsatile with a positive forward flow in systole followed by a short reverse flow and a further forward

STAGE 3

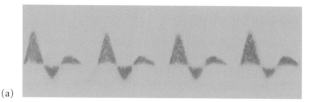

(a)

(b)

Fig. 4.21 (a) Doppler waveform from normal foot showing normal triphasic pattern. (b) Doppler waveform from neuroischaemic foot showing damped monophasic pattern.

flow in diastole, but in the presence of arterial narrowing the waveform shows a reduced forward flow and is described as 'damped and monophasic'. (Fig. 4.21a,b).

It is important to remember that a reduced pressure index is a significant predictive factor for cardiac events and heart deaths.

Transcutaneous oxygen tension (TcPo₂)

This measurement is a non-invasive method for monitoring arterial oxygen tension and reflects local arterial perfusion pressure. A heated oxygen-sensitive probe is placed on the dorsum of the foot. Normal $TcPo_2$ is greater than 40 mmHg. A level below 30 mmHg indicates severe ischaemia and indicates the need for further vascular assessment such as non-invasive angiography. However, levels can be falsely lowered by oedema and cellulitis.

Values in the foot can also be compared with those on the chest wall to derive a regional perfusion index, which is independent of fluctuations in systemic oxygen delivery, although commonly, the absolute pressure on the dorsum of the foot is used.

Toe pressures

Toe pressures can be measured using a special cuff and photoplethysmography. We regard a toe pressure of 30 mmHg or below as an indication of severe ischaemia and, in the presence of ulceration, requiring further investigations.

Angiography

If an ulcer has not progressed despite optimal treatment and ankle brachial pressure index is less than 0.5 or the Doppler waveform is damped and either $TcPo_2$ is less than 30 mmHg or toe pressure is less than 30 mmHg,

then duplex angiography should ideally be carried out. Such non-invasive procedures should be used first to examine the peripheral circulation and to detect areas of stenosis and occlusion.

Duplex angiography

Angiography can be carried out by an examination that combines the features of Doppler waveform analysis with ultrasound imaging to produce a picture of arterial flow dynamics and morphology. It is sometimes difficult to get good views of the tibial vessels in diabetic patients because of excessive calcification. Thus, duplex angiography is optimal in the iliac, femoral and popliteal vessels (Fig. 4.22). However, magnetic resonance angiography (MRA) and computed tomography (CT) angiography are alternative methods of imaging the peripheral circulation.

Magnetic resonance angiography

This technique uses magnetic resonance imaging to delineate arterial flow and disease.

There are two techniques of MRA:
- Time of flight MRA is dependent on a non-contrast

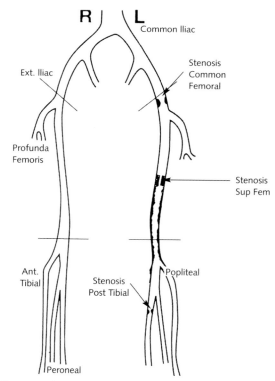

Fig. 4.22 Print-out of Duplex examination showing stenoses in the left common femoral artery, superficial femoral artery and posterior tibial artery.

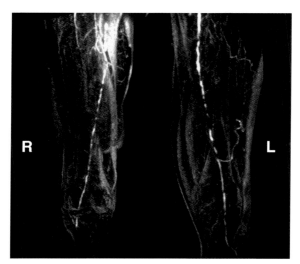

Fig. 4.23 Magnetic resonance angiography (MRA) showing multiple areas of stenosis and occlusion through the right and left superficial femoral arteries and in the left popliteal artery. (Courtesy of Dr Paul Sidhu.)

enhanced flow-sensitive magnetic resonance sequence. It is slow, lasting up to 2 hours, to cover the area from the bifurcation of the aorta to the distal lower extremity
- Gadolinium-enhanced MRA involves an intravenous injection of gadolinium contrast and a fast imaging that follows the passage of the contrast bolus through the arteries. (Fig. 4.23).

The advantage of MRA against conventional transfemoral angiography is that there is no need for an intra-arterial catheter. Further details of MRA are discussed in Chapters 5 and 6. Gadolinium should be avoided in patients with renal failure. Gadolinium containing MRI contrast agents have been associated in patients with renal failure, with Nephrogenic Systemic Fibrosis also known as Nephrogenic Fibrosing Dermopathy. The connective tissue in the skin lesions becomes thickened leading to joint contractures but there can also be systemic involvement of other organs including lungs, liver, muscles and heart. Five per cent of patients have a rapidly progressive clinical course.

Computed tomography angiography

CT angiography is a recently developed technique, which can be particularly useful to delineate the proximal vessels including the aorta but can also be used to assess the distal arteries. This technique has advantages over MRI in that patients with pacemakers and defibrillators may be imaged safely. Patients are less claustrophobic in the CT scanner. Its disadvantage is that iodinated contrast has to be given with the risk of renal impairment although

it is administered intravenously and therefore avoids intra-arterial injection. It also requires ionizing radiation.

Having carried out these non-invasive procedures to map out the arterial system, patients are discussed at a joint radiology/vascular meeting, to decide on appropriate intervention. It is now possible to focus treatment by performing transfemoral angiography, together with digital subtraction angiography, with the initial aim of carrying out angioplasty if possible.

Angioplasty

Angioplasty is tolerated well and can be carried out in very elderly patients. In suitable patients it is now possible to carry out transfemoral angiography and angioplasty as an outpatient procedure. A small-bore needle is used, and after the procedure the puncture site is closed by a special 'Perclose' technique which is a suture-mediated closure of the arterial access site. This allows the patient to sit up after 2 hours and to walk in 4 hours.

Contraindications for day-case angiography include:
- Myocardial infarction/cerebrovascular event within last 6 months
- Severe cardiac/respiratory disease
- Major surgery within last month
- Warfarin therapy
- Renal failure.

Preparations for transfemoral angiography and angioplasty

Patients taking metformin should stop this medication 2 days before the procedure and restart 2 days after, or when renal function returns to normal.

Insulin-dependent patients are placed first on the list in outpatient angiography and have their insulin after the procedure is finished.

It is important to keep the patient well hydrated.

Pre- and perioperative dopamine is no longer used. Instead, if patients have a raised serum creatinine then N-acetylcysteine 600 mg orally twice daily is given for 1 day pre procedure and up to 2 days post procedure (usually 48 hour total duration). Concurrent hydration is essential in these patients and renal function should be rechecked 24 hours post procedure.

Angioplasty is possible at several levels of the leg arterial system to obtain straight line flow to the foot. It is indicated for the treatment of isolated or multiple stenoses as well as short segment occlusions less than 10 cm in length in iliac, femoral and tibial arteries. Recent progress has resulted in long occlusions being satisfactorily angioplastied, either using long balloons or by the technique of subintimal angioplasty.

Overall, the use of angioplasty in this way has led to favourable outcomes. Complications are few and trash foot, caused by emboli to the distal circulation, is very rare after distal angioplasty.

CASE STUDY
Failed healing solved by angioplasty

A 69-year-old woman with type 2 diabetes for 12 years and end-stage renal failure treated by haemodialysis was referred to the diabetic foot clinic with a cold, red ischaemic left foot (Fig. 4.24). She was referred to the vascular laboratory: they were unable to measure her brachial pressure due to fistulas in both arms. However, her tibial vessels were monophasic pulsatile with high diastolic flow. She did not want further vascular investigations at this point. However, she returned to the foot clinic 2 weeks later with a sloughy ulcer deep to bone on the apex of her left hallux, a deep subungual ulcer on her left 3rd toe and a sloughy ulcer on her left heel. $TcPo_2$ tension of the right foot was 20 mmHg. She underwent duplex angiography followed by transfemoral angiography and angioplasty of an occlusion of the superficial femoral artery and stenosis of the anterior tibial artery. This achieved straight line arterial flow to her foot and her ulcers healed in 10 months.

Key points
- Angioplasty is the first-line treatment for peripheral arterial disease in the diabetic limb, where the intention is to obtain straight line arterial flow to the foot
- Measuring the pressure index may be impossible in patients on haemodialysis with fistulas
- $TcPo_2$ is a useful alternative method of quantitating ischaemia in these circumstances.

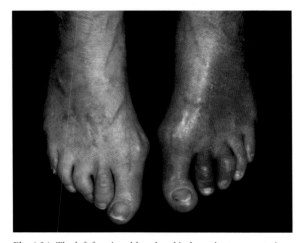

Fig. 4.24 The left foot is cold, red and ischaemic at presentation.

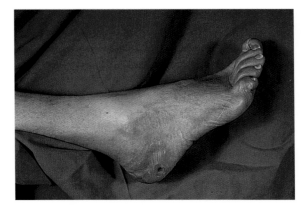

Fig. 4.25 This small painful ischaemic ulcer on the heel of a 90-year-old woman healed in 9 weeks following angioplasty.

CASE STUDY
Angioplasty in the elderly

A 90-year-old woman with type 2 diabetes of 20 years' duration developed a small painful ulcer on the lateral border of her right heel (Fig. 4.25). The foot was pulseless with a pressure index of 0.53. Pain around the ulcer kept her awake at night. She underwent angioplasty of a short stenosis of the superficial femoral artery, the pain improved and the foot healed in 9 weeks.

Key points
- Advanced age is not a contraindication for angioplasty
- Patients with painful ischaemic ulcers should be referred for vascular assessment without delay.

Arterial bypass

If lesions are too widespread for angioplasty, then arterial bypass may be considered. However, this is a major, sometimes lengthy, operation, and is not without risk. It is more often reserved to treat severe tissue destruction that cannot be managed without the restoration of pulsatile blood flow to the foot (see Chapter 6). However, in some patients, angioplasty may not be technically feasible and then arterial bypass should be considered if the ulcer does not respond to conservative treatment.

CASE STUDY
Distal bypass for ischaemic ulcer

A 62-year-old woman with type 1 diabetes of 12 years' duration wore tight shoes and developed an ulcer on the plantar surface of her forefoot after a nail penetrated her

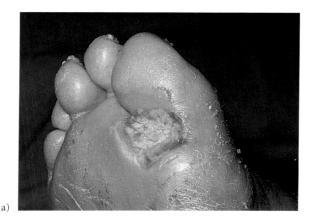

(a)

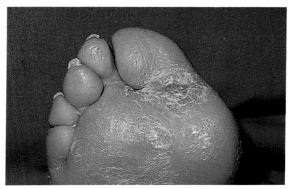

(b)

Fig. 4.26 (a) Large ischaemic ulcer, previously a penetrating injury, which failed to heal despite conservative care. (b) The same ulcer has healed in 14 weeks following femoral/anterior tibial bypass.

shoe. Despite regular podiatry, special shoes and antibiotics the ulcer failed to heal for 7 weeks and became larger (Fig. 4.26a). Her feet were pulseless and her pressure index was 0.42. She did not suffer from intermittent claudication or rest pain. Angiography showed a 10 cm occlusion of the superficial femoral artery and advanced disease of the proximal tibial arteries with reforming of the anterior tibial artery in the lower leg. She underwent femoral to anterior tibial bypass. The ulcer healed in 14 weeks (Fig. 4.26b).

Key points
- Patients with ischaemic ulceration which fails to heal or deteriorates should undergo angiography with a view to angioplasty or arterial bypass
- When angioplasty is not technically possible, arterial bypass should be considered if there is a suitable run-off vessel in the lower leg

- Intermittent claudication and rest pain are often absent in the ischaemic diabetic limb.

Hybrid procedures involving angioplasty and arterial bypass
Distal bypasses are more successful if they are relatively short and are carried out from the popliteal region to the ankle or foot. Patients may also have femoral artery disease and it is sometimes preferable if this is treated by angioplasty above the knee to allow a short 'jump' distal bypass below the knee. (See Chapter 6, p. 191)

Pain control
In general, the neuroischaemic foot is not painful; however, in a few cases when neuropathy is mild the patient suffers pain from the ulcer as well as rest pain in the foot, particularly at night. It is important to control this pain.
- An opioid such as dihydrocodeine, alone (30 mg every 4–6 hours) or in combination with a non-opioid analgesic, e.g. co-dydramol (dihydrocodeine 10 mg, paracetamol 500 mg, two tablets every 4–6 hours) may be useful in moderate pain
- Tramadol (50–100 mg every 4–6 hours) is an opioid derivative, which is often less sedating and less constipating than codeine
- Tricyclic antidepressants, for example dothiepin 50–100 mg at night, are useful at relieving rest pain in bed
- When pain is severe, it is important to give regular morphine therapy. Initially it is best to start with a short-acting preparation taken 4-hourly, and the patient can quickly titrate the dose necessary to relieve pain. After this, it is possible to advance to the modified slow-release preparations devised for twice-daily administration such as 10–20 mg every 12 hours, if no other analgesic or paracetamol has been previously prescribed. However, if it is replacing a weaker opioid analgesic, for example co-dydramol, the initial dose should be 20–30 mg every 12 hours. The doses should be gradually increased but the frequency kept at every 12 hours. If breakthrough pain occurs between the 12-hourly doses, then morphine, as oral solution (Oramorph 5–20 mg every 4 hours) or standard formulation tablets such as Sevredol 10–50 mg every 4 hours, can be given. It is now possible to give opioids by patches applied to the skin, which can last between 48 and 72 hours. These include fentanyl and buprenorphine patches.
- Beware of respiratory depression, to which diabetic patients with autonomic neuropathy can be susceptible. One of our patients with severe autonomic neuropathy underwent marked respiratory depression when she

took dihydrocodeine phosphate and almost stopped breathing

- Chemical sympathectomy by paravertebral injection of phenol is also used to relieve rest pain, although it does not increase peripheral blood flow
- Opiates will be retained by patients in renal failure, often leading to drowsiness, and the dose will need to be suitably reduced.

Metabolic control

A foot ulcer is an indication of multi-organ disease, which is associated with significant comorbidities and an ever present predisposition to infection. It is important to control blood glucose, blood pressure and lipids, and ask the patient to stop smoking. Patients with neuroischaemic ulcers should be on statin therapy as well as antiplatelet therapy. Diabetic patients who are over 55 years old and have peripheral vascular disease should also benefit from an angiotensin-converting enzyme (ACE) inhibitor to prevent further vascular episodes. When managing hypertension in the presence of leg ischaemia it is important to achieve a fine balance between maintaining a pressure that improves perfusion of the ischaemic limb while reducing the blood pressure enough to limit the risk of cardiovascular complications. However, β-blockers are not contraindicated in the neuroischaemic foot although it is preferable to use selective β-blockers.

Many patients will have evidence of cardiac failure in association with their widespread ischaemia. Aggressive treatment of the cardiac failure using ACE inhibitors, diuretics and β-blockers will improve tissue perfusion and also reduce swelling of the feet.

Renal impairment may also be present. Patients with renal impairment are very susceptible to dehydration. A short period of nausea and vomiting may lead to significant renal impairment and patients will need urgent replacement with intravenous fluids. These patients have very little renal reserve, and infection also leads to deterioration of renal function. They must therefore be kept under close surveillance during the treatment of ulceration, particularly the neuroischaemic patient. Just as these patients are susceptible to dehydration and prerenal failure, they are also susceptible to fluid overload which may be precipitated by the administration of excess intravenous fluids. This will lead to peripheral oedema, which is also a factor that reduces healing.

Systemic, metabolic or nutritional disturbances retard healing. The influence of blood glucose on wound healing is controversial. Diabetes is related to faulty wound healing, but this may be because of associated factors such as infection and macrovascular disease. Nevertheless, it is important to achieve good blood glucose control. Short-term metabolic control has been related to experimental wound healing. In the patient with type 2 diabetes, oral hypoglycaemic therapy will need to be optimized, but if this is not successful then insulin should be started.

Educational control

The care of ulcers in diabetic patients is fraught with problems. People with foot ulcers have a more negative attitude towards their feet compared to those people without ulcers, and they are also more depressed. Indeed depression is associated with an increased mortality in patients presenting with their first foot ulcers.

It is easy for health-care professionals to issue instructions to rest, take time off work, wear special shoes or casts and follow advice to the letter. In practice, many patients are unwilling or unable to follow advice.

People who live entirely on their own need to stand and walk to obtain the basic necessities of life. Where the patient lives on his own, has neuropathy and sometimes poor vision as well, it can be very difficult to detect deterioration early, or to do dressings properly.

Patients who lack protective pain sensation need to know that foot ulcers are a serious problem but that they will heal with optimal care. The following educational material—aimed directly at patients—seeks to clarify common misconceptions about ulcers and their management.

Education for patients with foot ulcers
Are foot ulcers a serious health problem?
Diabetic foot ulcers are a very serious health problem. It is essential to treat them quickly. They may not hurt, which makes them even more serious because you may be tempted to stick a plaster on and forget about them.

How are ulcers caused?
Any injury to your feet, no matter how tiny, may lead to an ulcer. If you have neuropathy it is easy to injure your foot without noticing. If you have a poor blood supply to your feet then ulcers can develop for no obvious reason. It is often nobody's fault that you have an ulcer: not yours and not the fault of the last person who treated the foot before you had the ulcer. People with ulcers sometimes feel angry and afraid and look for someone to blame. It is better to avoid these negative feelings.

Many ulcers develop when you injure your foot by knocking or cutting it or picking it, when patches of hard skin or callus on the foot become too thick, or when skin breaks down under a thickened toe nail. Often it is only when the hard skin is removed that the ulcer can be seen. The ulcer is not the fault of the person who removed the hard skin. It was there before. It is nobody's fault.

Other ulcers are due to carelessness. If people with numb feet and a poor blood supply walk barefoot, wear unsuitable shoes or fail to follow foot care advice then they will be very likely to develop ulcers.

How will I know if I have an ulcer?

You should check your feet every day for ulcers. You may feel no pain to warn you that you have a problem. You may see a discoloured area, a break in the skin or a sore place. You may see blood or pus, or notice that your sock is wet from discharge. If you cannot see clearly or reach your feet easily you should ask for help checking them. A mirror is helpful for seeing the underside of your feet.

How can a painless ulcer be a big problem?

Any injury to the foot is difficult to heal unless you rest it. If the wound is not painful then you will be tempted to carry on with life as normal. If you do this there is a great risk that the ulcer will fail to heal and will gradually get bigger. The longer an ulcer has been present the harder it will be to heal it, so it is essential to catch ulcers early and treat them quickly and effectively.

Why are foot ulcers dangerous?

Germs can enter your foot through any break in the skin such as an ulcer, a split, a graze, a blister or a sore place and cause infection. If you have neuropathy (nerve damage) you will not feel the infection as it takes hold. If the blood supply to your foot is poor you will be unable to fight the infection. Untreated infection can destroy a diabetic foot.

What are the signs that an ulcer is getting worse and what should I do about it?

Signs that things are getting worse are when the ulcer seems to be getting bigger or deeper, discharges more fluid than usual (blood or pus), develops swelling or colour changes in the skin around it, or starts to hurt or throb. If any of these occurs, you should go to the diabetic foot clinic at once.

What must I do to heal my foot quickly?

- You should ask for help (the same day) from your doctor, hospital or diabetic foot service. Insist that they look at the foot straight away: do not be fobbed off with an appointment in a few days
- Clean the ulcer with saline
- Cover the ulcer with a sterile dressing held in place with a light bandage
- Ask for help dressing the ulcer from your community nurse if you or your family have difficulty with this
- Keep right off the ulcer. Use crutches or a wheelchair and try not to put your foot to the ground
- Keep your foot up on a stool and cushion, sofa or bed
- Stay home from work or work from home if possible
- Do not go away on holiday with an open ulcer
- If you are offered special shoes or plaster cast treatment, remember that these heal ulcers very successfully.

Remember that a few days off work can heal an ulcer and prevent months of misery and long stays at home or in hospital.

If ulcers are healed quickly there will be less scarring and you will be far less likely to develop another ulcer in the future.

What other treatment will my ulcer need?

Ulcers are often surrounded or covered with dead tissue, callus and debris. If these are allowed to gather around the ulcer they will prevent it from healing and may make the ulcer get worse. The ulcer should be cleaned by cutting away all the unwanted tissue. It may be necessary to clean up the edges until they bleed. This sounds drastic and frightening but it is usually quite painless and is essential treatment if you want your ulcer to heal quickly. This treatment is called 'debridement'. Never try to debride your ulcer yourself: ask your podiatrist or doctor for help.

Another aspect of ulcer treatment is preventing pressure on the ulcer. This can be achieved by resting and elevating the foot, by using crutches or a wheelchair, or by wearing special footwear or casts as advised by the foot clinic.

How long do ulcers take to heal?

In a patient who attends a well-organized, multidisciplinary diabetic foot clinic and follows advice, diabetic foot ulcers should heal within 3 months.

What should I do if my ulcer fails to heal?

- Tell the foot clinic you are concerned and ask them why they think the ulcer is not healing
- Ask them if a second opinion might help
- Ensure you are being treated by an experienced multidisciplinary team. You should be seen by a doctor, a podiatrist and an orthotist (shoe expert)
- Follow their advice explicitly

- If any aspects of their advice are impossible for you to follow, tell them and ask for suggestions. There may be an alternative approach that will suit you better.

What short-term lifestyle changes would help?

- Ask your family or friends for help. People like to rally round in times of trouble, and you can repay them later. If you live alone you can ask your doctor or nurse to organize help
- Let your usual high standards slip a bit: do less
- Prioritize! Leave the housework and let the dust gather or get help with cleaning: it'll all be the same in a hundred years!
- Don't run around helping other people: they should be looking after you
- Don't stand at the stove: use quick and easy recipes or use ready-cooked or take-away food. Cooking can be hard on the feet. Make the family do the washing up or use disposable plates
- Fight the boredom factor: think about things you can do while you are sitting or lying down and ways of getting out and about without overloading your foot. Get your friends to come to you instead of going to them— and ask them to bring the refreshments with them! Get a wheelchair so that you can still go out without putting pressure on your foot ulcer
- Don't feel guilty. You are keeping off your feet in order to avoid future problems. Be sure that everyone knows that. If anyone criticizes you for being lazy ask them to talk to the diabetic foot service
- Keep your foot clinic appointments without fail. If you miss one, ask for another without delay
- Good control of your diabetes will help your ulcer to heal and help to prevent infection. If your diabetes is poorly controlled ask for help from the doctor or nurse.

What should I do if my foot ulcers keep coming back?

If you get recurrent ulcers, the following long-term lifestyle changes would help:

- Try to avoid jobs that involve long hours of walking or standing
- Work as close to home as possible: long journeys are bad for feet
- Get your car adapted to hand controls instead of foot pedals. Use a car with automatic gears
- Ask the foot clinic team for advice on preventing ulcers from coming back.

Should I drive with an ulcer?

Driving with an ulcer is better than walking, but not as good as resting.

What should I do if it is essential to drive?

If you need to drive you should:

- Stop frequently to rest and elevate the feet
- Avoid emergency stops!
- Consider having hand controls fitted to your car
- Enquire about a different design of foot pedal which will not pressurize the ulcerated area
- Always wear your hospital shoes for driving. (If shoes are large and bulky, the control pedals of the car may need to be adjusted or changed.)

What else should I be doing to help my foot heal and stay healed?

- If you enjoy sports, try to choose something like swimming which off-loads your feet
- Avoid situations where you are out of control. For example, if you go on holiday after your ulcer has healed then allow plenty of time at the airport, and organize a wheelchair if you have a history of recurring ulceration. If you go on a guided tour, ensure it will not involve long walks over rough ground
- Walk as little as possible
- Try to lose weight if you are overweight
- Be on the lookout for potential problems that have caused ulcers in the past or might cause a future problem. Radiators or hot pipes by the bed can burn your feet, worn-out shoes can rub sores and walking barefoot can injure you. Try to remember the hidden dangers in day-to-day life and think hard about how to avoid them
- Every time you injure yourself and cause an ulcer, try to work out the reason and take steps to prevent it in future. It sounds boring, but it isn't nearly as tedious as having foot ulcers
- Be prepared to drop everything and come to the foot clinic at the first sign of a foot problem.

Can I go on holiday with an ulcer?

Ideally you should not go on holiday until:

- The ulcer has healed and remained healed for at least a month
- Your footwear is adjusted
- Your footwear has been worn in and is trouble free
- You have received holiday foot care advice
- You know what to do and where to go if you get a foot problem on holiday.

What should I do if my own doctor or nurse wants to change the treatment?

Always ask them to discuss your treatment with the diabetic foot service.

Specific categories of ulcer

The rest of this chapter discusses the presentation and management of other categories of ulcer.

Bullae

Bullae are superficial fluid-filled sacs which develop when the skin is traumatized (Fig. 4.27). In acute vesicular tinea pedis, vesicles may become confluent and form large bullae. Large bullae may form when there is massive lower limb oedema, often secondary to cardiac or renal failure. In the neuropathic foot the first presentation of an ulcer is frequently as a blister under callus which should be drained and debrided (Fig. 4.28a–c).

Ischaemic ulcers on the margin of the foot can also begin with a bulla (Fig. 4.29).

When assessing a bulla the following should be ascertained:

- Is it tense or flaccid?
- What colour is it?
- What does it contain?
- What was the probable cause?

There are two schools of thought on the wisdom of deroofing blisters. Our practice is to drain tense bullae and all bullae more than 1 cm in diameter. This is because the hydrostatic pressure of a tense blister can damage the

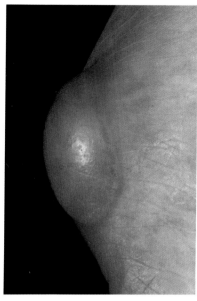

Fig. 4.27 This large bulla developed on the medial border of the 1st metatarsophalangeal joint associated with a hallux valgus deformity which was not accommodated in sufficiently wide shoes.

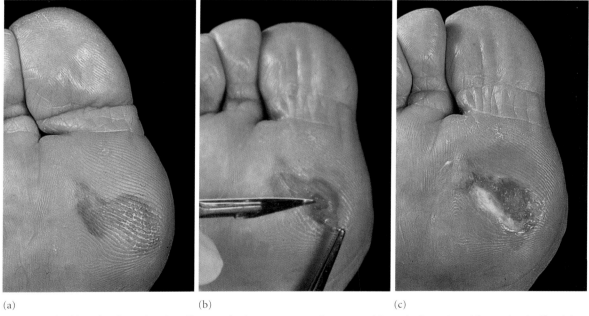

(a)   (b)   (c)

Fig. 4.28 (a) A blister has formed under callus over the first metatarsal head. (b) The roof of the blister is grasped in forceps and cut away with a scalpel together with associated callus. (c) After debridement the base of the neuropathic ulcer is revealed.

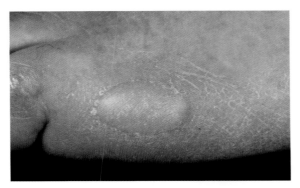

Fig. 4.29 The first presentation of this lesion was as a marginated bulla over the lateral border of the foot but it soon developed into an ischaemic ulcer.

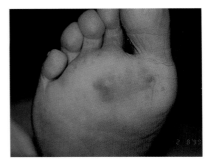

Fig. 4.30 A purple area has developed on the patient's forefoot where it was in contact with the footboard of the bed.

wound bed, while any blister more than 1 cm in diameter is likely to rupture spontaneously, and this is best done under aseptic conditions in the diabetic foot clinic.

Decubitus ulcers

Decubitus ulcers, which develop when the foot is exposed to unrelieved pressure, are common on the diabetic foot and especially on the heel. Patients who have been ill or immobilized are particularly vulnerable. Decubitus ulcers can develop in a short time.

Contributing causes include:
- Rough sheets
- Moisture
- Foreign bodies in the bed (biscuit crumbs, etc.)
- Patients attempting to move in the bed by putting excessive pressure on the heels
- Sliding down the bed so that feet are in contact with bed end
- Failing to provide pressure-relieving mattresses early enough
- Failing to turn helpless patients regularly
- Long periods on the operating table without protection can cause decubitus ulcers even in patients with no neuropathy and no ischaemia.

CASE STUDY
Decubitus ulcer

A 93-year-old woman with type 2 diabetes of 10 years' duration was admitted to hospital following a stroke. On admission her feet were intact. She slid down the bed and was found with her foot jammed against the footboard. A purple area developed where the foot had been in contact

with the footboard (Fig. 4.30). The footboard was removed and the purple area did not deteriorate further.

Key points
- Elderly immobile frail patients are very vulnerable to the development of pressure ulcers
- Remove footboards from the bed of frail, immobile patients who slide down the bed.

Management of heel ulcer
The first sign of a heel ulcer is localized erythema. If pressure is not relieved a 'blister' will develop, which fills first with clear fluid and subsequently with serosanguineous fluid. The base of the blister becomes blue and then black. If pressure is not relieved then deep necrosis may develop. Tense heel blisters should be opened and drained using aseptic precautions.

Urgent pressure relief should be organized. This can be achieved by:
- Regular turning and repositioning of immobile patients to relieve continuous local ischaemia over pressure points. The problems encountered trying to prevent bed sores in elderly, frail, unwell, immobile patients with oedematous legs should, however, not be underestimated
- The pressure relief ankle–foot orthosis (PRAFO) has a washable fleeced liner with an aluminium and polypropylene adjustable frame and a non-slip walking Neoprene base. The patient can wear this orthosis both lying down and walking to avoid pressure on the back of the heel (Fig. 4.31)
- Foam wedges are traditionally used to protect the heels. Heel-protector rings and special heel-relieving splints are available which suspend the heel to protect against further breakdown and allow the ulcer to drain

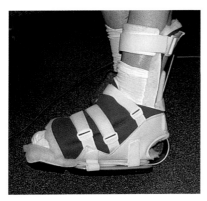

Fig. 4.31 The pressure relief ankle–foot orthosis (PRAFO) relieves pressure on the back of the heel.

- Heel ulcers often occur in the bedbound neuroischaemic foot and rapidly become infected and necrotic. Apart from pressure relief, the circulation should be investigated as described earlier to assess whether the patient is suitable for angioplasty and, failing this, bypass. When necrosis develops this will need either bedside or surgical debridement. If the ulcer is painful and the patient not fit enough for surgical debridement, then debridement with larvae can be offered to the patient. After debridement there is often a cavity which may respond to VAC therapy. Thus, heel ulcers in the neuroischaemic foot require a vigorous and multifocal approach employing different techniques, each of which may be appropriate at different times. Healing may be very slow in these circumstances but a long-term approach, initially in hospital and then by follow-up in the diabetic foot clinic can produce surprisingly good results

- Heel ulcers on the neuropathic foot can be healed with a total-contact cast (Fig. 4.32a,b).

The ulcer associated with Charcot's osteoarthropathy and deformity

When ulceration occurs over a bony prominence associated with a deformed Charcot foot, it is notoriously difficult to heal. Ulceration of the unstable hindfoot and ankle is a particularly serious problem. Ulceration is also a frequent complication of the rocker-bottom deformity and medial convexity of Charcot's osteoarthropathy.

Patients with bony prominences on deformed feet with Charcot's osteoarthropathy need regular removal of callus to prevent ulceration. We use the total-contact cast to treat most of these ulcers (Fig. 4.33a,b). A bespoke cast is usually necessary as few of these deformed, ulcerated feet will fit into an Aircast or other removable walker.

However, conservative measures may fail. If management in a cast does not achieve healing within 3 months, surgery should be considered. Exostectomy is indicated for the mid-foot Charcot's osteoarthropathy and internal stabilization of the ankle for the hindfoot ulcer which is not healing. The patient shown in Fig. 4.34a,b developed

Fig. 4.32 (a) This large heel ulcer had been present for 3 years. (b) The same ulcer healed in 9 weeks after a total-contact cast was applied.

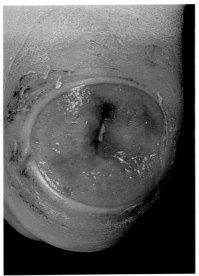

(a)

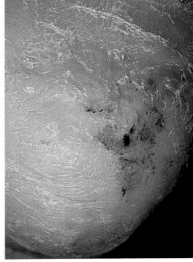

(b)

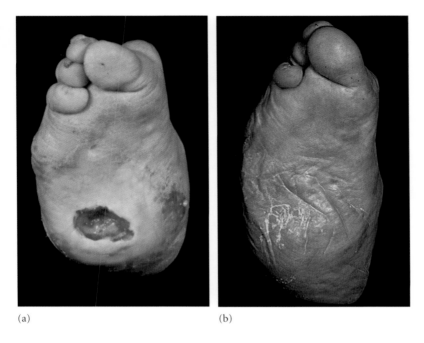

(a)   (b)

Fig. 4.33 (a) This foot with Charcot's osteoarthropathy and rocker-bottom deformity developed an indolent plantar ulcer. When this picture was taken the ulcer had been present for 6 years. (b) The same foot healed in 12 months. The patient had remained at work throughout the casting period and was very active, working as an architect and inspecting building sites.

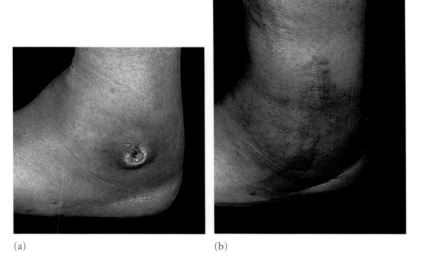

(a)   (b)

Fig. 4.34 (a) Indolent ulceration over the lateral malleolus in an unstable ankle with Charcot's osteoarthropathy of the hindfoot. (b) The ulcer has healed following internal fixation to stabilize the ankle. The healed surgical wound can be seen.

indolent ulceration over an unstable ankle with Charcot's osteoarthropathy of the hindfoot, but healed after he underwent internal fixation. Ulceration associated with Charcot deformity also responds well to the Taylor Spatial Frame as we have described in Chapter 3.

Ulcers over the Achilles tendon

This is another notoriously difficult site to heal. It is an unusual site for ulceration and is usually triggered by unsuitable footwear or is a pressure lesion in an immobile patient. When tendon is exposed in the base of the ulcer the advice of a surgeon should be sought. Our colleague, E. Maelor Thomas, a founder member of our diabetic foot clinic and an orthopaedic surgeon, always said that dead tendon was the worst kind of sequestrum and should always be excised from ulcers. We have used Hyaff to encourage granulation over healthy tendon.

Traumatic wounds
Puncture wounds
Puncture wounds are potentially serious injuries that may first appear as trivial superficial pinpoint wounds. These injuries are caused by a foreign body that may have penetrated the footwear as well as the foot. The foreign body (nail, needle, staple, glass, wooden splinter or other object) may inoculate bacteria into the wound resulting in severe infection. Some of the most serious foot infections we have seen have followed puncture wounds. In some cases the initial wound has fully healed but within a few days the 'volcano' has erupted with severe tissue destruction.

Treatment of puncture wounds is as follows:

- If possible, the foreign body should be inspected to see whether it is intact, or whether a piece has broken off which might remain in the foot
- The foot should be X-rayed and a radio-opaque foreign body sought. Even clear glass will usually show up
- Ultrasound of the foot is also a useful technique to detect foreign bodies.
- The wound should be probed and irrigated, although this may be difficult when the portal of entry is small. In neuropathic patients it may be possible to enlarge the wound to ensure thorough cleaning. Local anaesthesia may be required for sensate individuals
- Wide-spectrum antibiotics should be prescribed
- The wound should be inspected at frequent intervals
- The patient should be asked to report any pain, swelling, discomfort or systemic signs or symptoms immediately
- Tetanus prophylaxis may be needed.

Thermal trauma including burns
- Severe tissue damage and ulceration can be caused by thermal traumas.

CASE STUDY
Burns

A 25-year-old man with type 1 diabetes mellitus of 14 years' duration, profound neuropathy and end-stage renal failure treated with dialysis, slept in a bed next to a central heating radiator. During the night, in his sleep, his leg slipped against the radiator. He sustained full-

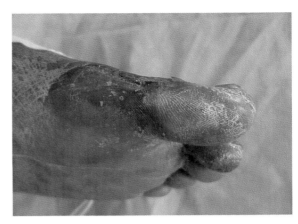

Fig. 4.35 Burn with leathery eschar.

thickness burns to his foot, but only attended the diabetic foot clinic when these became malodorous (Fig. 4.35). There was a leathery eschar with purulent discharge. He was admitted to hospital for intravenous antibiotics. The burns were surgically debrided and split-skin grafts applied from a donor site on his thigh. He healed in 5 months.

Key points
- We warn patients to position beds away from radiators
- The home environment should be adapted when patients develop neuropathy
- Full-thickness burns need skin grafting and specialist surgical care.

Superficial burns usually present as erythema or bullae and can be treated conservatively. Deep burns, which manifest themselves by white, devitalized tissue and subsequent eschar formation, need specialized care from a burns unit, as do all burns which are unhealed after 3 weeks. It can be difficult to assess the severity of recent burns to the diabetic foot as lack of pain may be due to diabetic neuropathy rather than full-thickness damage.

Recent burns should be seen at 48-hourly intervals until their depth is established and should be assessed by an expert burns clinic without delay if there is any suspicion that a burn is deep.

Burns are common in neuropathic patients and the cause should always be established and action taken to prevent repetition. Infection is a serious complication of burns in the diabetic foot and prophylactic antibiotics may need to be given (Fig. 4.36).

Partial thickness burns are allowed to heal by secondary intention, as are some small full-thickness burns. Extensive full-thickness wounds need skin grafting.

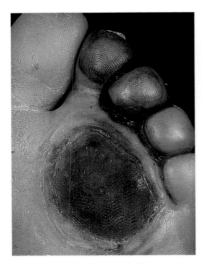

Fig. 4.36 Patient who soaked his foot in hot water. The resulting burns became secondarily infected leading to gangrene of the toes.

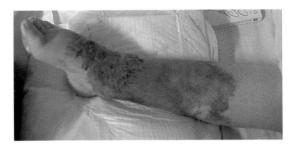

Fig. 4.37 This patient developed severe *Pasteurella multocida* infection after allowing a puppy to lick a blister.

Chemical burns may originate from proprietary remedies, including:
- Corn and callus removers, which contain strong acids or caustics
- Undiluted antiseptics applied directly to wounds
- Contact with noxious chemicals.

As with thermal burns, these can be difficult to assess. When corn cures have been used, as much macerated, acid-loaded callus as possible should be sharp debrided. Chemical burns should be cleansed with saline, covered with a dry dressing and reviewed within 48 hours. Extensive burns or burns when tissue devitalization is obvious at first presentation should be referred to a specialist burns unit.

Zoophilic traumas

Bites and scratches from domestic animals such as dogs and cats are common. (A case was reported from America of a pet dog which caused serious damage to his neuropathic owner's foot, by gnawing it and thus removing large pieces of tissue on more than one occasion.).

CASE STUDY
Pasteurella multocida infection

A 35-year-old woman with type 2 diabetes of 7 years' duration presented at Casualty with a grossly swollen leg with lymphoedema and pyrexia. She said that 2 days earlier a small blister had developed at the back of her ankle and she had allowed her new puppy to lick it. She was admitted for intravenous antibiotics. Swabs grew *P. multocida*, an organism commonly found in the saliva of cats and dogs. She was treated with co-amoxiclav (Fig. 4.37) and was discharged after 2 weeks but the lymphoedema never fully resolved.

Key points
- Animals should not be allowed to lick diabetic foot ulcers
- Severe lymphoedema following infection may never fully resolve
- Animal bites need tetanus prophylaxis. Deep bites may need surgical debridement
- Rat bites can be a problem in the insensate foot. Paul Brand recommended that neuropathic patients keep a cat and avoid eating in bed in case crumbs attract rats
- Insect stings can produce intensive erythema and oedema in the diabetic lower limb with local histamine release
- In tropical countries, ants sometimes infest wounds. Stings and bites from insects may cause ulcers.

Iatrogenic lesions
Common examples include:
- Tape applied to atrophic skin and ripped off
- Tight bandages. We have seen a 53-year-old woman with type 2 diabetes mellitus of 13 years' duration and oedematous feet, who sustained a burn to the dorsum of the foot. She applied a sterile dressing held in place by a bandage which completely encircled the foot and ankle, and made an appointment to be seen at the diabetic foot clinic. When the bandage was removed she had developed superficial necrosis from an overtight bandage and fluctuant oedema. The bandage was replaced with a light tubular bandage and the foot healed in 2 weeks

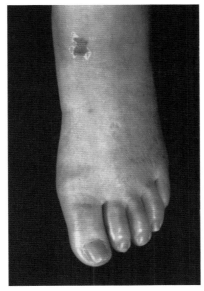 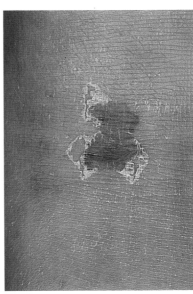

Fig. 4.38 (a) This patient developed necrosis on the front of the ankle from a bandage which became too tight when her oedema increased. (b) A close-up view of the iatrogenic lesion shown in (a). The conventional bandage was replaced with light tubular bandage which could accommodate her oedema.

(a)

(b)

- A further patient with cardiac failure developed a lesion in tight bandages (Fig. 4.38a, b)
- Bulky dressings taking up too much space in unadjusted footwear
- Injection of cortisone into painful heels. Cortisone injection can lead to ulceration and full-thickness necrosis which will need surgical debridement (Fig. 4.39a,b). We have also seen a case of extensive calcification of the soft tissues of the heel associated with pain and ulceration following a cortisone injection into the heel.

Artefactual ulcers

Some patients cause ulcers by pulling skin off their feet or applying noxious substances, or prevent ulcers from healing.

CASE STUDY
Artefactual ulcer

A 24-year-old woman with type 1 diabetes of 13 years' duration presented with an atypical lesion on the dorsum of the foot with irregular outlines (Fig. 4.40). She said she could not remember how it started but on further questioning by the dermatologists she agreed that she might have applied some lavatory bleach to a sore place on her foot.

Key points
- When a lesion is atypical and presents in an unusual site with irregular edges then artefactual disorder should be considered
- A dermatological opinion is useful in patients with possible artefactual ulcers
- Direct confrontation is unwise. A sympathetic psychiatrist should be involved.

Our patients with artefactual ulcers have been young and mostly female, and have suffered in the past from eating disorders or 'brittle' diabetes. Many such patients have numerous admissions with severe foot infections or ketotic episodes related to foot infections. This is a difficult condition to treat and involvement of a psychiatrist with a special interest in artefactual disorders may be useful. Patients who cause their own ulcers or deliberately prevent their ulcers from healing are aware of what they are doing but have little insight into their motives. They can injure themselves with impunity because of their neuropathy. Tamper-free dressings or unremovable casts probably provide the best means of achieving short-term healing, but the long-term outlook is poor. Confrontation and admonishment are unhelpful, as the patient will just go elsewhere for their care and will be at increased risk with clinicians who are not aware of what is going on. Many of these patients are profoundly hypochondriac and only feel safe and in control when they are causing the foot problem.

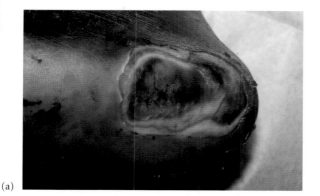

(a)

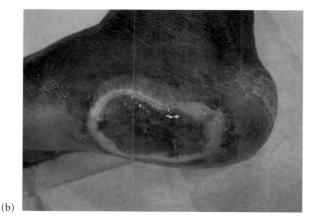

(b)

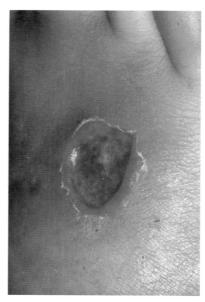

Fig 4.40 Lavatory cleaner was applied to the foot in this patient with peripheral neuropathy.

Fig. 4.39 (a) Plantar heel ulceration after cortisone injection pre-debridement. (b) Ulceration improving post debridement.

We have also seen a 41-year-old patient with 'brittle' type 1 diabetes mellitus of 24 years' duration, who had numerous hospital admissions for infected ulcers of the feet and legs. On one occasion his leg ulcers were grafted using split-skin grafts and the evening before his proposed discharge from hospital, the dressings were removed and the skin grafts scratched off. On two occasions during that admission, glass was broken on the ward and found in his foot ulcers. He was discharged, attended another hospital, and underwent bilateral below-knee amputations within 6 months.

Malignant ulcers

We have seen a number of cases of malignant tumours masquerading as diabetic foot ulcers. Several required more than one biopsy to confirm the diagnosis.

'Cauliflower' appearance and development within a scar were common factors (Fig. 4.41). We have also seen

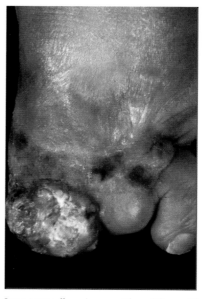

Fig. 4.41 Squamous cell carcinoma with cauliflower-like growth.

amelanotic malignant melanoma masquerading as subungual ulceration and basal cell and squamous cell carcinomas which were thought to be plantar warts.

Pigmented lesions which enlarge and develop satellite lesions, an irregular border, erosions or ulceration should

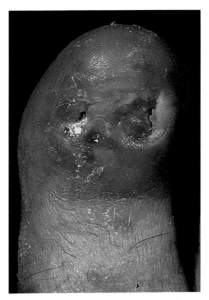

Fig. 4.42 This subungual lesion, shown 1 week following biopsy, was a squamous cell carcinoma.

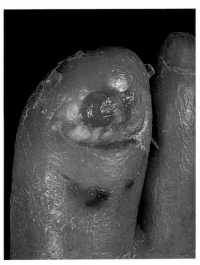

Fig. 4.43 This subungual ulcer failed to heal and was referred to the dermatologists. Biopsy revealed an amelanotic malignant melanoma.

be seen urgently by the dermatologist. These lesions could be malignant melanoma: the lower leg is a common site. Some melanomas are not associated with pigment.

Squamous cell carcinoma (Fig. 4.42), and rarely a basal cell carcinoma, may develop in an indolent diabetic foot ulcer or scar from previous ulcer or surgery.

CASE STUDY
Malignant melanoma

A 78-year-old man with type 2 diabetes of 5 years' duration was referred with a discharging subungual ulcer on his right hallux which had been present for 8 years. Pedal pulses were palpable. The footwear was narrow and insufficiently roomy, and he was asked to purchase shoes with a deep toe box which would not cause pressure on the nails.

The toe nail was cut back. The patient wore suitable shoes, and the ulcer improved, with less discharge, but failed to heal completely. An X-ray showed no signs of osteomyelitis.

When the foot failed to heal after 3 months, the patient was referred to the dermatology clinic for an opinion (Fig. 4.43). Although the dermatologists were not really suspicious that there was any neoplasia present because the area was not elevated, they felt that it would be wise to

check, and a biopsy was arranged. A malignant melanoma was diagnosed and the toe was amputated. The patient is alive and well 7 years later and has regular follow-up appointments with the dermatologists.

Key points
- Ulcers which fail to heal after full treatment should be regarded as suspicious lesions and referred to the dermatology clinic for biopsy
- Malignant melanomas may be amelanotic
- Malignant lesions may not be elevated.

PRACTICE POINTS

- An ulcer is a sign of multi-organ disease. The diagnosis of a neuroischaemic foot ulcer provides the opportunity to treat atherosclerotic risk factors so as to prevent myocardial infarction and stroke
- Ulcers need mechanical, wound, vascular, microbiological, metabolic and educational control
- Mechanical control consists of total-contact casts, Scotchcast boots, crutches, wheelchairs, Aircasts, PRAFOs, custom-made walking AFOs, rest and elevation as appropriate
- Wound control involves sharp debridement and dressings and may need advanced wound healing products or supplementary treatments

- To obtain vascular control it is necessary to assess the vascular status of all ulcerated feet. Neuroischaemic feet may need vascular intervention
- To achieve microbiological control, neuroischaemic feet, burns and puncture wounds will need early antibiotic therapy
- Optimizing control of blood glucose, blood pressure and blood lipids and helping patients to stop smoking will achieve good metabolic control to encourage ulcer healing
- Educational control involves teaching patients the need for rest, debridement, regular dressings and early reporting of problems, and explaining how lifestyle changes can prevent relapse.

FURTHER READING

Presentation and diagnosis

Apelqvist J, Larsson J, Agardh CD. Long-term prognosis for diabetic patients with foot ulcers. *J Int Med* 1993; **233**: 485–91.

Boyko EJ, Ahroni JH, Cohen V *et al.* Prediction of diabetic foot ulcer occurrence using commonly available clinical information: the Seattle Diabetic Foot Study. *Diabetes Care* 2006; **29**: 1202–7.

Cavanagh PR, Young MJ, Adams JE *et al.* Radiographic abnormalities in the feet of patients with diabetic neuropathy. *Diabetes Care* 1994; **17**: 201–9.

Edmonds ME, Foster AV. Diabetic foot ulcers. *BMJ* 2006; **332**: 407–10.

Lipscombe J, Jassal SV, Bailey S *et al.* Chiropody may prevent amputations in diabetic patients on peritoneal dialysis. *Perit Dial Int* 2003; **23**: 255–9.

Reiber GE, Vileikyte A, Boyko EJ *et al.* Causal pathways for incident lower-extremity ulcers in patients with diabetes from two settings. *Diabetes Care* 1999; **22**: 157–62.

Young MJ. Foot problems in diabetes. In Williams G, Pickup J (eds). *Textbook of Diabetes.* Blackwell Science Ltd, Oxford, UK, 2003, pp. 57.1–57.18.

Classification

Foster A, Edmonds M. Simple staging system: a tool for diagnosis and management. *Diabetic Foot* 2000; **2**: 56–62.

Grayson ML, Gibbons GW, Balogh K *et al.* Probing to bone in infected pedal ulcers. A clinical sign of underlying osteomyelitis in diabetic patients. *JAMA* 1995; **273**: 721–3.

Lavery LA, Armstrong DG, Peters EJ, Lipsky BA. Probe to bone test for diagnosing diabetic foot osteomyelitis: reliable or relic? *Diabetes Care* 2007; **30**: 270–4.

Margolis DJ, Allen-Taylor L, Hoffstad O, Berlin JA. Diabetic neuropathic foot ulcers: the association of wound size, wound duration, and wound grade on healing. *Diabetes Care* 2002; **25**: 1835–9.

Mechanical control

Armstrong DG, Short B, Espensen EH *et al.* Technique for fabrication of an 'instant total-contact cast' for treatment of neuropathic diabetic foot ulcers. *J Am Podiatric Med Assoc* 2002; **92**: 405–8.

Armstrong DG, Lavery LA, Wu S, Boulton AJ. Evaluation of removable and irremovable cast walkers in the healing of diabetic foot wounds: a randomized controlled trial. *Diabetes Care* 2005; **28**: 551–4.

Armstrong DG, Nguyen HC, Lavery LA *et al.* Off-loading the diabetic foot wound: a randomized clinical trial. *Diabetes Care* 2001; **24**: 1019–22.

Baumhauer JF, Wervey R, McWilliams J *et al.* A comparison study of plantar foot pressure in a standardised shoe, total contact cast and prefabricated pneumatic walking brace. *Foot Ankle Int* 1997; **18**: 26–33.

Beuker BJ, van Deursen RW, Prive P *et al.* Plantar pressure in off-loading devices used in diabetic ulcer treatment. *Wound Repair Regen* 2005; **13**: 537–42.

Boninger ML, Leonard JA. Use of bivalved ankle-foot orthosis in neuropathic foot and ankle lesions. *J Rehabil Res Dev* 1996; **33**: 16–22.

Burden AC, Jones GR, Jones R, Blandford RL. Use of the 'Scotchcast boot' in treating diabetic foot ulcers. *BMJ* 1983; **286**: 1555–7.

Bus SA, Ulbrecht JS, Cavanagh PR. Pressure relief and load redistribution by custom made insoles in diabetic patients with neuropathy and foot deformity. *Clin Biomech* 2004; **19**: 629–38.

Cavanagh PR, Owings TM. Nonsurgical strategies for healing and preventing recurrence of diabetic foot ulcers. *Foot Ankle Clin* 2006; **11**: 735–43.

Cavanagh PR, Lipsky BA, Bradbury AW, Botek G. Treatment for diabetic foot ulcers. *Lancet* 2005; **366**: 1725–35.

Chantelau E, Breuer U, Leisch AC *et al.* Outpatient treatment of unilateral diabetic foot ulcers with 'half shoes'. *Diabetic Medicine* 1993; **10**: 267–70.

Chantelau E, Leisch A. Footwear: uses and abuses. In Boulton AJM, Connor H, Cavanagh PR (eds). *The Foot in Diabetes*, 2nd edn. John Wiley & Sons, Chichester, UK, 1994, pp. 99–108.

Guse ST, Alvine FG. Treatment of diabetic foot ulcers and Charcot neuroarthropathy using the patellar tendon-bearing brace. *Foot Ankle Int* 1997; **18**: 675–7.

Holstein P, Lohmann M, Bitsch M, Jorgensen B. Achilles tendon lengthening, the panacea for plantar forefoot ulceration? *Diabetes Metab Res Rev* 2004; **20**(suppl 1): S37–40.

International Working Group on the Diabetic Foot (IWGDF). *International Consensus on the Diabetic Foot with Specific Guidelines on Footwear and Offloading.* Launched at the 5th International Symposium on the Diabetic Foot, May 2007.

Janisse DJ, Janisse EJ. Pedorthic and orthotic management of the diabetic foot. *Foot Ankle Clin.* 2006; **11**: 717–34.

Kalish SR, Pelcovitz N, Zawada S *et al.* The Aircast walking brace versus conventional casting methods. *J Am Podiatr Med Assoc* 1987; **77**: 589–95.

Katz IA, Harlan A, Miranda-Palma B *et al*. A randomized trial of two irremovable off-loading devices in the management of plantar neuropathic diabetic foot ulcers. *Diabetes Care* 2005; **28**: 555–9.

Knowles EA, Armstrong DG, Hayat SA *et al*. Offloading diabetic foot wounds using the Scotchcast boot: a retrospective study. *Ostomy Wound Manage* 2002; **48**: 50–3.

Mueller MJ, Diamond JE, Sinacore DR *et al*. Total contact casting in treatment of diabetic plantar ulcers controlled clinical trial. *Diabetes Care* 1989; **12**: 384–8.

Piaggesi A, Macchiarine S, Rizzo L *et al*. An off-the-shelf instant contact casting device for the management of diabetic foot ulcers: a randomized prospective trial versus traditional fiberglass cast. *Diabetes Care* 2007; **30**: 586–90.

Rome K. Orthotic materials: a review of the selection process. *Diabetic Foot* 1998; **1**: 14–19.

Tovey FI. The manufacture of diabetic footwear. *Diabetic Medicine* 1984; **1**: 69–71.

Wu SC, Crews RT, Armstrong DG. The pivotal role of offloading in the management of neuropathic foot ulceration. *Curr Diab Rep* 2005; **5**: 423–9.

Zimny S, Schatz H, Pfohlo U. The effects of applied felted foam on wound healing and healing times in the therapy of neuropathic diabetic foot ulcers. *Diabet Med* 2003; **20**: 622–5.

Wound control

Alvarez OM, Markowitz L, Wendelken M. Local care of diabetic foot ulcers In Veves A, Giurini JM, LoGerfo FW (eds). *The Diabetic Foot*, 2nd edn. Humana Press, New Jersey, USA, 2006, pp. 311–34.

Andros G, Armstrong DG, Attinger CE *et al*; Tucson Expert Consensus Conference. Consensus statement on negative pressure wound therapy (V.A.C. Therapy) for the management of diabetic foot wounds. *Ostomy Wound Manage* 2006; **Suppl**: 1–32.

Apelqvist J, Ragnarson Tennvall G. Cavity foot ulcers in diabetic patients; a comparative study of Cadexomer Iodine ointment and standard treatment. An economic analysis alongside a clinical trial. *Acta Derm Venereol* 1996; **76**: 231–5.

Armstrong DG, Salas P, Short B *et al*. Maggot therapy in 'lower-extremity hospice' wound care: fewer amputations and more antibiotic-free days. *J Am Podiatr Med Assoc* 2005; **95**: 254–7.

Armstrong DG, Lavery LA; Diabetic Foot Study Consortium. Negative pressure wound therapy after partial diabetic foot amputation: a multicentre, randomised controlled trial. *Lancet* 2005; **366**: 1704–10.

Baker N. Debridement of the diabetic foot: a podiatric perspective. *Int J Low Extrem Wounds* 2002; **1**: 87–92.

Bakker DJ. Hyperbaric oxygen therapy and the diabetic foot. *Diab Metab Res Rev* 2000; **16** (Suppl 1): S55–8.

Banwell PE, Teot L. Topical negative pressure (TNP): the evolution of a novel wound therapy. *J Wound Care* 2003; **12**: 22–8.

Bentley J, Bishai P, Foster A, Preece J. Clinical competence in sharp debridement: an innovative course. *Br J Community Nurs* 2005; **10**: S6–13.

Bowling FL, Salgami EV, Boulton AJ. Larval therapy: a novel treatment in eliminating methicillin-resistant *Staphylococcus aureus* from diabetic foot ulcers. *Diabetes Care* 2007; **30**: 370–1.

Caravaggi C, De Giglio R, Pritelli C *et al*. HYAFF 11-based autologous dermal and epidermal grafts in the treatment of non-infected diabetic plantar and dorsal foot ulcers: a prospective, multicenter, controlled, randomized clinical trial. *Diabetes Care* 2003; **26**: 2853–9.

Church JCT. Larval intervention in the chronic wound. *Eur Wound Manag Assoc J* 2001; **1**: 10–3.

Dini V, Romanelli M, Piaggesi A *et al*. Cutaneous tissue engineering and lower extremity wounds (part 2). *Int J Low Extrem Wounds* 2006; **5**: 27–34.

Edmonds M, Foster A. Hyalofill: a new product for chronic wound management. *Diabetic Foot* 2000; **3**: 29–30.

Edmonds ME, Foster AVM, McColgan M. Dermagraft: a new treatment for diabetic foot ulcers. *Diabetic Medicine* 1997; **14**: 1010–11.

Ehrenreich M, Ruszczak Z. Update on tissue-engineered biological dressings. *Tissue Eng* 2006; **12**: 2407–24.

Faglia E, Oriani G, Favales F *et al*. Adjunctive systemic hyperbaric oxygen therapy in treatment of severe prevalently ischemic diabetic foot ulcer. A randomized study. *Diabetes Care* 1996; **19**: 1138–43.

Fisken RA, Digby M. Which dressing for diabetic foot ulcers? *Pract Diabetes Int* 1996; **13**: 107–9.

Gentzkow GD, Iwasaki SD, Hershon KS *et al*. Use of dermagraft, a cultured human dermis, to treat diabetic foot ulcers. *Diabetes Care* 1996; **19**: 350–4.

Di mario c, Ossino AM, Trefiletti M. Lyophilized collagen in the treatment of diabetic ulcers. *Drugs Exp Clin Res* 1991; **17**: 371–3.

Hehenberger K, Kratz G, Hansson A, Brismar K. Fibroblasts derived from human chronic diabetic wounds have a decreased proliferation rate, which is recovered by the addition of heparin. *J Dermatol Sci* 1998; **16**: 144–51.

Jude EB, Apelqvist J, Spraul M, Martini J; the Silver Dressing Study Group. Prospective randomized controlled study of Hydrofiber(R) dressing containing ionic silver or calcium alginate dressings in non-ischaemic diabetic foot ulcers. *Diabet Med* 2007; **24**: 280–8.

Kalani M, Jorneskog G, Naderi N *et al*. Hyperbaric oxygen (HBO) therapy in treatment of diabetic foot ulcers. Long-term follow-up. *J Diab Comp* 2002; **16**: 153–8.

Lipkin S, Chaikof E, Isseroff Z, Silverstein P. Effectiveness of bilayered cellular matrix in healing of neuropathic diabetic foot ulcers: results of a multicenter pilot trial. *Wounds* 2003; **15**: 230–6.

Marston WA, Hanft J, Norwood P, Pollak R; Dermagraft Diabetic Foot Ulcer Study Group. The efficacy and safety of Dermagraft in improving the healing of chronic diabetic foot ulcers: results of a prospective randomized trial. *Diabetes Care* 2003; **26**: 1701–5.

Martin BR, Sangalang M, Wu S, Armstrong DG. Outcomes of allogenic acellular matrix therapy in treatment of diabetic foot wounds: an initial experience. *Int Wound J* 2005; **2**: 161–5.

Mason JM, O'Keefe C, McIntosh A *et al.* A systematic review of foot ulcer in patients with Type 2 diabetes mellitus. I. Prevention. *Diabetic Medicine* 1999; **16**: 801–12.

Mason JM, O'Keefe C, McIntosh A *et al.* A systematic review of foot ulcer in patients with Type 2 diabetes mellitus. II. Treatment. *Diabetic Medicine* 1999; **16**: 889–909.

Naughton G, Mansbridge J, Gentzkow G. A metabolically active human dermal replacement for the treatment of diabetic foot ulcers. *Artificial Organs* 1997; **21**: 1203–10.

Niezgoda JA, Van Gils CC, Frykberg RG, Hodde JP. Randomized clinical trial comparing OASIS Wound Matrix to Regranex Gel for diabetic ulcers. *Adv Skin Wound Care* 2005; **18**: 258–66.

Petrova N, Edmonds M. Emerging drugs for diabetic foot ulcers. *Expert Opin Emerg Drugs* 2006; **11**: 709–24.

Puttirutvong P. Meshed skin graft versus split thickness skin graft in diabetic ulcer coverage. *J Med Assoc Thai* 2004; **87**: 66–72.

Rayman A, Stansfield G, Woollard T *et al.* Use of larvae in the treatment of the diabetic necrotic foot. *Diabetic Foot* 1998; **1**: 7–13.

Rodeheaver GT. Wound cleansing, wound irrigation, wound disinfection. In Krasner DL, Rodeheaver GT, Sibbald RG (eds). *Chronic Wound Care: a clinical source book for healthcare professionals.* HMP Communications, Wayne, USA, 2001, pp. 273–85.

Roeckl-Wiedmann I, Bennett M, Kranke P. Systematic review of hyperbaric oxygen in the management of chronic wounds. *Br J Surg* 2005; **92**: 24–32.

Sherman RA. Maggot therapy for treating diabetic foot ulcers unresponsive to conventional therapy. *Diabetes Care* 2003; **26**: 446–51.

Steed DL and the Diabetic Ulcer Study Group. Clinical evaluation of recombinant human platelet-derived growth factor for the treatment of lower extremity diabetic ulcers. *J Vasc Surg* 1995; **21**: 71–81.

Steed DL, Donohoe D, Webster MW *et al.* Effect of extensive debridement and treatment on the healing of diabetic foot ulcers. *J Am Coll Surg* 1996; **183**: 61–4.

Tsang MW, Wong WK, Hung CS *et al.* Human epidermal growth factor enhances healing of diabetic foot ulcers. *Diabetes Care* 2003; **26**: 1856–61.

Veves A, Falanga V, Armstrong DG *et al.* Graftskin, a human skin equivalent, is effective in the management of noninfected neuropathic diabetic foot ulcers: a prospective randomised multicenter clinical trial. *Diabetes Care* 2001; **24**: 290–5.

Veves A, Sheehan P, Pham HT. A randomised, controlled trial of Promogran (a collagen/oxidized regenerated cellulose dressing) vs standard treatment in the management of diabetic foot ulcers. *Arch Surg* 2002; **137**: 822–7.

Microbiological control

Bergin SM, Wraight P. Silver based wound dressings and topical agents for treating diabetic foot ulcers. *Cochrane Database Sys Rev* 2006; **25**: CD005082.

Bowler PG, Duerden BI, Armstrong DG. Wound microbiology and associated approach to wound management. *Clin Microbiol Rev* 2001; **14**: 244–69.

Browne AC, Vearncombe M, Sibbald RG. High bacterial load in asymptomatic diabetic patients with neurotrophic ulcers retards wound healing after application of Dermagraft. *Ostomy Wound Manag* 2001; **47**: 44–9.

Chantelau E, Tanudjaja T, Altenhofer F *et al.* Antibiotic treatment for uncomplicated neuropathic forefoot ulcers in diabetes: a controlled trial. *Diabetic Medicine* 1996; **13**: 156–9.

Edmonds M, Foster A. The use of antibiotics in the diabetic foot. *Am J Surg* 2004; **187**: 25S–28S.

Rayman G, Rayman A, Baker NR *et al.* Sustained silver-releasing dressing in the treatment of diabetic foot ulcers. *Br J Nurs* 2005; **14**: 109–14.

Robson MC. Wound infection. A failure of wound healing caused by an imbalance of bacteria. *Surg Clin North Am* 1997; **77**: 637–50.

Robson MC, Mannari RJ, Smith PD, Payne WG. Maintenance of wound bacterial balance. *Am J Surg* 1999; **178**: 399–402.

Roghmann MC, Siddiqui A, Plaisance K, Standiford H. MRSA colonization and the risk of MRSA bacteraemia in hospitalized patients with chronic ulcers. *J Hosp Infect* 2001; **47**: 98–103.

Schmidt K, Debus ES, St Jessberger *et al.* Bacterial population of chronic crural ulcers: is there a difference between the diabetic, the venous, and the arterial ulcer. *Vasa* 2000; **29**: 62–70.

Wright JB, Lam K, Burrell RE. Wound management in an era of increasing bacterial antibiotic resistance: a role for topical silver treatment. *Am J Infect Control* 1998; **26**: 572–7.

Xu L, McLennan SV, Lo L *et al.* Bacterial load predicts healing rate in neuropathic diabetic foot ulcers. *Diabetes Care* 2007; **30**: 378–80.

Vascular control

American Diabetes Association. American Consensus Conference on Diabetic Foot. *Diabetes Care* 1999; **22**: 1354–60.

Carpenter JP, Baum RA, Holland GA, Barker CF. Peripheral vascular surgery with magnetic resonance angiography as the sole preoperative imaging modality. *J Vasc Surg* 1994; **20**: 861–71.

Clerici G, Fratino P, De Cata P *et al.* Extensive use of peripheral angioplasty, particularly infrapopliteal, in the treatment of ischaemic diabetic foot ulcers: clinical results of a multicentric study of 221 consecutive diabetic subjects. *J Intern Med* 2002; **252**: 225–32.

Faglia E, Dalla Paola L, Clerici G *et al.* Peripheral angioplasty as the first-choice revascularization procedure in diabetic patients with critical limb ischaemia: prospective study of 993 consecutive patients hospitalized and followed between 1999 and 2003. *Eur J Vasc Endovasc Surg* 2005; **29**: 620–7.

Kalani M, Brismar K, Fagrell B *et al.* Transcutaneous oxygen tension and toe blood pressure as predictors for outcome of diabetic foot ulcers. *Diabetes Care* 1999; **22**: 147–51.

Kroger K, Stewen C, Santosa F, Rudofsky G. Toe pressure measurements compared to ankle artery pressure measurements. *Angiology* 2003; **54**: 39–44.

Motomura H, Ohashi N, Harada T *et al.* Aggressive conservative therapy for refractory ulcer with diabetes and/or arteriosclerosis. *J Dermatol* 2006; **33**: 353–9.

Norgren L, Hiatt W, Dormandy J; TransAtlantic Inter-Society Consensus (TASC). Management of peripheral arterial disease (PAD). (TASC II). *J Vasc Surg* 2007; **45**: S5–S67.

Metabolic control

Armstrong DG, Nguyen HC. Improvement in healing with aggressive edema reduction after debridement of foot infection in persons with diabetes. *Arch Surg* 2000; **135**: 1405–9.

Black E, Vibe-Peterson J, Jorgensen L *et al.* Decrease of collagen deposition in wound repair in type 1 diabetes independent of glycaemic control. *Arch Surg* 2003; **138**: 34–40.

Heart Outcomes Prevention Evaluation Study investigators. The effects of ramopril on cardiovascular and microvascular outcomes in people with diabetes mellitus: results of the HOPE study and MICRO-HOPE sub study. *Lancet* 2000; **355**: 253–9.

Educational control

Day JL. Diabetic patient education: determinants of success. *Diabetes Metab Res Rev* 2000; **16** (Suppl 1): S70–4.

Haas LB Ahroni JH. Lower limb self management education In

Bowker JH, Pfeifer MA (eds). *Levin and O'Neals The Diabetic Foot.* Mosby, St Louis, USA, 2001, pp. 665–75.

Ismail K, Winkley K, Stahl D *et al.* Depression: A cohort study of people with diabetes and their first foot ulcer: the role of depression on mortality. *Diabetes Care* 2007; **30**: 1473–9.

Johnson M, Newton P, Goyder E. Patient and professional perspectives on prescribed therapeutic footwear for people with diabetes: a vignette study. *Patient Educ Couns* 2006; **64**:1–3.

Vileikyte L, Rubin RR, Leventhal H. Psychological aspects of diabetic neuropathic foot complications: an overview. *Diabetes Metab Res Rev* 2004; **20** (Suppl 1): S13–8.

Walsh CH, Soler NG, Fitzgerald *et al.* Association of foot lesions and retinopathy in patients with newly diagnosed diabetes. *Lancet* 1975; **1**: 878–80.

Special categories of ulcer

Armstrong DG, Lavery LA, Quebedeaux TL *et al.* Surgical morbidity and the risk of amputation due to infected puncture wounds in diabetic versus non diabetic adults. *South Med J* 1997; **90**: 384–9.

British Burns Association. *Referral Guidelines.* British Burns Association, London, UK, 2001.

du Vivier A. *Atlas of Clinical Dermatology.* Churchill Livingstone, London, UK, 2002.

Imtiaz KE, Khaleedi AA. Squamous cell carcinoma developing in necrobiosis lipoidica. *Diabet Med* 2001; **18**: 325–8.

Kalra B, Kalra S, Chatley G, Singh H. Rat bite as a cause of diabetic foot ulcer–a series of eight cases. *Diabetologia* 2006; **49**:1452–3.

Rogers JC, Armstrong DG, Boulton AJM *et al.* Malignant melanoma misdiagnosed as a diabetic foot ulcer. *Diabetes Care* 2007; **30**: 444–5.

5

Stage 4: the infected foot

Pursue him to his house and pluck him thence,
Lest his infection, being of catching nature,
Spread further . . .
(Coriolanus, III, i, William Shakespeare)

PRESENTATION AND DIAGNOSIS

William Shakespeare asks in Coriolanus, Act 5 Scene 4:

'Is't possible that so short a time
Can alter the condition of a man?'

In persons with diabetes, infection can destroy their foot and ruin their life in a remarkably short time: sometimes within just a few hours. In this chapter we describe the case of a patient with a fulminating *Streptococcus* group A infection who was apparently well at noon and very seriously ill 4 hours later, needing resuscitation and urgent treatment to save his life.

We have previously spoken of infection as a great destroyer of the diabetic foot and this is particularly the case in the neuroischaemic foot where the blood supply is insufficient to mount a good inflammatory response. Stage 4 is a highly significant staging post on the road to amputation for both neuropathic and neuroischaemic feet, and is usually involved in the final common pathway to amputation: more people undergo major amputation because of combined diabetes and infection than for all other causes. When someone is very ill it can be difficult to mobilize the services they need sufficiently quickly.

In this chapter we describe a system for managing infected diabetic feet, both in the outpatient diabetic foot clinic and on the wards. (We do not think it is ever appropriate to manage diabetic foot infection entirely in primary care unless there is also input from specialist multidisciplinary centres and the possibility of immediate access of the patient to the hospital if the patient deteriorates.)

Diabetic foot patients with late infections are often in immediate danger of losing life and limb. We also discuss the polymicrobial organisms associated with deep wound infections and detail the meticulous care these patients need. We have tried to illustrate these points with very detailed case studies. We hope that we have outlined a good case for multidisciplinary care, with daily input from medical and surgical teams for inpatients with severe infections.

Our aim has always been to devise a practical approach that can diagnose infections early and treat them rapidly and aggressively, and thus prevent amputations, remembering that all infections are worst in the neuroischaemic foot.

Our guiding principle is that we do not forget that 85% of major amputations in people with diabetes begin with a 'clean' ulcer.

In this second edition we have greatly simplified our system for managing the infected foot in diabetes, remembering that staging systems *based on treatment needed* are the most useful, and also not forgetting our useful adage, that the essentials of successful management at stage 4 (as at every different stage of the diabetic foot) are the usual triad: rapid presentation, rapid diagnosis and rapid treatment. When managing these very difficult and unstable feet, we are guided in our decision making by the following:
- Symptoms and signs of infection
- Results of properly taken wound swabs and tissue cultures
- Past and present knowledge of individual patients.

Spectrum of clinical presentations

There are three distinct stages in the natural history of infection in the diabetic foot. Each of these entities is distinguished by virtue of the treatment it needs:

A Practical Manual of Diabetic Foot Care, 2nd edition, Edmonds, Foster and Sanders.
Published 2008 Blackwell Publishing. ISBN 978-1-4051-61473

- Localized infection
- Spreading infection
- Severe infection.

We will now describe the presentation of each of these three entities of infection, illustrated with case studies, and then describe the management of these infections.

Localized infection

This refers to infection in the ulcer bed or immediately surrounding skin. This may present with purulent discharge and surrounding erythema, but often the classical signs of infection are diminished by the presence of neuropathy and ischaemia. Thus, the signs of infection may be very subtle. Galen's classical signs and symptoms of redness, heat, pain and loss of function may not be evident. However, early warning signs of infection and signs of deterioration should be searched for with great assiduity in all diabetic foot patients especially those with breaks in the skin.

We believe that if the practitioner waits for florid advanced signs of infection to develop then valuable time is lost. We act early upon the initial signs of infection. Local signs that an ulcer has become infected include any or all of the following:

- Pain
- Base of the ulcer changes from healthy pink granulations to yellowish or grey tissue (Fig. 5.1)
- Increased friability of granulation tissue (Fig. 5.2)
- Increased amount of exudate (Fig. 5.3)
- Exudate changes from clear to purulent
- Unpleasant smell
- Sinuses develop in an ulcer (Fig. 5.4)
- Edges may become undermined so that a probe can be passed under the skin

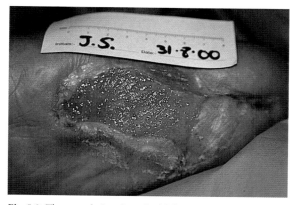

Fig. 5.2 The granulation tissue in this large ulcer has become friable and bleeds easily. This is an early sign of infection.

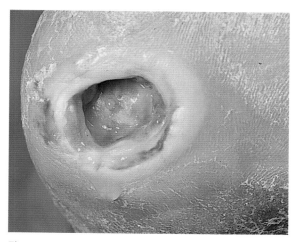

Fig. 5.3 An increased amount of exudate is dripping out of this neuropathic ulcer.

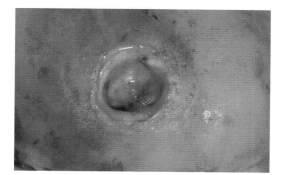

Fig. 5.1 Base of the ulcer has changed from healthy pink granulations to grey tissue.

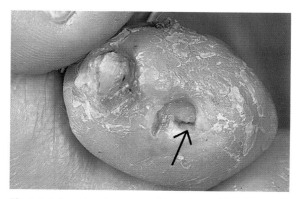

Fig. 5.4 A deep sinus has appeared in the base of this ulcer.

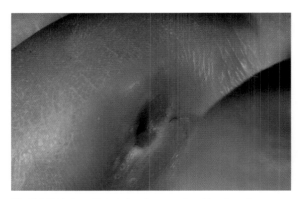

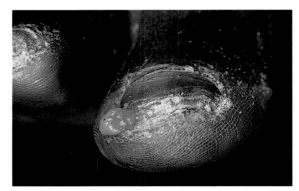

(a)

Fig. 5.5 This interdigital ulcer has associated local erythema.

• Bone or tendon becomes exposed in the base of the ulcer or can be reached if a probe is passed along a sinus. Where there is erythema of surrounding skin there will usually also be local signs of infection as described above. Localized erythema, warmth and swelling are usually associated with ulceration (Fig. 5.5), although the portal of entry of infection may be a corn, callus, blister, fissure, a problem beneath a nail, or any other skin break. In the darkly pigmented foot, cellulitis can be difficult to detect, but careful comparison with the other foot may reveal a tawny hue. Patients with retinopathy may not see the erythema of cellulitis. In localized infection, the colour alone of surrounding skin may have changed, becoming pink or red, but the texture of the surrounding skin does not change.

In most cases of localized infection, oral antibiotics are sufficient and patients do not usually need admission to hospital.

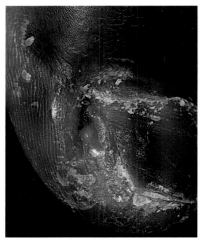

(b)

Fig. 5.6 (a) This patient complained of pain on the medial side of his toe. There was no swelling or cellulitis. The nail has been gently pared back and a small abscess is draining. (b) Abscess site post drainage.

CASE STUDY
Pain as the sole manifestation of infection in a neuroischaemic foot

A 77-year-old blind Afro-Caribbean man with type 2 diabetes of 22 years' duration, and peripheral vascular disease complained of pain in his right hallux and was brought to the foot clinic the same day (Fig. 5.6a). There was no swelling or cellulitis but pain was exacerbated by gentle pressure on the nail plate and a small area of nail plate close to the medial sulcus was very gently pared away to expose a small abscess under the nail which was drained (Fig. 5.6b). A deep swab was sent for culture and the abscess cavity was irrigated with normal saline and dressed with Melolin and Tubegauze; amoxicillin 500 mg tds and flucloxacillin 500 mg qds were prescribed. The wound swab grew *Staphylococcus aureus* and *Streptococcus* group B. The toe healed in 1 month.

Key points
• Pain may be the sole manifestation of infection in the diabetic neuroischaemic foot and is not always due to ischaemia. However, in the presence of sufficient neuropathy, pain may be absent in the infected neuroischaemic foot
• Pain from infection under the nail is exacerbated by gentle pressure on the nail plate
• A podiatrist can achieve successful drainage of infection without causing further trauma to the ischaemic toe
• Infection in the neuroischaemic foot may not be associated with swelling.

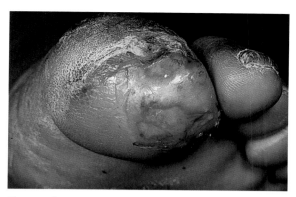

Fig. 5.7 Ulceration at the apex of the hallux with cellulitis.

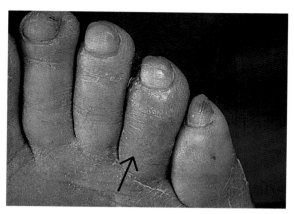

Fig. 5.8 The first sign of infection: 4th toe becomes slightly pink.

CASE STUDY
Pain as the sole early warning of infection

An 82-year-old woman with type 2 diabetes of 38 years' duration, profound peripheral neuropathy and a previous history of neuropathic ulceration, complained of pain in her hallux at a routine foot clinic appointment. There was no history of trauma. On visual examination and palpation, nothing abnormal was detected, X-ray was unremarkable, and she was apyrexial. She was Afro-Caribbean with heavy pigmentation. She was advised to keep a close eye on the toe and return immediately if it deteriorated and to return in 48 hours for review. When she came back 2 days later she had an infected ulcer on the apex of the toe, severe unilateral oedema and cellulitis spreading up the leg (Fig. 5.7). She was admitted to hospital and given intravenous amoxicillin 500 mg tds, flucloxacillin 500 mg qds, metronidazole 500 mg tds and ceftazidime 1 g tds. The toe healed in 2 weeks.

Key points
- Pain may have been the first symptom of infection in this neuropathic foot
- Elderly neuropathic patients complaining of new pain of unknown aetiology with no other clinical signs or symptoms should be rechecked within 48 hours
- It is difficult to detect cellulitis in pigmented skin.

Early warning signs of infection and signs of deterioration should be searched for with great assidulity in all diabetic foot patients (Fig. 5.8), especially those with breaks in the skin.

CASE STUDY
Infection not noted by patient

A 53-year-old woman with type 1 diabetes of 25 years' duration, proliferative retinopathy with reduced vision, peripheral neuropathy and hallux rigidus developed a neuropathic ulcer under callus on the plantar surface of her right hallux. She was warned of the usual danger signs of deterioration (redness, warmth, swelling, pain, purulent discharge) but did not return to clinic until her routine appointment. Callus had grown over the ulcer preventing drainage and the toe had become cellulitic (Fig. 5.9a,b). Callus was debrided and pus drained (Fig. 5.9c). A deep wound swab was taken and oral amoxicillin 500 mg tds and flucloxacillin 500 mg qds were prescribed. She was reviewed the next day. The toe had not improved and she was admitted for bedrest and intravenous antibiotics according to our protocol, namely amoxicillin 500 mg tds, flucloxacillin 500 mg qds, metronidazole 500 mg tds and ceftazidime 1 g tds. The swab taken at her outpatient clinic visit grew *Staphylococcus aureus* and *Streptococcus* group B. The metronidazole and ceftazidime were stopped when this result became available. She was discharged after 4 days and the ulcer healed in 6 weeks.

Key points
- Patients with impaired vision and neuropathy cannot be relied upon to detect signs of infection such as cellulitis
- Lack of discharge does not necessarily mean that an ulcer is healed: it can indicate that callus has sealed it off, preventing drainage. If this happens the foot can deteriorate rapidly
- *Staphylococcus aureus* and *Streptococcus* group B in combination can act synergistically to produce a rapidly spreading infection.

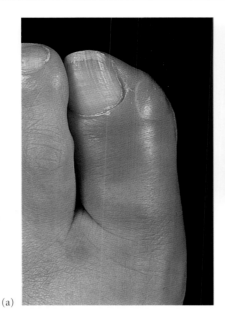

(a)

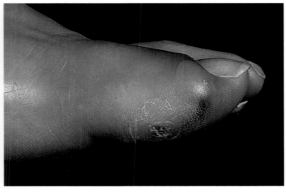

(b)

(c)

Fig. 5.9 (a) Cellulitis of the right hallux. (b) Cellulitis of the right hallux and a collection of pus under callus. (c) Callus debrided and pus drained.

Spreading infection

Sepsis has progressed to give signs of spreading infection emanating from the ulcer such as diffuse spreading erythema, oedema, lymphangitis and lymphadenitis and in addition, there will usually be local signs of infection as described above. In the erythematous skin, wrinkles disappear, and when the infection is resolving there is scaling.

The portal of entry of infection may be a corn, callus, blister, fissure or any other skin break. This condition should be treated with systemic antibiotics. It can sometimes be treated with intramuscular antibiotics and bedrest at the patient's home under close surveillance by relatives and frequent visits from the community nurse. However, where the cellulitis is extensive, or in the ischaemic foot, intravenous antibiotics and hospital admission will be needed for patients with spreading infection.

CASE STUDY
Lymphangitis in an Afro-Caribbean skin

A 35-year-old Afro-Caribbean woman with type 2 diabetes of 10 years' duration treated with insulin, and severe neuropathy with a vibration threshold at the hallux over 35 volts, presented unwell with nausea and shivering. She had no fever and felt no pain in the foot. She had noted an ulcer on her left 5th toe for the previous week but had not sought help because of the absence of pain. On examination she had an ulcer of the left 5th toe with a streak of lymphangitis spreading up the dorsum of the foot (Fig 5.10). This was not immediately obvious because of her dark skin, but was revealed on close inspection and comparison with the other foot. She was admitted to hospital and given intravenous amoxicillin 500 mg tds, flucloxacillin 500 mg qds, metronidazole 500 mg tds and ceftazidime 1 g tds. Ulcer swab grew *Staphylococcus aureus* and *Streptococcus* group B. Metronidazole and ceftazidime were stopped and amoxicillin and flucloxacillin continued. Infection resolved within 5 days, and she was discharged for follow-up in the diabetic foot clinic. The ulcer was shallow but took a month to heal.

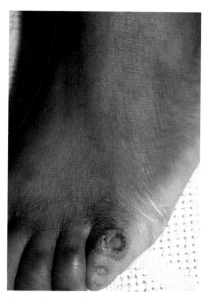

Fig. 5.10 Ulcer of the left 5th toe with a streak of lymphangitis spreading up the dorsum of the foot in an Afro-Caribbean woman.

Key points

- Lymphangitis is an important sign of spreading sepsis but may be obscured in a dark skin
- There may be no pyrexia and no pain in cases of spreading infection of the diabetic foot
- Absence of pain in response to infection leads to late presentations
- Infection retards healing.

CASE STUDY
Infection in a pregnant woman

A 32-year-old woman with type 1 diabetes of 19 years' duration, who was 28 weeks pregnant, noted a blister on the plantar aspect of the first toe associated with swelling and cellulitis (Fig 5.11a, b). The blister was drained to reveal an ulcer. Deep wound swab grew *Staphylococcus aureus*, *Streptococcus* group B and *Citrobacter koseri*. She had neuropathy but no ischaemia. She was admitted and given intravenous ceftriaxone 1 g daily and healed quickly (Fig. 5.11c). She was followed up in the diabetic foot clinic.

Key points

- Diabetic foot disease in pregnancy is rare: we have seen only four patients in 25 years
- Antibiotics that are safe in pregnancy are shown in Table 5.1

Table 5.1 Antibiotics that can be taken in pregnancy

The following antibiotics have no known association with birth defects or other pregnancy-related complications:

Amoxicillin
Co-amoxiclav
Flucloxacillin
Metronidazole (although there is some controversy about taking it by mouth in the first trimester)
Cephalosporins including cephalexin, cefadroxil and cefuroxime
Clindamycin
Erythromycin

Table 5.2 Antibiotics safe in breastfeeding

Amoxicillin
Azithromycin
Cefaclor
Cefuroxamine
Cephalexin
Cephradine
Clarithromycin
Co-amoxiclav
Co-fluampicil

Erythromycin

Flucloxacillin
Penicillin V

Trimethoprim

- Polymicrobial infections can occur in superficial infections
- Table 5.2 shows antibiotics that can be taken by breast-feeding women.

Severe infection

This refers to ulcers with extensive deep soft tissue infection and also infected feet with blue or purple discolouration of tissues. These people need intravenous antibiotics, immediate hospital admission and an urgent surgical opinion regarding the necessity of surgical drainage and, if the foot is neuroischaemic, appropriate assessments of the possibility of vascular reconstruction. This stage may also be associated with septicaemia, with the patient presenting with hypotension and organ failure.

In the presence of neuropathy pain and throbbing may be absent, but if present this is a danger sign, usually indicating serious infection with pus within the tissues. Palpation may reveal fluctuance, suggesting abscess formation. There may be bulging of the plantar surface of the

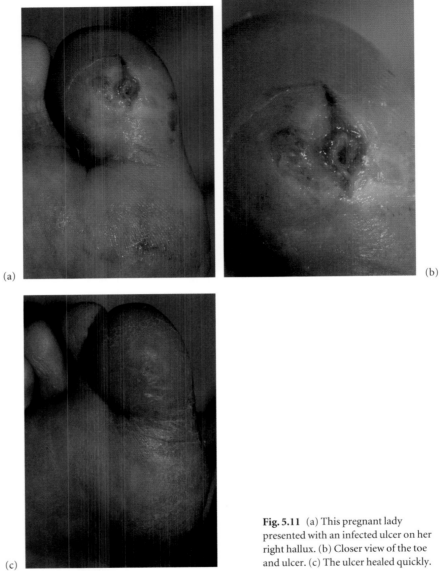

(a)

(b)

(c)

Fig. 5.11 (a) This pregnant lady presented with an infected ulcer on her right hallux. (b) Closer view of the toe and ulcer. (c) The ulcer healed quickly.

foot. Discrete abscesses are relatively uncommon in the infected diabetic foot. Often there is a generalized sloughing of the ulcer and surrounding subcutaneous tissues, which eventually liquefy and disintegrate. In late infection there is swelling and the tissues may be sloughing and breaking down and blistered, or fluctuant, and often never recover but become necrotic and need surgical removal.

Severe infection can also present as a blueish-purple discolouration when there is inadequate supply of oxygen to the soft tissues. This is caused by increased metabolic demands of infection and a reduction of blood flow to the skin, secondary to a septic vasculitis of the cutaneous circulation. Purple blebs may indicate subcutaneous necrosis. Blue discolouration can occur in both the neuropathic and also the neuroischaemic foot, particularly in the toes, and in the neuroischaemic foot must not be automatically attributed to worsening ischaemia.

Systemic symptoms and signs may be present in the patient with late infection whose foot has extensive diffuse cellulitis, deep soft tissue infection or blue discolouration. Signs of severe infection may include drowsiness, shivering, tachycardia, hypotension, reduced body temperature ($< 35°C$) or high fever ($> 40°C$).

However, systemic signs and symptoms are notoriously absent in many severe infections of the diabetic foot. Among patients hospitalized for late infections only 12–35% have significant fever and only 50% of episodes of severe cellulitis will provoke a fever or leucocytosis. However, when a fever is present it usually indicates a severe infection, and the deep spaces of the foot are usually involved with tissue necrosis, severe cellulitis and possible bacteraemia.

Severe infections are often polymicrobial and both Gram-positive and Gram-negative organisms are present together with anaerobes. Severe subcutaneous infection by Gram-negative and anaerobic organisms produces gas, which may be detected by palpating crepitus on the lower limb and can be seen on X-ray. The presence of gas does not automatically mean that the classical gas gangrene organism *Clostridium perfringens* is present.

CASE STUDY
Late infection associated with a cast rub

A 50-year-old man with type 1 diabetes for 30 years and a renal transplant, suffered a spontaneous rupture of his Achilles tendon and was treated in another hospital in a plaster cast. He noted staining from discharge within the cast and came up to the diabetic foot clinic. The cast was removed, revealing infected ulceration from the cast

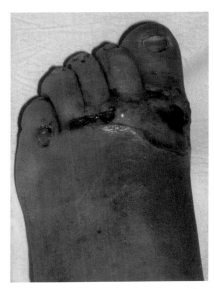

Fig. 5.12 This infection complicated a rub from a total contact cast.

rubbing against the foot (Fig. 5.12). He was admitted for intravenous antibiotics: amoxicillin 500 mg tds, flucloxacillin 500 mg qds, metronidazole 500 mg tds and ceftazidime 1 g tds. The deep wound swab grew *Staphylococcus aureus* and the antibiotics were reduced to flucloxacillin 500 mg qds. After the cellulitis settled, another cast was applied.

Key points
- People with type 1 diabetes and renal transplant with associated immunosupression may be particularly susceptible to ulceration and infection
- Practitioners should take extra care when casting diabetic patients with neuropathy
- Staining on casts is a valuable warning sign that should never be ignored
- Spontaneous rupture of the Achilles tendon is associated with diabetes and renal failure.

Severe infection may be associated with puncture wounds which are notoriously deceptive and may lead to very severe tissue loss if underestimated.

CASE STUDY
Infected puncture wound

A 55-year-old diabetic man with type 1 diabetes of 40 years' duration and rheumatoid arthritis for 10 years treated with sulphasalazine went on holiday and walked barefoot on the beach. He then noticed swelling of his heel, which also became painful. He was severely neuropathic and was unaware of having injured himself. He returned to our diabetic foot clinic where we noted erythema and swelling associated with a puncture injury (Fig. 5.13a–c).

He was admitted and treated initially with quadruple therapy: amoxicillin 500 mg tds, flucloxacillin 500 mg qds, metronidazole 500 mg tds and ceftazidime 1 g tds. X-rays were normal and did not show evidence of a radio-opaque foreign body. He was pyrexial and his C-reactive protein was elevated at 69.2 mg/L. Deep wound swab

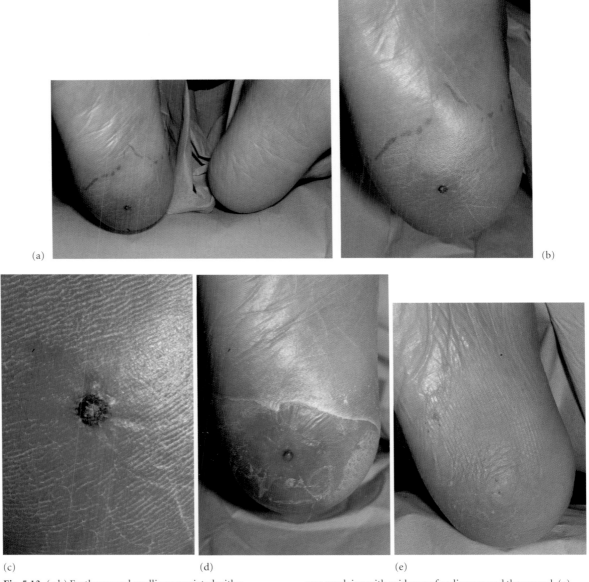

(a)

(b)

(c)

(d)

(e)

Fig. 5.13 (a,b) Erythema and swelling associated with a puncture injury. Initial limit of erythema delineated by pen markings. (c) Close-up view of puncture injury. (d) Ten days later, after treatment with intravenous antibiotics, the erythema was resolving with evidence of scaling around the wound. (e) One week further on, the cellulitis had resolved considerably and the puncture wound was healed.

grew *Staphylococcus aureus* and the antibiotics were reduced to flucloxacillin 500 mg qds. The multidisciplinary team discussed the necessity for surgical drainage. At that time he had no specific evidence of a collection of pus or osteomyelitis and it was decided to treat him conservatively but to review the situation on a daily basis. He made slow progress and the antibiotic was changed to clindamycin 600 mg qds. The erythema then slowly resolved and he was showing evidence of scaling around the wound (Fig. 5.13d). In view of his multiple immunosuppression by his diabetes, his rheumatoid arthritis and his sulphasalazine, it was decided to prolong his intravenous antibiotic therapy, and 1 week further on the cellulitis had resolved considerably and the puncture wound was healed (Fig. 5.13e).

Key points

- Diabetic patients are immunosuppressed and do not respond appropriately to infection. This is exacerbated when the patient has other autoimmune diseases or is on immunosuppressant therapy. Diabetic patients with foot infections in such circumstances demand very close surveillance
- The response to infection is delayed in such patients and they often need prolonged courses of intravenous antibiotics
- Puncture wounds are notoriously deceptive and should always be taken very seriously. A surgical opinion is essential. Practitioners should not be deceived by the seemingly trivial sign of a small puncture injury. Infection is often present at the base of the wound but then gradually takes hold. Puncture wounds often need admission as sepsis may be already apparent. Even when they are treated in the diabetic foot clinic and not admitted, these patients should be reviewed every 2 to 3 days, despite the benign appearance of their foot
- When dealing with puncture wounds always remember the mighty volcano, Krakatoa!

CASE STUDY
Late infection following 'bathroom surgery'

This was a case of severe infection caused by 'bathroom surgery' in a 60-year-old patient with type 2 diabetes of 15 years' duration who tried to cut his own nails. He cut a chunk of tissue out of his toe along with the nail and ignored the injury for a week. When he finally reached the clinic, referred by his general practitioner with sepsis, he lay on the couch and exhibited classic 'belle indifference', being quite unconcerned. However, there was cellulitis and swelling of the dorsum of the foot and first toe (Fig. 5.14a,b) with ulceration of the apex of the toe (Fig. 5.14c). His wound swabs grew *Staphylococcus aureus* and *Klebsiella*. He was neuroischaemic and, unusually, had iliac disease. He was a smoker. He was admitted, initially treated with our usual intravenous quadruple regime: amoxicillin 500 mg tds, flucloxacillin 500 mg qds, metronidazole 500 mg tds and ceftazidime 1 g tds and this was rationalized to flucloxacillin and ceftazidime when the results of culture were available. He underwent angioplasty of the iliac arteries. The cellulitis quickly resolved and he was followed up in the diabetic foot clinic; the toe healed within 6 weeks.

Key points

- Belle indifference is common in patients with neuropathy
- High-risk diabetic patients should not be expected to cut their own nails and should be warned of the dangers of undertaking 'bathroom surgery'
- Although tibial disease is the most prevalent form of peripheral arterial disease in diabetes, iliac disease is occasionally found in diabetic patients, particularly in smokers. It responds very well to angioplasty and also stenting.

CASE STUDY
Hidden depths—unsuspected soft tissue infection complicating apparently superficial heel ulceration under callus

A 56-year-old man with type 2 diabetes of 12 years' duration and peripheral neuropathy trod on a nail while walking barefoot. The wound healed after 6 days, but the heel developed a callus which became painful after 2 weeks so he sought advice from the diabetic foot clinic. The callus was debrided and the underlying skin appeared to show superficial ulceration only (Fig. 5.15a). However, when the heel was palpated the patient complained of pain, and careful inspection revealed a deep sinus from which a bead of pus could be expressed (Fig. 5.15b). He was admitted for intravenous antibiotics, a surgical opinion was sought and he underwent extensive operative debridement of infected sloughy tissue the same day (Fig. 5.15c). The large residual defect healed after 7 months (Fig. 5.15d).

Key points

- Puncture wounds can lead to deep infections
- Pain on palpation in the ulcerated neuropathic foot is often a symptom of severe underlying infection

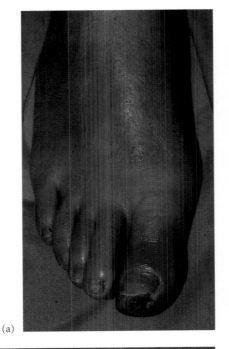

(a)

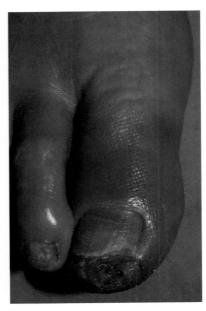

(b)

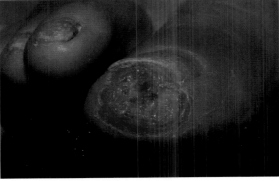

(c)

Fig. 5.14 (a) Cellulitis of the dorsum of the foot and 1st toe. (b) Close-up view of the cellulitic 1st toe. (c) Ulceration of the apex of the 1st toe.

- Careful palpation may express pus and reveal a deep sinus
- Puncture wounds may be complicated by cellulitis and lead to this presentation. Bacteria are inoculated at the base of the puncture wound and then track back towards the surface of the skin, with infection eventually manifesting itself as a cellulitis and extensive deep soft tissue infection.

All diabetic foot infections, whether localized, spreading or severe, can develop and progress with great rapidity, and for this reason we advocate daily checking of all diabetic foot ulcers by the patient or carer. Furthermore, any

of the above three presentations may be complicated by underlying osteomyelitis.

Osteomyelitis

Clinically, osteomyelitis may be suspected when a sterile probe inserted into the base of the ulcer penetrates to bone. This may happen in an apparently clean, uninfected ulcer, but osteomyelitis must still be suspected. X-ray and magnetic resonance imaging (MRI) are helpful in the diagnosis of osteomyelitis, which may be confirmed in theory by a positive bone culture or bone biopsy showing bone death, inflammation and repair. Bone biopsy is

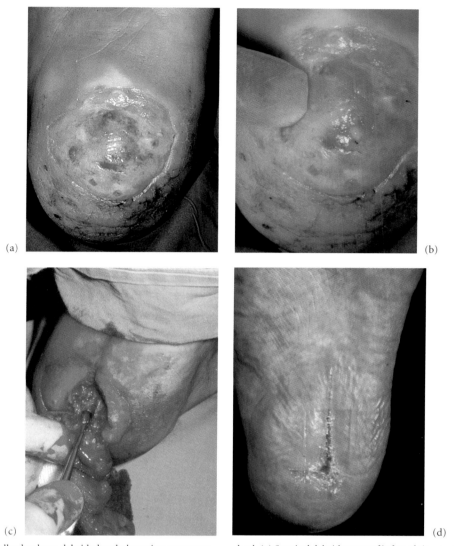

Fig. 5.15 (a) Callus has been debrided and ulceration appears to be shallow. (b) Palpation extrudes a bead of pus from deep in the heel. (c) Surgical debridement of infected tissues. (d) The foot healed after surgical debridement.

often not very practical, and then the diagnosis is made on clinical and radiological grounds.

- Osteomyelitis should be suspected when a sterile probe penetrates to bone. Usually osteomyelitis will present in association with soft tissue infection. Occasionally it may present as probing to bone in an apparently clean, non-infected ulcer. It may present as obvious fragmentation of the bone within the ulcer bed which is easily visible

- It is most commonly diagnosed on X-ray (Fig. 5.16a,b). Loss of cortex, fragmentation and bony destruction on X-ray are signs of osteomyelitis. These changes may take 10–14 days to develop
- MRI is the best imaging technique to diagnose osteomyelitis and can demonstrate oedema and abscesses in bone. However bone oedema may also be present in Charcot's osteoarthropathy
- Chronic osteomyelitis of a toe has a swollen, red, sausage-like appearance (Fig. 5.17).

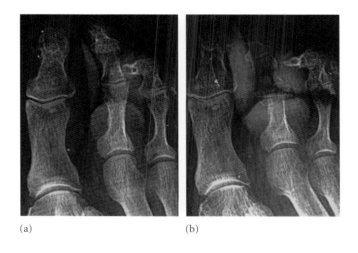

(a)   (b)

Fig. 5.16 (a) The X-ray shows intact distal phalanx of the 2nd toe. (b) Destruction of the distal phalanx 2 weeks later indicative of osteomyelitis.

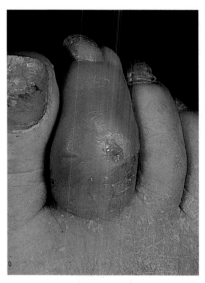

Fig. 5.17 'Sausage toe' with ulceration and cellulitis indicates osteomyelitis.

Rarely, we have seen metastatic infection from a primary infection in the foot.

CASE STUDY
Bacterial discitis of the lumbar spine as a complication of longstanding neuropathic ulceration in a foot with Charcot's osteoarthropathy

A 55-year-old man with insulin-treated type 2 diabetes of 15 years' duration, peripheral neuropathy and impaired liver function due to previous hepatitis B infection presented late with acute Charcot's osteoarthropathy of the right foot. Two years subsequently he developed neuropathic ulceration of the left 2nd toe. The ulcer became infected and he was admitted to hospital for intravenous antibiotics and underwent a ray amputation. He was discharged after 3 weeks. His left foot became red, swollen and warm, and Charcot's osteoarthropathy was diagnosed. He declined a total-contact cast but said that he would rest the foot as much as possible. (Two nights later one of the authors saw him in Central London at a Promenade Concert hiding behind a pillar so as not to be seen and reprimanded for not resting!) He developed a rocker-bottom deformity with a neuropathic ulcer over the bony prominence, and re-presented with severe infection and spreading cellulitis. He was admitted for intravenous antibiotics and surgical debridement of the foot, with removal of infected soft tissue (Fig. 5.18). Three months later, he complained of severe pain in the region of his lumbar spine. An MRI scan revealed infection of the disc between the 4th and 5th lumbar vertebrae, which was treated with long-term antibiotics and resolved.

Key points
- Metastatic infection can develop from a primary infection in the foot
- Presentation of metastatic infection may be delayed.

Differential diagnosis of the cellulitic foot

Charcot's osteoarthropathy and cellulitis
It is important to distinguish between the red, hot, swollen foot of Charcot's osteoarthropathy and the red, hot,

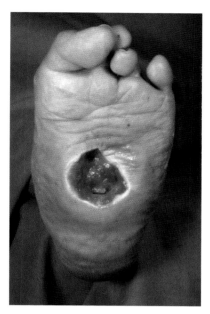

Fig. 5.18 The patient has undergone surgical debridement of his infected foot with rocker-bottom deformity and plantar ulceration.

swollen cellulitic foot. The oedema of Charcot's osteoarthropathy responds more rapidly to elevation than does that of the infected foot. In a recent series of 25 Charcot feet with acute presentation, C-reactive protein (CRP) was normal in 50% of the cases and only moderately elevated in the remainder. Thus a normal or only slightly raised CRP in a patient with a red, hot, swollen foot is suggestive of Charcot's osteoarthropathy. Infection and Charcot's osteoarthropathy can sometimes be present together in the same foot. If in doubt, treat for both.

CASE STUDY
Relapse of Charcot's osteoarthropathy or infection?

A 60-year-old woman with type 1 diabetes of 42 years' duration who had bilateral Charcot's osteoarthropathy affecting both feet and 12 years' previous history of ulcers and infections, was referred to the foot clinic with a hot, swollen left ankle and erythema over the medial malleolus. Both her feet were intact. The left foot was very painful on weightbearing. A provisional diagnosis of infection was made although we could not be sure that this was not a relapse of Charcot's osteoarthropathy. She

was given intravenous vancomycin 1 g bd, ceftazidime 1 g tds, metronidazole 500 mg tds and oral fucidin 500 mg tds as she had recently had an MRSA infection. The ankle initially appeared to settle, but after 3 days she developed severe pain in the left foot and ankle at rest, with a fever of 39°C and rigors. She went to theatre and a soft tissue abscess communicating with the subtalar joint was drained. A swab showed pus cells but no growth. She healed in 4 months, but came back to the foot clinic again with a severely infected toe on her other foot after 2 weeks.

Key points
- Patients with Charcot's osteoarthropathy can occasionally relapse with increased swelling and warmth of the involved foot
- It may be difficult to distinguish between relapsed Charcot's osteoarthropathy and infection in an intact foot. If in doubt, treat for both
- Clinical progress needs to be closely monitored with daily review for specific signs of infection

Ischaemia and cellulitis
In the neuroischaemic foot, it may be difficult to differentiate between the erythema of cellulitis and the redness of ischaemia. It is helpful to elevate the leg. The redness of ischaemia is usually cold and is most marked on dependency: it will disappear upon elevation of the limb, whereas cellulitis will remain. The erythema associated with inflammation is warm, although a very ischaemic foot may become deceptively warm when it is infected.

Erythema also occurs secondary to traumas, including insect stings, where it is associated with histamine release.

Investigations

Microbiological investigations
We believe that it is important to make a microbiological diagnosis and ascertain the organisms that are responsible for the infection. This involves either taking a deep ulcer swab or tissue scrapings after debridement. It is preferable to obtain a tissue specimen and this is relatively straightforward in a neuropathic foot. However, in a neuroischaemic foot, taking a tissue specimen is more difficult, especially when tissue perfusion is severely limited. In these circumstances, an ulcer swab taken after debridement is acceptable and can still give valuable results.

How to take a deep ulcer swab/curettings:
- The ulcer is debrided of surrounding callus and superficial slough
- The ulcer is washed out with sterile normal saline
- The base of the wound is then scraped with a scalpel blade and the scrapings sent for culture without delay. If scraping is not possible then a deep swab is taken from the base of the ulcer.

If the patient subsequently undergoes operative debridement, then deep infected tissue rather than a swab should be sent to the laboratory.

Bone fragments removed by debridement should be sent for culture.

Blood cultures should also be taken if there is fever and systemic toxicity.

Laboratory investigations

Blood should be taken for:
- Full blood count
- Urea, creatinine and electrolytes
- Liver function tests
- C-reactive protein (CRP).

Although the white blood count is only raised in 50% of infections, we find that the CRP is nearly always elevated in diabetic foot infections and is a valuable guide to the severity of infection and a useful way of judging a positive response to treatment.

Radiological investigations

With all the above presentations of infection, it is important to X-ray the foot to detect
- Signs of osteomyelitis
- Gas in the deep tissues
- Radio-opaque foreign body.

In the initial stages of osteomyelitis, X-ray may be normal. Signs of osteomyelitis such as localized loss of bone density or cortical outline may not be apparent for at least 14 days.

MRI may be useful to look for the presence of osteomyelitis and also to detect collections of fluid in the foot. Intravenous injection of gadolinium-containing contrast agent heightens the sensitivity of the diagnosis of these clinical features. However, this contrast should not be used in patients with renal failure. The sequences employed in MRI for detection of soft tissue and bony abnormalities may include T1, short tau inversion recovery (STIR) and postgadolinium with fat suppression.

T1 sequence

This shows pathology in specific anatomy. Bone marrow which is normal is bright, and abnormal marrow is dark.

STIR sequence

Normal marrow is dark. Abnormal marrow is bright. Fluid collections become bright.

Postgadolinium with fat suppression sequence

Gadolinium concentrates in areas of inflammation and results in a hyperintense signal on T1 images. As fat is hyperintense on T1 sequence, images are acquired using a fat suppression technique. Normal marrow in the foot is predominantly composed of fat. Thus it is hypointense on the fat-suppressed images. Any bright or high signal after injection of gadolinium with fat suppression technique applied represents a focus of inflammation.

The main MRI finding in osteomyelitis is an abnormal marrow signal which is dark on T1 images and bright on STIR images. After injection of gadolinium the abnormal marrow enhances as shown by a bright focus on the fat suppressed T1 images. Further signs of osteomyelitis include cortical disruption and periosteal reaction. An MRI which is negative excludes osteomyelitis.

An abscess presents as a focal low T1 signal but a high STIR lesion. Following the injection of gadolinium on fat suppressed T1 images there is a low signal in the centre of the abscess.

However, MRI has notable limitations. MRI of the septic diabetic foot can show a number of false-positive diagnoses. An abnormal marrow signal can be seen with Charcot's osteoarthropathy and fractures. The acute phase of Charcot's osteoarthropathy may show the same enhancing marrow oedema that is impossible to separate from osteomyelitis.

CASE STUDY
MRI and osteomyelitis

A 55-year-old man with type 2 diabetes of 15 years' duration had ulceration of the right first hallux and surgical debridement in which part of the proximal phalanx was removed. Postoperatively the wound did not heal. X-ray showed slight irregularity of the cortex of the proximal phalanx (Fig. 5.19a). MRI was carried out. This showed essentially a normal response on T1 (Fig. 5.19b) and STIR sequences (Fig. 5.19c), and the gadolinium sequence (Fig. 5.19d) did not show increased uptake. He was continued on his antibiotics but the ulcer did not heal and X-ray (Fig. 5.19e) was repeated after a further 8 weeks. This showed increasing cortical irregularity and MRI now showed definite signs of osteomyelitis (Fig. 5.19f,g) with increased uptake of gadolinium in the proximal phalanx (Fig. 5.19h). The patient then underwent further surgery to remove the infected bone and the wound healed.

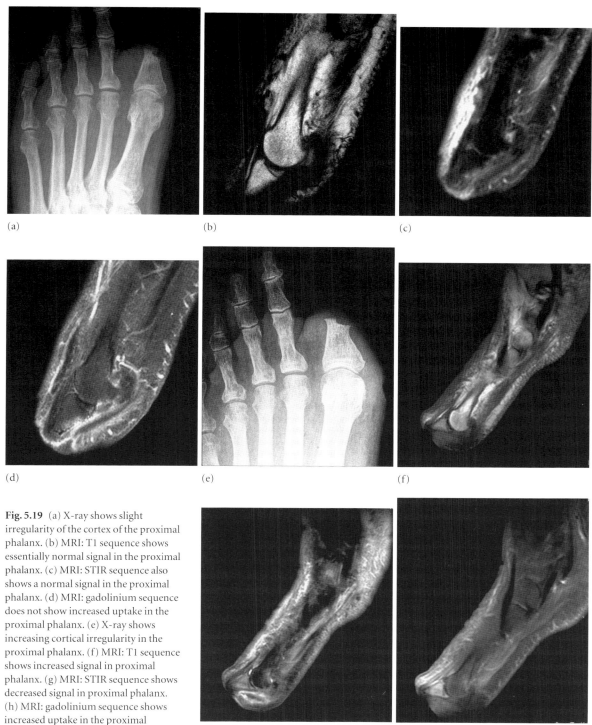

Fig. 5.19 (a) X-ray shows slight irregularity of the cortex of the proximal phalanx. (b) MRI: T1 sequence shows essentially normal signal in the proximal phalanx. (c) MRI: STIR sequence also shows a normal signal in the proximal phalanx. (d) MRI: gadolinium sequence does not show increased uptake in the proximal phalanx. (e) X-ray shows increasing cortical irregularity in the proximal phalanx. (f) MRI: T1 sequence shows increased signal in proximal phalanx. (g) MRI: STIR sequence shows decreased signal in proximal phalanx. (h) MRI: gadolinium sequence shows increased uptake in the proximal phalanx.

Key points

- When an ulcer is not healing, underlying osteomyelitis should be suspected
- When X-ray does give a definite diagnosis of osteomyelitis, MRI is a useful investigation to detect infection in the bone
- Prolonged antibiotic therapy can be successful in treating osteomyelitis but when the ulcer does not heal after a 3-month course of antibiotics and there is evidence of osteomyelitis on imaging then the infected bone should be removed surgically.

CASE STUDY
Diabetic foot infection and MRI

A 62-year-old man with type 2 diabetes of 3 years' duration developed an ulcer of the right 1st toe which had been present for 6 months when first seen in the foot clinic. He then had cellulitis and a markedly swollen 1st toe. X-ray was normal. Deep wound swab revealed *Streptococcus* group B. He was treated with amoxicillin 500 mg tds and gentamicin 5 mg/kg daily, both intravenously. The temperature resolved but the cellulitis was slow to improve. Because of the persistent swelling of the right 1st ray, the patient underwent an MRI to assess the presence of osteomyelitis and a possible collection of fluid. The images were T1, and STIR and T1 postgadolinium with fat suppression to assess presence of fluid collections. There was oedema within the marrow of the head of the 1st metatarsal. There was cortical loss on its volar aspect and enhancement of the marrow in this region (Fig. 5.20a,b). This indicated osteomyelitis of the metatarsal head.

There was a small collection of fluid between the extensor hallucis longus tendon and the metatarsophalangeal joint/proximal phalanx of the big toe (Fig. 5.20c–e). The decision whether to debride the foot and carry out a 1st ray amputation was difficult but in view of the resolution of his fever (Fig. 5.20f) and the improvement in the soft tissues clinically, intravenous antibiotic therapy was continued and the patient's ulcer eventually healed without surgery.

Key points

- It is difficult to diagnose osteomyelitis in the cellulitic foot as the X-ray is often initially normal
- MRI can indicate signs of marrow oedema which suggest osteomyelitis
- Group B *Streptococcus* is an important pathogen in the diabetic foot. It may need aggressive treatment with high-dose penicillin therapy such as amoxicillin 1 g tds.

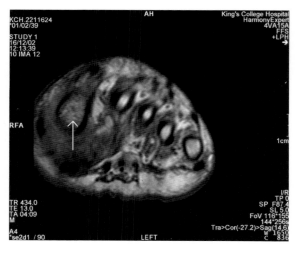

(a)

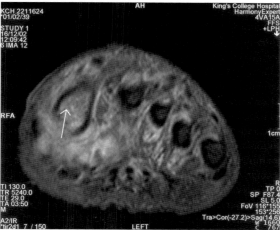

(b)

Fig 5.20 (a) T1 sequence shows reduced signal in 1st metatarsal head compared with other metatarsal heads. (b) Increased uptake on STIR sequence in 1st metatarsal head compared with other metatarsal heads. (Courtesy of Dr David Elias.)

In severe cases, gentamicin 5 mg/kg daily can be added for synergy
- Osteomyelitis may be managed conservatively, especially when the soft tissue sepsis is responding to intravenous antibiotic therapy.

CASE STUDY
Extensive deep soft tissue infection with abscess revealed by MRI

A 65-year-old man with type 2 diabetes of 10 years' duration tripped and fell on the pavement. He had no pain at

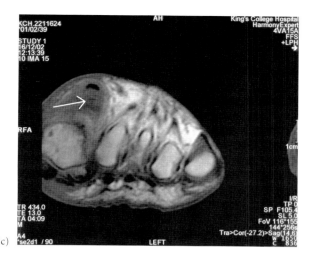

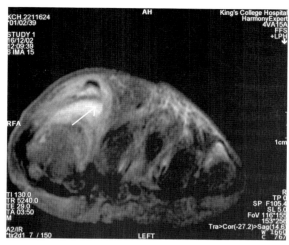

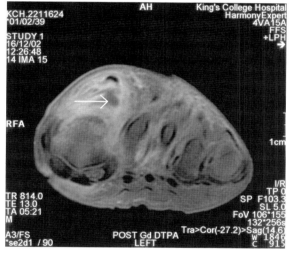

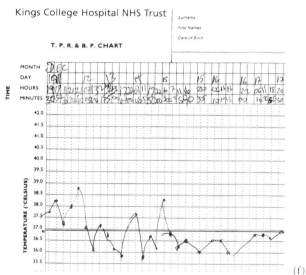

Fig. 5.20 (*cont'd*) (c) MRI T1 sequence shows normal uptake in soft tissues under extensor hallucis longus tendon. (d) Increased uptake on STIR sequence. (e) A small collection of fluid under the extensor hallucis longus tendon (postgadolinium). (f) Temperature chart showing resolution of fever.

the time but he noticed swelling the next day and was sent for an X-ray by his general practitioner. The X-ray revealed that he had fractured the necks of his left 2nd, 3rd and 4th metatarsals and he was treated with a below-knee walking plaster. He sustained ulceration on the plantar surface of the foot over the 2nd and 3rd metatarsal heads and the cast was removed. He was referred to the diabetic foot clinic. The left foot was swollen and cellulitic and he had rigors. Clinically there was no obvious abscess, but he had a fever. A deep wound swab grew *Staphylococcus*

aureus. He was treated with intravenous amoxicillin 500 mg tds, flucloxacillin 500 mg qds, metronidazole 500 mg tds and ceftazidime 1 g tds. His left foot remained oedematous with pus discharging from the plantar lesion. He became increasingly unwell and went into renal failure. An MRI then showed an inflammatory mass with communication through to the plantar surface of the foot at metatarsophalangeal joint level. On the dorsal aspect of the foot a fluid collection was seen suggesting an abscess (Fig. 5.21a–c). He underwent surgical debridement and

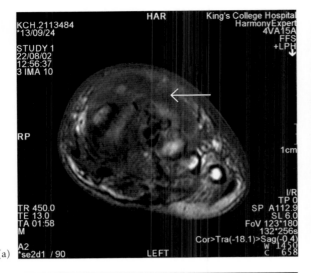

(a)

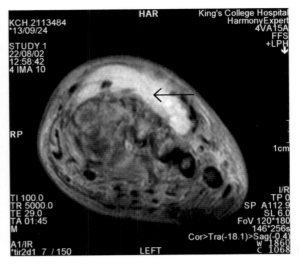

(b)

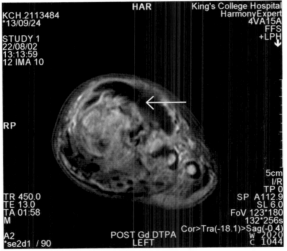

(c)

Fig. 5.21 (a) T1 sequence shows inflammatory mass but normal uptake in dorsum of foot. (b) High uptake in the dorsum on STIR sequence. (c) Collection of fluid on the dorsum (postgadolinium). (With thanks to Dr David Elias and Dr Huw Walters.)

20 mL of pus was drained from the foot. Postoperatively he needed haemodialysis but the swelling of the foot gradually improved, and the ulcer healed. His renal function improved and he came off dialysis.

Key points

- Deep infection with soft tissue involvement can be associated with severe systemic upset and in some cases with renal failure
- The decision to carry out surgical debridement of a diabetic foot is a difficult one. It is often made on clinical grounds alone. The main indications are an abscess or extensive sloughing of subcutaneous tissue
- An MRI may be helpful in locating fluid collections.

MANAGEMENT OF INFECTION

Infection in the diabetic foot needs full multidisciplinary treatment. It is vital to achieve:

- Microbiological control
- Wound control
- Vascular control
- Mechanical control
- Metabolic control
- Educational control.

Microbiological control

The aim of this section is to enable clinicians to make

rapid and effective decisions regarding the management of infection in the diabetic neuropathic and neuro-ischaemic foot, and to control it rapidly.

The key questions that need to be answered for each individual patient with infection are as follows:
- Which antibiotics should be prescribed?
- Will antibiotics alone control the infection or will surgery also be necessary?

Principles of antibiotic treatment
- The microbiology of the diabetic foot is unique. Infection can be caused by Gram-positive aerobic, and Gram-negative aerobic and anaerobic bacteria, singly or in combination (Table 5.3)
- As there may be a poor immune response from the diabetic patient, even bacteria normally regarded as skin commensals may cause severe tissue damage. This includes Gram-negative organisms such as *Citrobacter, Serratia, Pseudomonas* and *Acinetobacter*. When Gram-negative bacteria are isolated from a deep ulcer swab or curettings they should not, therefore, be regarded as automatically insignificant
- When a positive culture is found, it is then possible to focus antibiotic therapy according to sensitivities of the bacteria cultured (Table 5.4)
- However, at initial presentation we believe that it is important to prescribe a wide spectrum of antibiotics for three reasons:
  (a) it is impossible to predict the number and type of organisms from the clinical presentation
  (b) there is no way of predicting who will develop a rapidly ascending infection which becomes limb-threatening and even life-threatening
  (c) diabetic patients are immunosuppressed. The neuropathy and ischaemia of the diabetic foot reduces the local resistance to invading bacteria. As Louis Pasteur said: 'The germ is nothing. It is the terrain in which it grows that is everything'.

Table 5.3 Bacteria isolated from the diabetic foot

Gram-positive	Gram-negative
Staphylococcus aureus	*Klebsiella*
Streptococcus	*Escherichia coli*
Enterococcus	*Enterobacter*
	Pseudomonas
Anaerobes	*Citrobacter*
Bacteroides	*Morganella morganii*
Clostridium	*Serratia*
Peptostreptococcus	*Acinetobacter*
Peptococcus	*Proteus*

Duration of antibiotic therapy will depend on the clinical progress of the foot and ulcer, tissues involved, severity of the initial infection and also on individual factors relating to the patient.

The route by which therapy is given will depend on the severity of the infection. We use oral therapy for localized infections, intramuscular or intravenous therapy for spreading infections and intravenous therapy for severe infections. Intestinal absorption is unreliable in these circumstances.

It is important to have a working knowledge of the principal bacteria and their local antibiotic sensitivities including awareness of the prevalence of resistant organisms. However, in every patient, individual sensitivities of each organism isolated on culture should be sought to guide rational antibiotic therapy. There should be close cooperation between the microbiology laboratory and the diabetic foot service.

Staphylococcus aureus
This is the commonest pathogen in the diabetic foot and flucloxacillin is the ideal treatment. Clindamycin can also be used but beware of antibiotic-induced colitis especially in the elderly and postoperative patients. Erythromycin may increase the risk of myositis from statin therapy. When taking erythromycin, patients should be advised to stop their statin therapy temporarily.

Rifampicin and fucidin are also good antistaphylococcal agents, but they should not be given alone as resistance will develop rapidly. They should each be accompanied by a further antistaphylococcal agent.

Methicillin-resistant Staphylococcus aureus (MRSA)
MRSA is associated with the whole spectrum of clinical presentations of diabetic foot infections and commonly occurs in patients who have been in hospital. It can be simply a commensal with no signs of invasive infection but it can also cause severe infections, osteomyelitis and bacteraemia. The frequency of MRSA infections is increasing in the diabetic foot. However, MRSA infections are not necessarily more pathogenic than conventional *Staphylococcus aureus* infections. They do frequently cause more extensive tissue destruction because they are often not diagnosed until late. This is an important reason to maintain frequent bacteriological surveillance on all ulcers in diabetic feet. Hospital-acquired MRSA is multi-resistant to all beta lactam antibiotics and to a varying extent, macrolides, fluoroquinolones and aminoglycosides.

There is a new strain of MRSA that is found in the community, so-called community-acquired MRSA. This has

Table 5.4 Antibiotics for treating the infected foot

Microorganism	Antibiotic treatment	
	Oral	IV
Staphylococcus aureus	Flucloxacillin 500 mg qds Sodium fusidate 500 mg tds Clindamycin 300 mg tds Rifampicin 300 mg tds	Flucloxacillin 500 mg qds Gentamicin 5 mg/kg/day (according to levels) Clindamycin 150–600 mg qds
Methicillin-resistant *Staphylococcus aureus* (MRSA)	Sodium fusidate 500 mg tds Trimethoprim 200 mg bd Rifampicin 300 mg tds Linezolid 600 mg bd	Vancomycin 1 g bd (according to levels) Teicoplanin 400 mg daily Linezolid 600 mg bd Tigecycline initially 100 mg then 50 mg bd Daptomycin 4 mg/kg once daily Quinupristin/dalfopristin 7.5 mg/kg/8 hrly
	Doxycycline 100 mg daily (first dose 200 mg)	
Streptococcus	Amoxicillin 500 mg tds Flucloxacillin 500 mg qds Clindamycin 300 mg tds Erythromycin 500 mg qds	Amoxicillin 500 mg tds Clindamycin 150–600 mg qds
Enterococcus	Amoxicillin 500 mg tds	Amoxicillin 500 mg tds Vancomycin 1 g bd (according to levels)
Anaerobes	Metronidazole 400 mg tds Clindamycin 300 mg tds	Metronidazole 500 mg tds Clindamycin 150–600 mg qds
Coliforms (*E. coli*, *Proteus*, *Klebsiella*, *Enterobacter*)	Ciprofloxacin 500 mg bd Cefadroxil 1 g bd Trimethoprim 200 mg bd	Ciprofloxacin 200 mg bd Ceftazidime 1–2 g tds Ceftriaxone 1–2 g daily Gentamicin 5 mg/kg/day (according to levels) Piperacillin–tazobactam 4.5 g tds Meropenem 500 mg–1 g tds Ticarcillin/clavulanate 3.2 g tds Ertapenem 1 g daily Tigecycline initially 100 mg then 50 mg bd
Pseudomonas	Ciprofloxacin 500 mg bd	Ceftazidime 1–2 g tds Gentamicin 5 mg/kg/day (according to levels) Piperacillin–tazobactam 4.5 g tds Meropenem 500 mg–1 g tds Ticarcillin/clavulanate 3.2 g tds
Stenotrophomonas maltophilia	Trimethoprim/sulphmethoxazole 960 mg bd	Trimethoprim/sulphmethoxazole 960 mg bd Ticarcillin/clavulanate 3.2 g tds

bd, twice daily; tds, three times daily; qds, four times daily.
Intramuscular antibiotics.
Ceftriaxone 1 g daily im to treat Gram-positives and Gram-negatives.
Teicoplanin 400 mg daily im to treat Gram-positives including MRSA.
Teicoplanin initially should be given as 400 mg 12 hourly for three doses, as a loading regimen.
Imipenem w. cilastatin 500 mg bd im to treat Gram-positives, Gram-negatives and anaerobes.
Ertapenem 1 g in 3.2 mL of 1% lidocaine daily.

been associated with outbreaks in groups of individuals with close contact in institutions such as prisons but can then be transferred to hospitals. These MRSA do not have the multi-resistance of the hospital-acquired MRSA but nevertheless can rapidly progress to severe infections. Approximately two-thirds possess the Panton-Valentine leukocidin (PVL) toxin, which acts to form pores in the cell membrane of mononuclear cells and polymorpho-nuclear cells and can lead to severe tissue necrosis. Also beware that one-third of hospital-acquired MRSA can express the PVL toxin.

MRSA can lead to invasive infection and in these circumstances it is best to give vancomycin intravenously with dosage to be adjusted according to serum levels, or teicoplanin. These antibiotics may need to be accompanied by either sodium fusidate or rifampicin orally. Linezolid is also active against MRSA and has good soft tissue and bony penetration. It is well absorbed. It is necessary, however, to check the platelet count regularly as there may be some marrow suppression with this antibiotic. Courses should not exceed 28 days. The combination of antibiotics quinupristin and dalfopristin can be used when an MRSA infection has not responded to other antibacterials. Daptomycin and tigecycline may also be used in MRSA infections. MRSA can also be treated with clindamycin but sensitivity needs to be confirmed as MRSA resistance to clindamycin has emerged. If MRSA is isolated in localized infections, oral therapy can be given with two of the following: sodium fusidate 500 mg tds, rifampicin 300 mg tds, trimethoprim 200 mg bd or doxycycline 100 mg daily, according to sensitivities.

Streptococcus group A, B, C, E, F and G

Streptococcus group B is the commonest and can cause severe infection in the diabetic foot although C, E, F and G can infect the foot. *Streptococcus* group A rarely causes infection but when it does it causes a severe blistering cellulitis and tissue destruction.

The *Streptococcus milleri* group of organisms are beta haemolytic streptococci that can cause abcesses in the foot.

Streptococci can be treated with amoxicillin. Clinda-mycin, rifampicin and erythromycin may also be also active against streptococci.

Enterococcus

Enterococcus faecalis is rarely pathogenic. It may be selected out by cephalosporin treatment. If it is causing definite infection then it may be treated with amoxicillin. *Enterococcus faecium* may need vancomycin.

Vancomycin-resistant enterococcus (VRE) is a problem with hospitalized patients previously treated with antibiotics (especially patients in renal failure). It is necessary to assess whether it is actually causing tissue destruction as it is normally not pathogenic. However, in the immuno-compromised diabetic patient, especially in the ischaemic foot, it may be responsible for infection and should therefore be treated with appropriate antibiotics as suggested by culture sensitivities.

Anaerobes

These are commonly found in deep infections but anaerobes are also a feature of many chronic wounds even when they are superficial. They are associated with necrotic wounds. Anaerobes can act synergistically with Gram-positive and Gram-negative aerobes to cause severe tissue destruction.

Metronidazole is the treatment of choice. Clinda-mycin and co-amoxiclav (amoxicillin/clavulanic acid) also have anti-anaerobic activity. Meropenem, piperacillin/tazobactam and ertapenem are also active against anaerobes.

Gram-negative organisms

Klebsiella, Escherichia coli, Proteus, Enterobacter, Citrobacter, Serratia and other Gram-negative bacteria can be definitely pathogenic in the diabetic foot especially when they are in a pure growth or as part of a polymicrobial deep infection. Oral agents that are available to treat Gram-negatives are ciprofloxacin and trimethoprim. Parenteral agents include ceftazidime, aminoglycosides, meropenem, piperacillin/tazobactam, ticarcillin/clavulanate, tigecycline and ertapenem. It is crucial to obtain sensitivity patterns with Gram-negative organisms and not depend on empirical therapy alone.

Recently, Gram-negative bacteria have acquired various resistance patterns through the development of certain enzymes and this is relevant to the choice of antibiotic therapy.

Organisms have developed extended-spectrum beta lactamases which are known as ESBLs. By this means, they have developed resistance to extended-spectrum (third generation) cephalosporins (e.g. ceftazidime, cefotaxime, and ceftriaxone) but not to carbapenems (e.g. meropenem or imipenem). ESBL enzymes are most commonly produced by two bacteria: *Escherichia coli* and *Klebsiella pneumoniae*. Another group of lactamases are AmpC β-lactamases, which are typically encoded on the chromosomes of many Gram-negative bacteria including *Citrobacter, Serratia and Enterobacter* species where expression is usually inducible.

Thus, organisms considered susceptible by *in vitro* testing can become resistant during treatment with cephalosporins. Carbapenems are the only reliable beta lactam drugs for the treatment of severe *Enterobacter* infections.

Pseudomonas

There are many members of the genus *Pseudomonas*. *Pseudomonas aeruginosa* is an important human opportunist bacterium in the diabetic foot. It can be responsible for a spectrum of presentations from superficial colonization of ulcers to extensive tissue damage, including osteomyelitis, septic arthritis and bacteraemia. It may be sensitive to ciprofloxacin as an oral agent. Otherwise parenteral therapy is necessary and includes ceftazidime, aminoglycosides, meropenem, piperacillin/tazobactam, and ticarcillin/clavulanate.

CASE STUDY
Necrosis caused by pseudomonal infection

A 45-year-old woman with type 1 diabetes of 20 years' duration and renal failure treated by haemodialysis, and a previous right below-knee amputation also had marked oedema of her left leg, which was particularly noticeable just before dialysis. She had observed areas of blackened skin (Fig. 5.22). The cause of this was not obvious but swabs were taken and showed pure growth of *Pseudomonas aeruginosa*. She received anti-pseudomonal therapy consisting of gentamicin and ceftazidime and the lesions slowly resolved.

Key points

- Discolouration due to *Pseudomonas* is usually green but it can also cause blackening of the infected tissues which have become necrotic

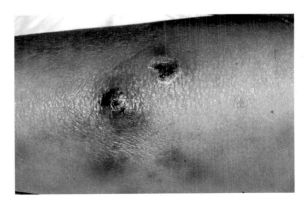

Fig. 5.22 Blackened areas of skin caused by infection with *Pseudomonas aeruginosa*.

- *Pseudomonas* is often regarded as a commensal and is thought not to cause tissue destruction in the diabetic foot. However, we have seen many cases of pseudomonal infections which have needed focused antibiotic therapy to achieve healing
- As *Pseudomonas* can have a high resistance to antibiotics, cultures are essential to achieve appropriate antibiotic therapy.

Stenotrophomonas maltophilia

This Gram-negative bactera is found in aqueous environments. It was initially classified as *Pseudomonas maltophilia*. It has now become the type species of the genus *Stenotrophomonas*. It is resistant to many broad-spectrum antibiotics (including all carbapenems), and is usually resistant to aminoglycosides, antipseudomonal penicillins, and antipseudomonal third-generation cephalosporins. It often acts as a colonizer. However, if isolated from a purulent wound, *S. maltophilia* may be the cause of the patient's wound infection. Many strains of *S. maltophilia* are sensitive to co-trimoxazole and ticarcillin/clavulanate.

Practical notes on antibiotics used in the diabetic foot infections
Antibiotics used mainly against Gram-positive organisms
Amoxicillin

This antibiotic is active against streptococci but is inactivated by penicillinases that are produced by *Staphylococcus aureus* and by Gram-negative bacteria such as *Escherichia coli*.

Co-amoxiclav

This is a combination of amoxicillin and clavulanic acid. The latter is a beta lactamase inhibitor, thus widening the spectrum of activity of co-amoxiclav against beta lactamase producing bacteria that are resistant to amoxicillin including staphylococci, anaerobes and Gram-negative bacteria. The risk of liver toxicity is six times greater with amoxiclav compared with amoxicillin.

Flucloxacillin

This antibiotic is not destroyed by pencillinases and thus it is effective against penicillin-resistant staphylococci. When given intravenously, its dosage may be increased to 2 g qds in staphylococcal bacteraemia or osteomyelitis.

Erythromycin and clarithromycin

They have a similar spectrum to penicillin and are thus useful against staphylococci and streptococci in patients who are allergic to penicillin. There is an increased risk of myositis and rhabdomyolysis if the patient is on statin therapy. Thus, statin therapy should be stopped for the duration of erythromycin therapy. If the patient develops intolerance to erythromycin, particularly gastrointestinal side-effects, then clarithromycin may be used.

Fucidin

This is active against penicillin-resistant staphylococci. It has good bone penetration and is useful in osteomyelitis. Resistance to it develops quickly if it is given alone and therefore it should be given with another antistaphylococcal agent. It is useful in combination therapy to treat MRSA infections. Liver function should be monitored if therapy is prolonged and it should be given with caution in patients with liver disease.

Doxycycline

This antibiotic can be used in treating MRSA infections. It should be used with caution in patients with hepatic impairment.

Rifampicin

This is active against staphylococci and streptococci and has good soft tissue and bone penetration. Patients should be warned that if they develop nausea, vomiting or malaise they should report this immediately as it may reflect liver dysfunction, which is a well described but rare side-effect of rifampicin therapy. It should be given with caution in patients with existing liver disease. Patients should be warned that their body secretions will turn red. Rifampicin should not be given alone because resistance can develop rapidly.

Clindamycin

This has very good soft tissue and bone penetration and is active against staphylococci, streptococci and anaerobes including *Bacteroides fragilis*. However, historically it has been linked with antibiotic-associated colitis caused by *Clostridium difficile* infections although this can occur with many antibiotics.

Vancomycin

This is usually given intravenously. It is active against Gram-positive organisms and is usually used for MRSA infections. Blood levels should be monitored and trough levels should be less than 15 mg/L.

Teicoplanin

This is a glycopeptide antibiotic which is active against Gram-positive organisms including MRSA. It can be given intravenously but also intramuscularly. This is a convenient therapy to be given at home.

Linezolid

Linezolid is active against Gram-positive organisms, including MRSA and vancomycin-resistant enterococci. It can be given orally or intravenously. It may cause marrow suppression and regular platelet counts are advisable. It should not be given for more than 28 days.

Daptomycin

This is a lipopeptide antibacterial active against Gram-positive organisms including MRSA. It is given intravenously and has good soft tissue penetration. Weekly creatine phosphokinase levels should be monitored.

Quinupristin/dalfopristin

This is a combination of two antibiotics, quinupristin and dalfopristin, which work synergistically against Gram-positive organisms including MRSA.

Trimethoprim

It has reasonable soft tissue penetration and is active against Gram-positive and -negative bacteria. It is also useful in combination therapy against MRSA.

Antibiotics used mainly against Gram-negative organisms

Ciprofloxacin

This is useful against Gram-negative organisms and has good soft tissue and bone penetration. It has only moderate activity against Gram-positive organisms. It is relatively well tolerated but occasionally can give neurological side-effects and can rarely predispose to hypoglycaemia in certain patients.

Septrin

This is a combination of trimethoprim and sulphmethoxazole. This is occasionally used to treat resistant Gram-negative organisms such as *Stenotrophomonas maltophilia* but should only be used if other antibiotics against Gram-negative organisms are not appropriate.

Ceftriaxone

This is a useful antibiotic that can be given either intravenously or intramuscularly when it is administered as 1 g in 3.5 mL of 1% lidocaine. It needs to be given only once a day. This can be given in the community on a once daily basis. It has a wide spectrum of activity but is not active against MRSA or *Pseudomonas*.

Ceftazidime

This is useful as an initial agent to cover Gram-negative infections as it is usually active against *Pseudomonas*. If the dosage is not reduced in renal impairment, then the patient may develop muscular twitching and even fits.

Piperacillin/tazobactam

This antibiotic is given intravenously. It has a wide spectrum of activity including Gram-positive and Gram-negative organisms such as *Pseudomonas* and anaerobes. It may be useful against bacteria with extended-spectrum beta lactamases.

Ticarcillin/clavulanic acid

This is given intravenously and is active against *Pseudomonas*, and other Gram-negative bacteria including *Proteus* spp. and *Bacteroides fragilis*.

Imipenem with Cilastin

It is a carbapenem with broad-spectrum activity against Gram-positive and Gram-negative organisms including anaerobes. Imipenem is partly inactivated in the kidney and this is blocked by cilastin. It should be used with caution in renal failure as it may cause fits.

Meropenem

This also has a wide spectrum of activity including usually *Pseudomonas*. Meropenem is given intravenously and has less frequently caused central nervous system side-effects including fits compared with imipenem. It is also useful against bacteria with ESBLs.

Ertapenem

This is given once daily and is useful against Gram-positive and Gram-negative organisms and also anaerobes. In a recent study it was shown to be equivalent in action with piperacillin/tazobactam in treating infected diabetic feet. It is not active against *Pseudomonas* or against *Acinetobacter*. It is useful against bacteria with ESBLs and AmpC-producing Gram-negative bacteria. It may be given intramuscularly as 1 g diluted with 3.2 mL of 1% lidocaine.

Tigecycline

This is a broad-spectrum glycylcycline antibiotic that is structurally similar to tetracycline antibiotics. It is useful in infections caused by Gram-positive organisms, including MRSA, *Staphylococcus aureus*, vancomycin-resistant enterococci, streptococci, Gram-negative organisms including those with ESBLs and anaerobes including *Bacteroides*

fragilis. Strains of *Proteus* spp. and *Pseudomonas aeruginosa* may be resistant.

Aminoglycosides.

These include amikacin, gentamicin, netilmicin and tobramycin. Gentamicin is the aminoglycoside of choice in the UK. It is active against some Gram-positive organisms and many Gram-negative organisms. Important side-effects are ototoxicity and nephrotoxicity. These side-effects are dose-related and thus extreme care should be taken with dosage. Gentamicin should be administered with strict blood level monitoring and the trough level should be less than 1 mg/L.

Antibiotics used against anaerobic organisms

Metronidazole

This is useful against anaerobic bacteria. Patients must be warned not to take alcohol.

Antibiotics, pseudomembranous colitis and *Clostridium difficile*

Infection with *Clostridium difficile*, leading to pseudomembranous colitis, is an increasing complication of antibiotic therapy. It usually presents with diarrhoea, but also abdominal discomfort and vomiting may occur. Pseudomembranous colitis is always worse in elderly patients: many do not have fever even though they have colitis. Any patient who develops diarrhoea whilst taking antibiotics should be assessed immediately. The ideal step is to stop the antibiotics and take a faecal specimen for culture and sensitivity and for detection of *C. difficile* toxin. However, the foot lesion must be examined to assess the extent of infection. If infection is still present then the risk to the patient of stopping the antibiotics must be carefully weighed against the risk of progression of a *C. difficile* infection. If the patient has diarrhoea but still has an extensive infection then he should be admitted to hospital. A CT scan of the abdomen is useful to illustrate the extent of the disease throughout the colon. The CT scan can show colonic wall changes but not changes in the mucosa. Certain antibiotics such as the cephalosporins and ciprofloxacin are more prone to lead to *C. difficile* infections and these should therefore be stopped; if antibiotics are considered absolutely necessary then piperacillin/tazobactam is more acceptable in this situation. Treatment is metronidazole 400 mg tds orally or vancomycin 125 mg qds orally. It is important to note that intravenous vancomycin is not active in the gut against *C. difficile* and neither does intravenous metronidazole have a major effect on this organism. The patient should also be given live yoghurt. If the patient does not respond to these conservative measures then a surgical opinion as to the necessity for a colectomy should be obtained.

Recently, new strains of *C. difficile* appear to be more virulent, with ability to produce greater quantities of toxins. Type 027 produces much more of the toxins than most other types because a mutation has knocked out the gene that normally restricts toxin production. It causes a greater proportion of severe disease and appears to have a higher mortality. It also seems to be particularly capable of spreading between patients.

There are three important components to the prevention and control of *C. difficile* disease:
• Prudent antibiotic prescribing to reduce the use of broad spectrum-antibiotics
• Isolation of patients with *C. difficile* diarrhoea
• Good infection control and nursing including handwashing (not relying solely on alcohol gel as this does not kill the spores) and wearing gloves and aprons, especially when dealing with bed pans. There should be enhanced environmental cleaning and use of a chlorine-containing disinfectant where there are cases of *C. difficile* disease to reduce environmental contamination with the spores.

Antibiotic adjustments for patients in renal failure
(Table 5.5)
Renal impairment is common in diabetic foot patients, and commonly used drugs can give rise to problems in diabetic patients with reduced renal function for the following reasons:
• Failure to excrete a drug or its metabolites may lead to toxicity
• Sensitivity to some drugs is increased even if elimination is unimpaired
• Many side-effects are poorly tolerated by people in end-stage renal failure
• Some drugs cease to be effective when renal function is impaired.
Many of these problems can be avoided by reducing the dose or by using alternative drugs.

The level of renal function below which a dose must be reduced depends on whether the drug is eliminated entirely by renal excretion or is partly metabolized, and on how toxic it is.

For many drugs with only minor or no dose-related side-effects, very precise modification of the dose regimen is unnecessary. However, if even minor renal impairment is considered likely on clinical grounds, renal function should be checked before prescribing antibiotics.

Indications for surgery
Antibiotics alone may be unable to control infection and it is necessary to decide whether adjunctive surgery is necessary. In severe episodes of cellulitis, the ulcer may be complicated by extensive infected subcutaneous soft tissue. At this point, the tissue is not frankly necrotic but has started to break down and liquefy. It is best for this tissue to be removed operatively. The definite indications for urgent surgical intervention are:
• A large area of infected sloughy tissue
• Localized fluctuance and expression of pus
• Crepitus with gas in the soft tissues on X-ray
• Blue or purplish discolouration of the skin.

Management of the three presentations of infection
Treatment is discussed for the three presentations of infection, in neuropathic feet and in neuroischaemic feet, both as initial treatment and follow-up.

Infection in the neuroischaemic foot is often more serious than in the neuropathic foot which has a good arterial blood supply. Also, patients with neuroischaemic feet often have cardiac and renal complications which impair the response to infection. We regard a positive ulcer swab in a neuroischaemic foot as having serious implications, and this influences antibiotic policy. We describe our approach which we believe to be successful in our clinical setting. However, such an approach needs to be sensitive to local prevalence of bacteria and their antibiotic sensitivities.

Localized infection
Neuropathic feet
Initial plan. We give amoxicillin 500 mg tds, flucloxacillin 500 mg qds and metronidazole 400 mg tds because streptococci, staphylococci and anaerobes are the most likely organisms. We believe that anaerobes are a common feature of superficial as well as deep infections, but may not always be isolated because of restriction on the length of time of incubation of cultures. If the patient is allergic to penicillin, we substitute clarithromycin 500 mg bd for amoxicillin.

When the ulcer extends deeply to fascia or tendon, we add either ciprofloxacin 500 mg bd or trimethoprim 200 mg bd to cover Gram-negative organisms. We send a deep swab or curettings for culture. It is important to know the organisms that are causing the infection so that antibiotics can be used accurately to target the causative

Table 5.5 Antibiotic dosage in renal failure

Antibiotic	Dose for normal renal function	Mild impairment (serum Cr 120–200 μmol/L)	Moderate impairment (serum Cr 200–400 μmol/L)	Severe impairment (serum Cr > 400 μmol/L)
Amikacin	iv 7.5 mg/kg/bd	Give 7.5 mg/kg daily; redose < 5 mg/L	Give 7.5 mg/kg daily; redose < 5 mg/L	Give 7.5 mg/kg daily; redose < 5 mg/L
Amoxicillin	iv/po 500 mg tds	No change	No change	500 mg bd
Benzylpenicillin	iv 1.2 g qds	No change	75% of normal dose	Maximum 3.6 g daily
Cefadroxil	po 0.5–1 g bd	0.5–1 g bd	0.5–1 g od	0.5–1 g od
Ceftazidime	iv 1–2 g tds	1 g 12 hrly	0.5–1 g 24 hrly	0.5–1 g 48 hrly
Ceftriaxone	iv 1–4 g daily	No adjustment	No adjustment	1–2 g od
Cefuroxime	iv 750 mg to 1.5 g tds	No adjustment	750 mg to 1.5 g bd	750 mg bd
Ciprofloxacin	iv 100–400 mg bd po 250–750 mg bd	No adjustment po max 500 mg bd	iv 100–200 mg bd po max 500 mg bd	iv 100–200 mg bd po max 500 mg bd
Clindamycin	iv 150–600 mg qds po 150–450 mg qds	No adjustment No adjustment	No adjustment No adjustment	No adjustment No adjustment
Co-trimoxazole	iv 960 mg bd po 960 mg bd	iv 480 mg bd po 480 mg bd	iv 480 mg bd po 480 mg bd	iv 480 mg bd po 480 mg bd
Daptomycin	iv 4 mg/kg once daily	No adjustment	No adjustment	iv 4 mg/kg every 48 h
Doxycycline	po First day 200 mg then 100 mg daily	No adjustment	No adjustment	No adjustment iv 500 mg daily
Ertapenem	iv 1 g daily	iv 1 g daily	iv 500 mg daily	iv 500 mg daily
Erythromycin	iv 500 mg qds po 500 mg qds	No adjustment	No adjustment	iv 500 mg tds po 500 mg tds
Flucloxacillin	iv 500 mg qds po 500 mg qds	No adjustment No adjustment	No adjustment No adjustment	500 mg tds 500 mg tds
Gentamicin	iv 5 mg/kg/once daily	1.5–2 mg/kg redose < 1 mg/L	1.5–2 mg/kg redose < 1 mg/L	1.5–2 mg/kg redose < 1 mg/L
Meropenem	iv 500 mg to 1 g tds	500 mg to 1 g 12 hrly	250–500 mg 12 hrly	250–500 mg 24 hrly
Metronidazole	iv 500 mg tds po 400 mg tds	No adjustment No adjustment	No adjustment No adjustment	No adjustment No adjustment
Quinupristin and dalfopristin	iv 7.5 mg/kg/8 hrly	No adjustment	No adjustment	No adjustment
Rifampicin	po 600 mg bd	No adjustment	No adjustment	No adjustment
Sodium fusidate	iv 500 mg tds po 500 mg tds	No adjustment No adjustment	No adjustment No adjustment	No adjustment No adjustment
Tazocin	iv 2.25–4.5 g tds	2.25–4.5 g tds	2.25–4.5 g bd	2.25–4.5 g bd
Teicoplanin	iv load with 400 mg 12 hrly iv × 3 then 400 mg daily	Load first then 200 mg once daily	Load first then 200 mg alt. days	Load first then 200 mg 3x/week
Tigecycline	iv initially 100 mg then 50 mg bd	No adjustment	No adjustment	No adjustment
Trimethoprim	po 100–200 mg bd	200 mg bd then half dose	Normal dose for 3 days then half dose	Normal dose for 3 days then half dose
Vancomycin	iv 1 g bd trough < 15 mg/L	Give 1 g; redose when level < 15 mg/L	Give 1 g; redose when level < 15 mg/L	Give 1 g; redose when level < 15 mg/L

Table 5.5 (*cont'd*)

Antibiotic	HD	CAPD	CAVH
Amikacin	Give 7.5 mg/kg daily; redose < 5 mg/L	Give 7.5 mg/kg daily; redose < 5 mg/L	Give 7.5 mg/kg daily; redose < 5 mg/L
Amoxicillin	500 mg bd	500 mg bd	500 mg tds
Benzylpenicillin	Maximum 3.6 g daily	Maximum 3.6 g daily	50% of normal dose
Cefadroxil	0.5–1 g od	0.5–1 g od	0.5–1 g od
Ceftazidime	0.5–1 g 48 hrly	0.5–1 g 48 hrly	1–2 g od
Ceftriaxone	1–2 g od	1–2 g od	1–2 g od
Cefuroxime	750 mg bd	750 mg bd	750 mg bd
Ciprofloxacin	iv 100–200 mg bd po max 500 mg bd	iv 100–200 mg bd po max 500 mg bd	iv 200 mg bd po max 500 mg bd
Co-trimoxazole	iv 480 mg bd po 480 mg bd	iv 480 mg bd po 480 mg bd	iv 480 mg bd po 480 mg bd
Clindamycin	No adjustment	No adjustment	No adjustment
Daptomycin	4 mg/kg every 48 h	4 mg/kg every 48 h	Not available
Doxycycline	No adjustment	No adjustment	No adjustment
Ertapenem	iv 500 mg od	Not available	Not available
Erythromycin	iv 500 mg tds po 500 mg tds	iv 500 mg tds po 500 mg tds	iv 500 mg tds po 500 mg tds
Flucloxacillin	500 mg tds	500 mg tds	500 mg qds
Gentamicin	1.5–2 mg/kg redose < 1 mg/L	1.5–2 mg/kg redose < 1 mg/L	1.5–2 mg/kg redose < 1 mg/L
Meropenem	250–500 mg 24 hrly	250–500 mg 24 hrly	250–500 mg 12 hrly
Metronidazole	No adjustment	No adjustment	No adjustment
Quinupristin and dalfopristin	No adjustment	No adjustment	No adjustment
Rifampicin	No adjustment	No adjustment	No adjustment
Sodium fusidate	No adjustment	No adjustment	No adjustment
Tazocin	2.25–4.5 g bd	2.25–4.5 g bd	2.25–4.5 g tds
Teicoplanin	Load first then 200 mg 3×/week	Load first then 200 mg 3×/week	Load first then 200 mg alt. days
Tigecycline	No adjustment	No adjustment	No adjustment
Trimethoprim	Half normal dose	Half normal dose	Half normal dose
Vancomycin	Give 1 g; redose when level < 15 mg/L	Give 1 g; redose when level < 15 mg/L	Give 1 g; redose when level < 15 mg/L

CAPD, continuous ambulatory peritoneal dialysis; CAVH, continuous arteriovenous haemofiltration; Cr, creatinine; HD, haemodialysis; iv, intravenously; od, po, orally; once daily; bd, twice daily; qds, four times daily; tds, three times daily.

organisms. We do not agree that it is unimportant to know the organisms. If there is not a good response to antibiotic therapy and the patient deteriorates and no swab has been taken, it is then difficult to be accurate in antibiotic therapy. Meanwhile, time has been lost while the patient continues to deteriorate.

Follow-up plan. If no signs of infection and no organisms are isolated, we stop antibiotics.

If no signs of infection are present but organisms (after od once daily) are isolated, we focus antibiotics and review the patient in 1 week.

If signs of infection are present but no organisms are isolated, we continue antibiotics as above.

If signs of infection are present and organisms are isolated, we focus antibiotics according to sensitivities.

If MRSA is grown, but there are no signs of infection we use topical mupirocin 2% ointment if sensitive. Patients

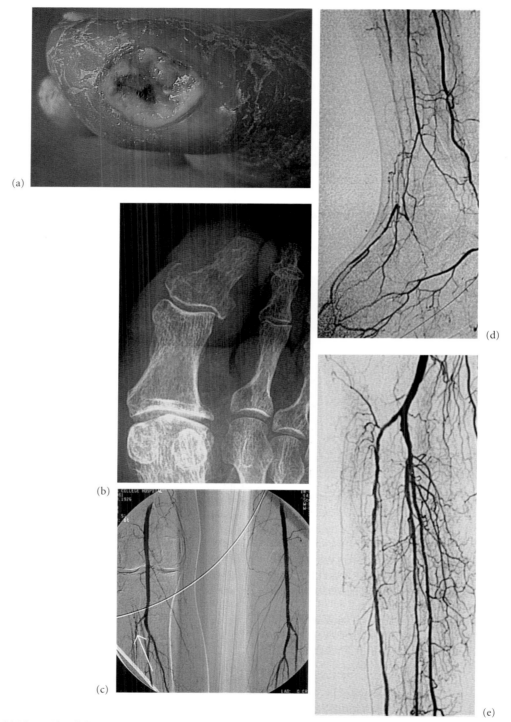

Fig. 5.25 (a) Ulcer with cellulitis on toe spreading to the foot. (b) X-ray was initially normal. (c) Stenosis at origin of anterior tibial artery. (d) Occlusions of anterior tibial artery. (e) Angioplasty of anterior tibial artery.

Table 5.5 (cont'd)

Antibiotic	HD	CAPD	CAVH
Amikacin	Give 7.5 mg/kg daily; redose < 5 mg/L	Give 7.5 mg/kg daily; redose < 5 mg/L	Give 7.5 mg/kg daily; redose < 5 mg/L
Amoxicillin	500 mg bd	500 mg bd	500 mg tds
Benzylpenicillin	Maximum 3.6 g daily	Maximum 3.6 g daily	50% of normal dose
Cefadroxil	0.5–1 g od	0.5–1 g od	0.5–1 g od
Ceftazidime	0.5–1 g 48 hrly	0.5–1 g 48 hrly	1–2 g od
Ceftriaxone	1–2 g od	1–2 g od	1–2 g od
Cefuroxime	750 mg bd	750 mg bd	750 mg bd
Ciprofloxacin	iv 100–200 mg bd po max 500 mg bd	iv 100–200 mg bd po max 500 mg bd	iv 200 mg bd po max 500 mg bd
Co-trimoxazole	iv 480 mg bd po 480 mg bd	iv 480 mg bd po 480 mg bd	iv 480 mg bd po 480 mg bd
Clindamycin	No adjustment	No adjustment	No adjustment
Daptomycin	4 mg/kg every 48 h	4 mg/kg every 48 h	Not available
Doxycycline	No adjustment	No adjustment	No adjustment
Ertapenem	iv 500 mg od	Not available	Not available
Erythromycin	iv 500 mg tds po 500 mg tds	iv 500 mg tds po 500 mg tds	iv 500 mg tds po 500 mg tds
Flucloxacillin	500 mg tds	500 mg tds	500 mg qds
Gentamicin	1.5–2 mg/kg redose < 1 mg/L	1.5–2 mg/kg redose < 1 mg/L	1.5–2 mg/kg redose < 1 mg/L
Meropenem	250–500 mg 24 hrly	250–500 mg 24 hrly	250–500 mg 12 hrly
Metronidazole	No adjustment	No adjustment	No adjustment
Quinupristin and dalfopristin	No adjustment	No adjustment	No adjustment
Rifampicin	No adjustment	No adjustment	No adjustment
Sodium fusidate	No adjustment	No adjustment	No adjustment
Tazocin	2.25–4.5 g bd	2.25–4.5 g bd	2.25–4.5 g tds
Teicoplanin	Load first then 200 mg 3×/week	Load first then 200 mg 3×/week	Load first then 200 mg alt. days
Tigecycline	No adjustment	No adjustment	No adjustment
Trimethoprim	Half normal dose	Half normal dose	Half normal dose
Vancomycin	Give 1 g; redose when level < 15 mg/L	Give 1 g; redose when level < 15 mg/L	Give 1 g; redose when level < 15 mg/L

CAPD, continuous ambulatory peritoneal dialysis; CAVH, continuous arteriovenous haemofiltration; Cr, creatinine; HD, haemodialysis; iv, intravenously; od, po, orally; once daily; bd, twice daily; qds, four times daily; tds, three times daily.

organisms. We do not agree that it is unimportant to know the organisms. If there is not a good response to antibiotic therapy and the patient deteriorates and no swab has been taken, it is then difficult to be accurate in antibiotic therapy. Meanwhile, time has been lost while the patient continues to deteriorate.

Follow-up plan. If no signs of infection and no organisms are isolated, we stop antibiotics.

If no signs of infection are present but organisms (after od once daily) are isolated, we focus antibiotics and review the patient in 1 week.

If signs of infection are present but no organisms are isolated, we continue antibiotics as above.

If signs of infection are present and organisms are isolated, we focus antibiotics according to sensitivities.

If MRSA is grown, but there are no signs of infection we use topical mupirocin 2% ointment if sensitive. Patients

Table 5.6 MRSA eradication protocol

Barrier nurse

Topical protocol for 5 days

Mupirocin 2% nasal ointment every 8 h. If MRSA resistant to mupirocin, then use chlorhexidine hydrochloride cream every 8 hours

Tricolsan 2% liquid soap for body and hair washing once daily

2 days protocol free

Repeat swabs three times at 48-hour intervals

If MRSA negative, no further treatment necessary

If MRSA positive, re-treat with 5 days topical protocol and repeat swabs at 48-hour intervals until three sets of negative swabs are obtained

should undergo an MRSA eradication protocol to remove it from carrier sites (Table 5.6). If MRSA is isolated with signs of infection, oral therapy with two of the following should be given: sodium fusidate 500 mg tds, rifampicin 300 mg tds, trimethoprim 200 mg bd or doxycycline 100 mg daily, according to sensitivities.

In this follow-up plan, the difficult decision is when there are no signs of infection present but organisms are isolated.

Some organisms may be commensals; however, if there are Gram-positive organisms or anaerobes or a pure growth of Gram-negative organisms we regard this as a significant result and microbiological evidence of infection.

Neuroischaemic feet
Initial plan. Regardless of the depth of the wound we aim to cover aerobic Gram-positive, aerobic Gram-negative and anaerobic infections, and thus we give amoxicillin 500 mg tds, flucloxacillin 500 mg qds, metronidazole 400 mg tds and ciprofloxacin 500 mg bd or trimethoprim 200 mg bd. If the patient is allergic to penicillin, we substitute clarithromycin 500 mg bd for amoxicillin and flucloxacillin.

We use this therapy for both superficial and deep infections because Gram-negative organisms may be a feature of infections in the ischaemic foot whether the ulcer is superficial or deep.

We send deep swabs or tissue (where possible) for the reasons already described above.

Follow-up plan. If there are no signs of infection and no organisms are grown, we consider stopping antibiotics. However, if the patient is severely ischaemic, with pressure index below 0.5, we continue antibiotics until the ulcer is healed.

If there are no signs of infection but organisms are present, we focus the antibiotics according to sensitivities.

If signs of infection are present but no organisms are grown, we continue to give broad-spectrum antibiotics as above.

If signs of infection are still present and organisms are grown, we focus the antibiotics according to sensitivities.

If MRSA is isolated with signs of infection, oral therapy with two of the following is given: sodium fusidate 500 mg tds, rifampicin 300 mg tds, trimethoprim 200 mg bd or doxycycline 100 mg daily, according to sensitivities.

If there is surrounding erythema then it should be traced to allow early recognition of extension of erythema, which indicates that antibiotic therapy needs adjustment.

Spreading infection
Neuropathic feet and neuroischaemic feet
Initial plan. In an ideal world these patients would be admitted to hospital and given intravenous antibiotic therapy as follows: amoxicillin 500 mg tds, flucloxacillin 500 mg qds, metronidazole 500 mg tds and ceftazidime 1 g tds. For patients who are allergic to penicillin we substitute clarithromycin 500 mg bd for amoxicillin and flucloxacillin. The reason for this regime is because spreading infections are often polymicrobial.

Other broad-spectrum parenteral therapies which may also be used, depending on local antibiotic policies, include:

• Ciprofloxacin and clindamycin
• Ticarcillin/clavulanate
• Piperacillin/tazobactam
• Meropenem
• Ertapenem
• Tigecyline.

If admission to hospital is not possible then a useful therapy is intramuscular ceftriaxone 1 g in 3.5 mL of 1% lidocaine once daily together with metronidazole either 1 g rectally tds or 400 mg tds orally. Ceftriaxone is a useful wide-spectrum antibiotic with a prolonged period of activity making it suitable for once a day administration. This regime is suitable for neuropathic and neuroischaemic patients, but anticoagulant therapy is a contraindication to intramuscular injections. Other useful intramuscular antibiotics include teicoplanin to treat Gram-positive organisms including MRSA and imipenem with cilastatin and ertapenem to treat Gram-positives, Gram-negatives and anaerobes.

Alternatively, it is possible to give intravenous therapy at home. This may be administered by a Hickman line

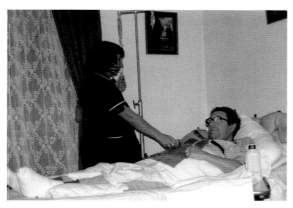

Fig. 5.23 Intravenous antibiotics administered through a Hickman line in the patient's home.

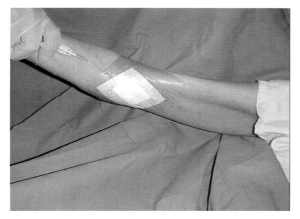

Fig. 5.24 Peripherally inserted central catheter (PICC) line inserted into an antecubital vein.

(Fig. 5.23) inserted through the subclavian vein or a peripherally inserted central catheter (PICC) line (Fig. 5.24), which is inserted into an antecubital fossa vein and guided under X-ray control into a central vein.

Our experience has been that fungal bacteraemias can be a common complication of Hickman lines and thus we now predominantly use the PICC line although these can also be associated with fungal bacteraemias.

Follow-up plan. The infected foot should be inspected daily to gauge the initial response to antibiotic therapy.

Appropriate antibiotics should be selected when sensitivities are available.

- If no organisms are isolated and yet the foot remains severely cellulitic, then a repeat deep swab or tissue should be taken but the quadruple antibiotic therapy as above should be continued
- If MRSA is isolated, give vancomycin 1 g iv bd, dosage to be adjusted according to serum levels, or teicoplanin 400 mg iv 12-hourly for three doses and then 400 mg daily. These antibiotics may need to be accompanied by either sodium fusidate 500 mg tds or rifampicin 300 mg tds orally (according to sensitivities)
- Intravenous antibiotic therapy can be changed to the appropriate oral therapy when the signs of infection have resolved
- Patients should be followed up weekly in the diabetic foot clinic and antibiotic therapy adjusted as described above.

CASE STUDY
Care of a neuroischaemic ulcer with diffuse spreading erythema

A 79-year-old man with type 2 diabetes of 5 years' duration with hypertension and steroid-treated polymyalgia rheumatica was referred from his local hospital with neuroischaemic ulceration of his right hallux and diffuse spreading cellulitis involving the forefoot (Fig. 5.25a). The ulcer had been present for 3 weeks, had first appeared to be a blood blister and had a moist sloughy base. A probe inserted into the ulcer touched bone. X-ray was initially normal (Fig. 5.25b). He was treated with amoxicillin 500 mg tds, flucloxacillin 500 mg qds, metronidazole 500 mg tds and ceftazidime 1 g tds. Tissue was sent for culture and grew MRSA and mixed anaerobes. Antibiotic therapy was changed to vancomycin 1 g bd and metronidazole was continued. Pedal pulses were impalpable and transcutaneous oxygen tension was 31 mmHg. He underwent digital subtraction angiography which showed stenosis and occlusions of the anterior tibial artery (Fig. 5.25c,d). He underwent angioplasty, dilating stenoses and occlusions along the anterior tibial artery on to the dorsalis pedis artery (Fig. 5.25e,f) following which his transcutaneous oxygen tension rose from 31 to 47 mmHg. Repeat X-ray showed fracture through the proximal phalanx of the great toe (Fig. 5.25g). But as the ulcer was continuing to improve and soft tissue infection was resolving he continued on conservative therapy with Hyaff applied to the ulcer and a Scotchcast boot. The ulcer healed after 9 months (Fig. 5.25h) and there was reasonable resolution of the bony changes to the proximal phalanx although there was resorption of bone of the distal phalanx (Fig. 5.25i).

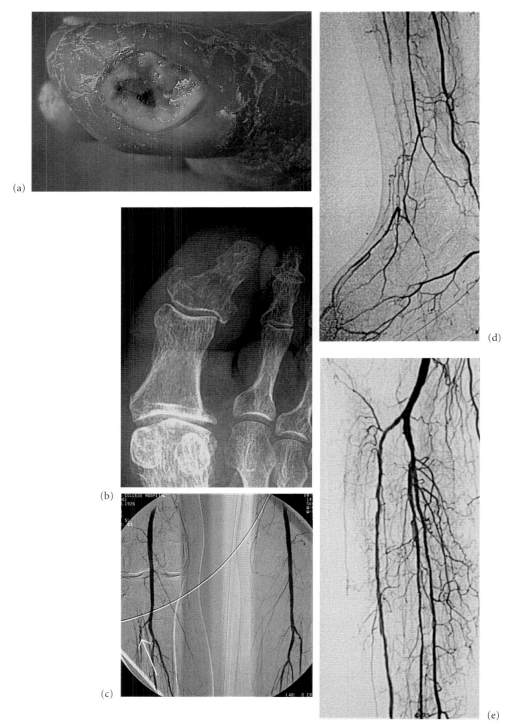

Fig. 5.25 (a) Ulcer with cellulitis on toe spreading to the foot. (b) X-ray was initially normal. (c) Stenosis at origin of anterior tibial artery. (d) Occlusions of anterior tibial artery. (e) Angioplasty of anterior tibial artery.

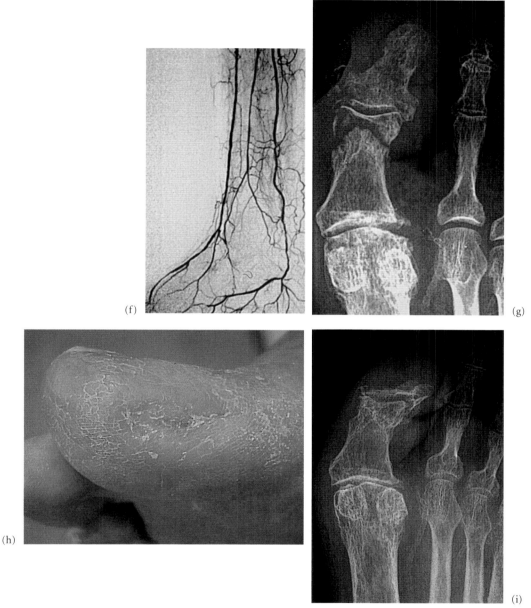

(f)

(g)

(h)

(i)

Fig. 5.25 (*cont'd*) (f) Straight-line flow of anterior tibial artery to the foot. (g) Fracture through proximal phalanx of greater toe. (h) Ulcer healed after 9 months. (i) Healing of fracture.

Key points

- Angioplasty can be a valuable adjunct to treatment for infection in the neuroischaemic foot
- Even if the improved blood supply is temporary and the artery restenoses after a few weeks or months, the management of infection will have benefited from the increased perfusion
- Initial culture was crucial in this case indicating MRSA which necessitated a change in antibiotic treatment
- Osteomyelitis can sometimes be treated conservatively.

Severe infection

Neuropathic feet and neuroischaemic feet

Initial plan. Intramuscular therapy with ceftriaxone is not sufficient therapy for severe infections, and every attempt should be made to give intravenous therapy in hospital as described for patients with spreading infection. However, various antibiotic regimes have been used in severe infections. Clinical and microbiological response rates have been similar in trials of various antibiotics and no single agent or combination of agents has emerged as most effective. If the patient shows signs of systemic sepsis such as systolic pressure < 100 mmHg or tachycardia > 125/min, then it may be advisable to give also an immediate dose of gentamicin 5 mg/kg. It has a wide spectrum of action against Gram-positive and Gram-negative organisms and it has a significant post-antibiotic effect for 24 hours.

However, patients in this group may well need surgical debridement as well as intravenous antibiotic therapy. If there is a large area of infected sloughy tissue, localized fluctuance and expression of pus, crepitus with gas in the soft tissues on X-ray or blue or purplish discolouration of the skin then, in addition to antibiotic therapy, debridement should be considered urgently. If the blue or purple discolouration is noted and treated promptly then it may resolve and the skin return to a normal colour. However, if intervention is late the blue discolouration indicating compromised oxygen supply to the skin will lead to necrosis and the foot moves to stage 5.

It is important to explore the possibility of revascularization in the infected neuroischaemic foot. Improvement of perfusion will not only help to control infection, but also promote healing of wounds if operative debridement is necessary. However, revascularization is not possible in all ischaemic feet.

Follow-up plan. This is the same as described for spreading infections.

CASE STUDY
A rare case of group A streptococcal infection with severe tissue loss in a neuroischaemic foot

A 79-year-old man with type 2 diabetes of 22 years' duration, who also had cardiac failure, severely impaired renal function and osteoarthritis of the hips, traumatized the dorsum of his foot leading to skin breakdown. This was treated at home with regular visits from the community nurse. He developed infection suddenly and acutely, on a Sunday. He was seen by the nurse at midday and his foot was deemed satisfactory. However, over the subsequent

4 hours his foot became swollen and red and he became acutely unwell. He called the emergency ambulance and was taken to Casualty. He had a high fever. He was treated with amoxicillin 500 mg tds, flucloxacillin 500 mg qds, metronidazole 500 mg tds and ceftazidime 1 g tds, insulin and fluids, all given intravenously. His foot showed extensive ulceration over the dorsal and medial aspects with surrounding cellulitis (see Fig. 5.26a,b). The wound swabs grew group A *Streptococcus*, but he quickly recovered from the episode of sepsis. His pulses were not palpable and he underwent duplex angiography, which showed total occlusion of the superficial femoral artery. He had a very severe fixed flexion deformity of both hips and it was not possible to carry out transfemoral angiography. His foot was debrided on the ward by the podiatrist (Fig. 5.26c,d) and he then underwent VAC therapy for the dorsal and medial wound which responded well to this therapy (Fig. 5.26e,f). After 12 weeks the wound was granulating well and he was discharged home to be followed up in the diabetic foot clinic (Fig.5.26g,h).

Key points
- Infection can spread rapidly, particularly through the dorsum of the foot, and can lead to severe systemic illness within a few hours
- The commonest streptococcal infection in the diabetic foot is caused by group B. However, group A, though rarely seen, can cause devastating infection and systemic upset. This demands rapid assessment, diagnosis and intervention
- Not all patients can be revascularized. The VAC pump is useful in encouraging granulation in the ischaemic wound, particularly when it is not possible to increase perfusion by a revascularization procedure.

CASE STUDY
Blue discolouration in a neuroischaemic foot

A 48-year-old man with type 1 diabetes mellitus of 20 years' duration, peripheral neuropathy, background retinopathy and no proteinuria presented with a 1-week history of malaise, high blood glucose and a 2-day history of discomfort and redness of the right foot. There was no history of trauma. There was an area of erythema over the dorsum and both medial and lateral aspects of the right foot, which was also oedematous. There was no break in the skin (Fig. 5.27a).

Body temperature was 39.2°C, pulse 104 regular, foot pulses absent, chest clear, abdomen normal. Haemoglobin 11.4 g/dL, white blood count (WBC) 17.3×10^9/L,

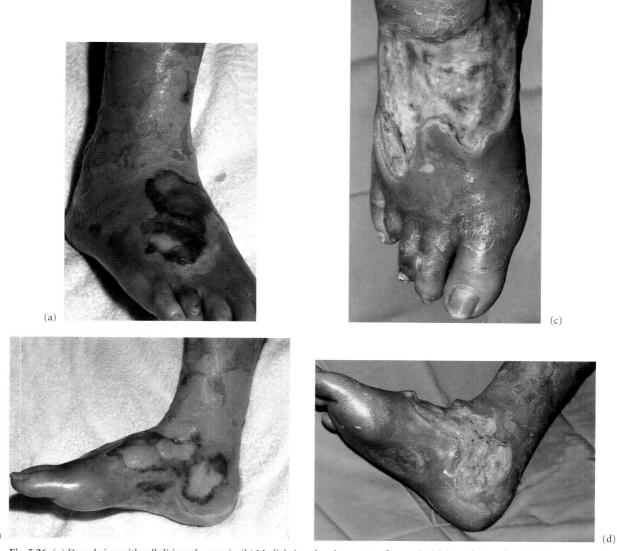

Fig. 5.26 (a) Dorsal view with cellulitis and necrosis. (b) Medial view showing extent of necrosis. (c) Dorsal view after debridement. (d) Medial view after debridement.

erythrocyte sedimentation rate (ESR) 105, HbA$_1$ 13% and glucose 18.6 mmol/L (335 mg/dL). X-ray of the foot was normal. Blood cultures showed no growth. There was no open lesion to take a swab.

Doppler studies in both legs showed a very high ankle/brachial pressure index (above 1.5) indicative of calcification. The foot artery waveforms were damped, indicating reduced blood flow. A clinical diagnosis of cellulitis in a neuroischaemic foot was made. The other much less likely diagnosis was an acute onset of Charcot's osteoarthropathy. However, it is unusual for Charcot's osteoarthropathy to be associated with such a high body temperature, which is much more suggestive of sepsis.

He was treated with quadruple intravenous antibiotic therapy (amoxicillin 500 mg tds, flucloxacillin 500 mg

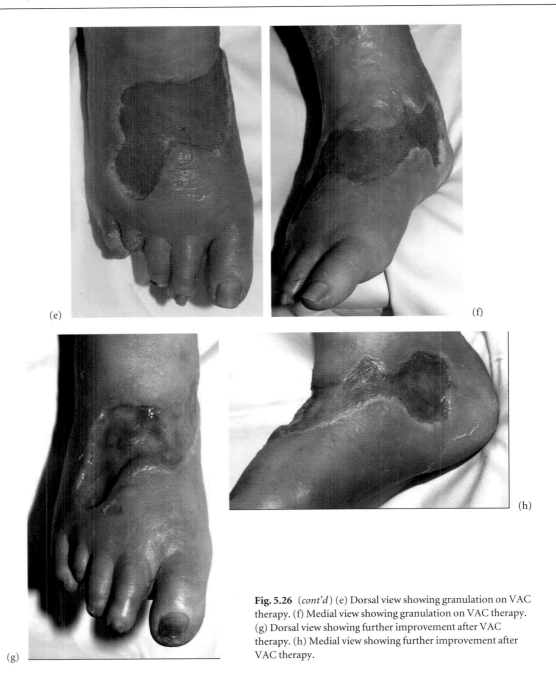

Fig. 5.26 (*cont'd*) (e) Dorsal view showing granulation on VAC therapy. (f) Medial view showing granulation on VAC therapy. (g) Dorsal view showing further improvement after VAC therapy. (h) Medial view showing further improvement after VAC therapy.

qds, metronidazole 500 mg tds and ceftazidime 1 g tds) to provide a wide-spectrum cover, and commenced on sliding scale intravenous insulin. By the next day, body temperature had fallen to 37.2°C but there was no improvement in the cellulitis. There were spikes of fever on the evening of the second and third days (Fig. 5.27b). The area of cellulitis did not regress, but there was no evidence of a collection of pus. A surgical opinion was obtained and confirmed that there was no indication for surgery.

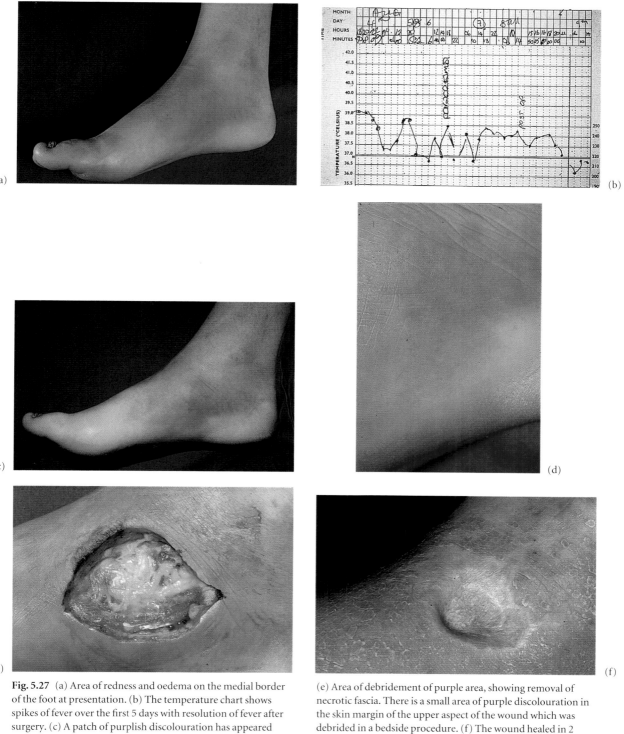

Fig. 5.27 (a) Area of redness and oedema on the medial border of the foot at presentation. (b) The temperature chart shows spikes of fever over the first 5 days with resolution of fever after surgery. (c) A patch of purplish discolouration has appeared within the cellulitis. (d) Close-up view of purple discolouration.

(e) Area of debridement of purple area, showing removal of necrotic fascia. There is a small area of purple discolouration in the skin margin of the upper aspect of the wound which was debrided in a bedside procedure. (f) The wound healed in 2 months after split-skin graft.

On the fourth day of the admission the patient was still pyrexial. He also had a rigor. The ceftazidime was withdrawn and intravenous gentamicin 80 mg tds started. (This was before once-daily dosing had come in.) The most common organism isolated in diabetic foot infections is *Staphylococcus aureus* and gentamicin is active against *Staphylococcus* as well as providing Gram-negative cover.

On the fifth day the patient remained pyrexial and within the area of erythema a patch of purplish discolouration was noted (Fig. 5.27c,d). In very severe cases of cellulitis, blueish-purplish discolouration of the skin indicates subcutaneous necrosis. The patient underwent surgical debridement of the area of discolouration. Subcutaneous necrosis and pus were noted. There was a wide excision of an ellipse of skin and subcutaneous tissue. Histology showed fibrous connective tissue, fat and necrotic debris showing extensive necrosis with haemorrhage.

Tissue and pus were sent for culture. Both grew *Staphylococcus aureus*. Antibiotic therapy specifically for *Staphylococcus aureus* was prescribed including rifampicin 600 mg bd, flucloxacillin and gentamicin. One day after the debridement an area of skin at the margin of the wound developed blue discolouration (Fig. 5.27e) and was debrided in a bedside procedure. The patient's temperature resolved within 2 days.

In view of the Doppler studies, the patient underwent a transfemoral angiogram which showed a 90% stenosis just distal to the origin of the right posterior tibial artery with a diffusely diseased common femoral artery. He underwent angioplasty of the posterior tibial artery 10 days after the surgical debridement. Finally a split-skin graft was applied and the wound healed in 2 months (Fig. 5.27f).

Key points

- The patient had been feeling generally ill with 'flu-like symptoms': this may be the first sign of a foot infection
- Severe infection can develop in an apparently intact foot
- Patients need close daily supervision with input from medical and surgical teams
- If fever does not resolve then further intervention is necessary
- Following surgical debridement, wounds in patients with subcutaneous necrosis should be inspected every day to detect any extension of the necrotic area. Any area developing blue discolouration of the skin should be excised.

CASE STUDY
Severe infection in a neuropathic foot

A 62-year-old African man, with type 2 diabetes of 14 years' duration, presented to Casualty with a very swollen left foot with marked bullae formation and cellulitis (Fig. 5.28a). He had noted swelling of the foot for a week and this had started whilst he was in Nigeria. His foot pulses were palpable. He had a pyrexia of 38.4°C, a high white cell count of 17.0×10^9/L, and his CRP was 200 mg/L. His blood glucose was 25 mmol/L. He was admitted to hospital, given amoxicillin 500 mg tds, flucloxacillin 500 mg qds, metronidazole 500 mg tds and ceftazidime 1 g tds intravenously, and also given intravenous insulin. He was taken to theatre and underwent radical surgical debridement to remove all of the infected tissue. A specimen of this tissue grew *Proteus mirabilis* and *Escherichia coli*. He was initially treated with quadruple antibiotic therapy which was then focused to amoxicillin and ceftazidime, and he made a complete recovery. He was left with a considerable loss of tissue cover on the dorsum. A week later a VAC pump was used to stimulate formation of a bed of granulation tissue (Fig. 5.28b), after which he was successfully skin grafted (Fig. 5.28c).

Key points

- Some of the worst diabetic foot infections we have seen began in tropical climates and many particularly affected the dorsum of the foot
- Infections of this site can lead to extensive soft tissue destruction with sloughing and necrosis which needs urgent surgical debridement
- With the appropriate antibiotic therapy and early surgical debridement, these neuropathic feet often do well even after a very late presentation
- The bacteriology of these lesions is often polymicrobial, including Gram-negative bacteria, and thus, wide-spectrum antibiotic therapy should be given in the first instance.

Osteomyelitis

Osteomyelitis can complicate any of the above infective presentations.

Initial treatment

- Usually antibiotics will be given for the associated soft tissue infection
- When soft tissue infection is not present but a diagnosis of osteomyelitis is made clinically, an empirical regime

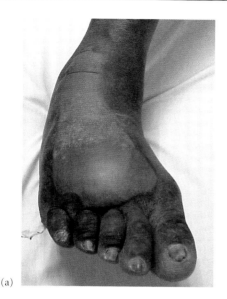

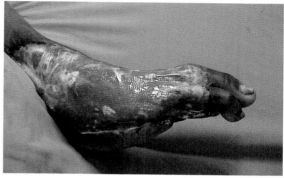

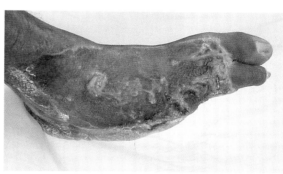

Fig. 5.28 (a) Very swollen foot at presentation with an enormous dorsal bulla. (b) Foot after radical surgical debridement and treatment with VAC therapy to stimulate formation of a bed of granulation tissue. (c) Foot after a successful skin graft.

(a)

(b)

(c)

with good bone penetration should be given such as rifampicin 300 mg tds and ciprofloxacin 500 mg bd

- On review, antibiotic selection is guided by the results of cultures from deep swabs, tissue curettings or bone fragments removed from the ulcer. Some centres base their antibiotic selection on formal bone biopsy carried out through intact skin, although this may be difficult to obtain and is not without risk in the neuroischaemic foot. However, sinus tract or ulcer culture results may be helpful. It is useful to choose appropriate antibiotics with good bone penetration, such as sodium fusidate 500 mg tds, rifampicin 300 mg tds, clindamycin 300 mg tds and ciprofloxacin 500 mg bd.

Follow-up plan

- Antibiotics should be given for at least 12 weeks. Parenteral therapy has in the past been given for up to 6 weeks followed by oral therapy for 6 weeks. However, it may be possible to limit the parenteral therapy to 2 weeks and follow this with appropriate oral antibiotics for up to 10 weeks (if the infected bone is resected then a shorter course of antibiotics such as 4 weeks may be necessary). Conservative therapy is often successful, and is associated with resolution of cellulitis and healing of the ulcer. Indeed the eventual duration of antibiotic therapy may be determined by the progress towards healing of the associated ulcer. If the soft tissues are responding to antibiotic therapy, then usually the underlying osteomyelitis resolves

- However, if, after 3 months treatment, the ulcer persists, with continued probing to bone that is fragmented on X-ray, we favour resection of the underlying bone, which may entail toe amputation or removal of a metatarsal head.

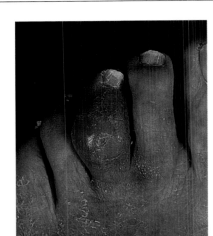

Fig. 5.29 Sausage toe with small ulcer on the dorsum.

CASE STUDY
Conservative treatment of osteomyelitis

A 76-year-old woman with type 2 diabetes of 10 years' duration was referred to the diabetic foot clinic by Casualty. She had an erythematous right 2nd toe with fusiform swelling (sausage toe) and a sloughy ulcer with a draining sinus which probed to bone (Fig. 5.29). Cellulitis extended onto the dorsum of the foot. She had been aware of redness and swelling of the toe for 3 days and the foot had begun to throb over the previous 24 hours.

Pedal pulses were absent. She was sent for X-ray (unremarkable), and for vascular assessment which showed monophasic pulsatile waveforms and elevated indices due to arterial calcification. A deep swab was sent for culture and grew *Staphylococcus aureus*. The ulcer was debrided and dressed with a foam dressing. Quadruple oral antibiotics were prescribed initially: oral amoxicillin 500 mg tds, flucloxacillin 500 mg qds, metronidazole 400 mg tds and ciprofloxacin 500 mg bd; and then narrowed down to fucidin 500 mg tds and flucloxacillin 500 mg qds. Although repeat X-ray after 2 weeks showed lucency of the terminal phalanx compatible with osteomyelitis, the ulcer healed in 3 weeks. The fusiform swelling remained but the erythema resolved after 3 months.

Key points
- Fusiform swelling (sausage toe) and erythema are frequently associated with osteomyelitis and X-rays are needed to confirm the extent of the infection in the bone and monitor progress
- Erythema may take several weeks to settle if infection was severe
- 'Sausage toe' may resolve with antibiotics: surgery is not always necessary for osteomyelitis
- In some centres osteomyelitis is treated by definitive bone resection followed by 4–6 weeks of parenteral or equivalent therapy.

Adjuvant therapy

Additional measures may improve resolution of infection. Granulocyte colony stimulating factor (GCSF) may improve outcome: a recent meta-analysis of studies with GCSF showed that it resulted in fewer amputations. Hyperbaric oxygen also reduces the rate of amputations but only in the ischaemic foot. Both need further study.

Wound control

Diabetic foot infections are almost always more extensive than would appear from initial examination and surface appearance. It is wise to perform an initial debridement in the diabetic foot clinic so that the true dimensions of the lesion can be revealed and samples obtained for culture. Often callus may be overlying the ulcer and this must be removed to reveal the extent of the underlying ulcer and allow drainage of pus and removal of infected sloughy tissue.

Wound care of ulcers with localized infection
Ulcers with local signs of infection including cellulitis should have podiatric debridement as described below.

Podiatric debridement of neuropathic ulcers
- All callus surrounding the wound is removed by sharp debridement
- If the ulcer is subungual, overlying nail is cut back to expose the base of the ulcer
- Undermined areas detected by probing are cut out
- Sloughy or discoloured areas of the wound bed are sharp debrided down to healthy bleeding tissue. Local discolouration of the wound bed is often a marker for an underlying track or fluctuant area containing pus. Sometimes the track has not yet broken through to the surface and the only indication of its presence is that the tissue of the wound bed which overlies the track may be a different colour, often greyish or purple. The discoloured area should be debrided away using scalpel and forceps to explore the underlying area

- Where a wound sinus is present and is very small it may be enlarged with a scalpel in order to aid drainage and enable tissue to be taken. The sinus may appear as an obvious hole in the wound bed or as a tiny slit, which is easily overlooked
- Sometimes the edges of the slit are pouting, the ulcer is very wet, and on palpation, pus or serous fluid emerges from the sinus. Fluctuant areas are drained. If pus is present it is collected in a syringe or small sterile pot for culture
- The ulcer is cleaned with normal saline. Tissue scrapings or deep swab are taken from the base of the ulcer and sent to the laboratory for culture
- Extent of cellulitis is marked with a spirit-based fibre pen so that any extension can be noted next time the dressing is lifted
- A sterile, absorbent, easily lifted dressing held in place with a light tubular bandage is applied
- The patient is instructed not to walk but to rest and elevate the foot and use crutches or wheelchair
- The dressing is lifted every day for wound inspection and to check the extent of the cellulitis. Callus or slough which reforms is sharp debrided at frequent intervals (not longer than 1 week).

Podiatric debridement of neuroischaemic feet

Neuroischaemic feet with signs of local infection or cellulitis are treated as above but with some important differences which are described below.

- Debridement is far less aggressive than for the neuropathic foot
- Accretions of slough in the wound bed are gently debrided with scalpel and forceps but great care is taken not to damage viable tissue
- If deep sinuses are located by probing, they should not be enlarged unless there is a very obviously fluctuant area associated with the sinus. In these circumstances the advantages of draining pus outweigh the danger of damaging ischaemic tissues
- Undermined edges are not removed
- If a halo of very thin dry callus develops around the ulcer it is very carefully debrided
- If the ulcer is subungual, overlying nail is very gently pared away so that the ulcer can drain
- The patient is sent to the hospital immediately if the foot deteriorates.

Dressing regimes for ulcers with localized infection

Regular dressing changes are important for all infected diabetic foot ulcers. Exudate may cause maceration and irritation of the tissues surrounding the ulcer. At dressing change, infected ulcers and surrounding areas should be carefully cleansed with saline and dried before a fresh dressing is applied. Simple, non-adherent dressings which are easily lifted are best. Any dressing which might prevent the free flow of exudate from an infected foot, or clog up a discharging sinus, should be avoided. Dressings should always be changed before 'strike-through' occurs.

CASE STUDY
Infection masked by irregular dressing changes

An 84-year-old man with type 2 diabetes of 12 years' duration, a previous above-knee amputation and a neuroischaemic foot developed a shallow ischaemic ulcer on his 2nd toe (Fig. 5.30) and a dressing was applied and changed at weekly intervals. Between dressing changes the ulcer deteriorated and became sloughy and deep with associated cellulitis, although the patient felt no pain. He was admitted to hospital for intravenous antibiotics. Vascular intervention was not feasible. The ulcer took 13 months to heal.

Key points
- Patients who lack protective pain sensation should have regular and frequent wound inspections
- We avoid using dressings which cannot be lifted frequently on patients without protective pain sensation

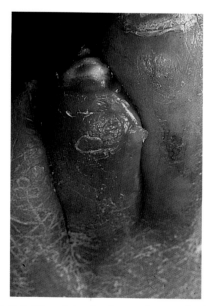

Fig. 5.30 Cellulitis and sloughy ulcer on dorsum of 2nd toe.

- Healing of previously infected lesions is very protracted in neuroischaemic patients.

Wound care of ulcers with spreading infections

Spreading infections should respond to parenteral antibiotics but the patient needs frequent review to detect evidence of spreading infection. An outline of the area of cellulitis may be drawn on the foot with a spirit-based pen so that extension of the cellulitic area can be detected quickly.

Wound care of ulcers with severe infections

In these patients, who have extensive deep soft tissue infection, often with cellulitis with blue-black discolouration, the ulcer may be complicated by sloughy infected soft tissue. It is best for this tissue to be removed operatively.

The definite indications for urgent surgical intervention (as described above) are:

- A large area of infected sloughy tissue
- Localized fluctuance and expression of pus
- Crepitus with gas in the soft tissues on X-ray
- Purplish discolouration of the skin, indicating subcutaneous necrosis.

We have repeated these indications here as we believe that they are so important. In these circumstances surgical debridement is always necessary in either neuropathic and neuroischaemic feet. However, if the foot is neuroischaemic, surgical debridement needs to be accompanied by an assessment of the arterial perfusion to the foot to evaluate the healing potential of surgical wounds. These patients will need timely vascular investigation.

CASE STUDY
Neuropathic foot complicated by extensive deep soft tissue infection needing a wide excision and skin grafting

A 43-year-old man with type 1 diabetes of 17 years' duration noticed swelling of the foot after treading on a piece of plastic which resulted in a break in the skin on the plantar aspect of the forefoot. After 5 days, he became unwell, and presented to Casualty with a high blood glucose 29 mmol/L (522 mg/dL). There was small breakdown over the plantar aspect of 4th metatarsal head but marked cellulitis over the dorsum of the foot with blue-black discolouration over the lateral aspect (Fig. 5.31a).

The patient was admitted and treated with intravenous insulin and initially quadruple intravenous antibiotics, amoxicillin 500 mg tds, flucloxacillin 500 mg qds, metronidazole 500 mg tds and ceftazidime 1 g tds. Tissue specimen grew *Aerococcus viridans* and mixed anaerobes. The necrotic area over the lateral aspect of the dorsum broke down to exude pus (Fig. 5.31b) and the patient underwent surgical debridement to drain the pus and remove sloughy tissue from the dorsum of the foot (Fig. 5.31c).

He was treated with VAC therapy and finally underwent skin grafting to achieve complete healing (Fig. 5.31d).

Key points

- Dorsal phlegmon is a diffuse inflammatory process spreading through the dorsum of the foot with formation of pus and purulent exudate

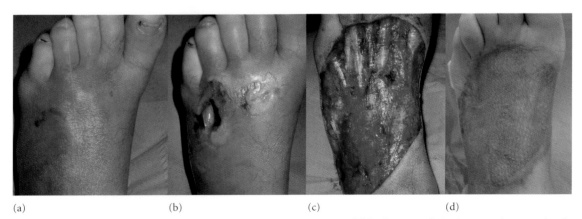

(a) (b) (c) (d)

Fig. 5.31 (a) Marked cellulitis over the dorsum with blue-back discolouration over the lateral aspect. (b) The necrotic area over the lateral aspect of the dorsum broke down to exude pus.

(c) Surgical debridement to drain the pus and remove sloughy tissue from the dorsum of the foot. (d) Skin grafting to achieve complete healing.

- The portal of entry is usually a web space lesion or a plantar lesion, through which infection spreads to the dorsum of the foot
- Dorsal phlegmon requires wide surgical excision.

Preoperative preparation for neuropathic and neuroischaemic patients needing surgical debridement

On admission, these patients should be regarded as medical and surgical emergencies.

Preparation for surgery

The following investigations should be carried out:
- Full blood count and typing
- Serum electrolytes and creatinine
- Blood glucose
- Liver function tests
- Electrocardiogram (ECG)
- Chest X-ray.

Patients should be medically stable prior to surgery.

Hyperglycaemia is usually present and patients with both type 1 and type 2 diabetes should be treated with an intravenous insulin sliding scale (Table 5.7).

If patients have nephropathy there may be abnormal fluid retention and electrolyte disturbances which should be considered when prescribing the intravenous therapy. Basic cardiovascular risk should be assessed from the history, physical examination and simple investigations such as ECG and chest X-ray. Enquiry for myocardial infarction, angina, coronary artery bypass and congestive cardiac failure should be made. The high-risk patient will need close cardiovascular monitoring, and the anaesthetic technique can also be varied according to the risk of the patient.

Table 5.7 Insulin sliding scale. Adjust volume of fluids according to clinical state of patient

50 units soluble human insulin in 50 mL 0.9% sodium chloride

Blood glucose (mmol/L)	Infusion rate (units/h)
< 4	0.5
4.1–9	1
9.1–15	2
15.1–19.9	4
> 20	Review and call doctor

Fluids
If blood glucose > 15 mmol/L give sodium chloride 0.9%
If blood glucose ≤ 15 mmol/L give glucose 5%

For high-risk patients, perioperative use of β-blockers is now established, and this is discussed further in Chapter 6 where vascular surgery is covered. The anaesthetist must be aware that virtually all of these patients will have autonomic as well as peripheral neuropathy, and respiratory reflexes may be diminished. Postoperative respiratory arrests have been reported. Careful anaesthetic attention, particularly in the recovery room, is necessary.

Rarely type 1 diabetic patients may present with diabetic ketoacidosis complicating their diabetic foot infection. This should be treated before the patient goes to the operating theatre.

Emergency surgery to the foot usually consists of debridement or minor amputation. It is often difficult to assess how much debridement will be necessary and in some cases debridement may need to be accompanied by amputation of a toe or ray. Consent for these procedures should therefore be obtained prior to operation.

The anaesthetist should understand that debridement of the foot is not a rapid procedure such as a usual incision and drainage for abscess, and therefore should anticipate at least 40 minutes operating time.

During surgery

- It is important that a meticulous wound exploration is carried out, with removal of infected sloughy tissue and laying open of all sinuses. It is rare to find a well-defined abscess
- The usual presentation is of heavily infected sloughy, grey tissue which needs to be removed down to healthy, bleeding tissue
- All dead tendon and necrotic tissue should be removed. Wide excision is necessary: small incisions with drains should be avoided
- Fragmented infected and non-bleeding bone should be removed
- Deep infected tissue should be sent urgently to the microbiology laboratory
- The wound should not be sutured but left to heal by secondary intention.

After surgery

- Continue the insulin pump postoperatively until infection is resolving. Then transfer to short-acting insulin three times daily with long-acting insulin at night
- When debridement results in a large postoperative wound, then VAC therapy can be used to accelerate healing. It is advisable to wait 24 hours before applying VAC therapy to make sure all postoperative bleeding has ceased.

- When the postoperative wound is particularly sloughy, wound irrigation with a sodium hypochlorite solution (2% Milton) may be useful in the neuropathic foot. A one in 50 dilution of the concentrated 1% weight in volume solution of sodium hypochlorite is made by adding 20 mL of concentrated sodium hypochlorite to 980 mL of sterile water. Approximately 300–400 mL are irrigated through the wound, making sure to swab the edges of the wound and surrounding skin with normal saline at the end of the procedure to prevent skin drying and irritation. Milton irrigation should be stopped when the wound is no longer sloughy or infected (usually within 5 days)
- We find a simple dressing regime of non-adherent dressing bulked out with gauze and held in place by a tubular bandage is best. It is very quick and simple to lift, and enables regular and frequent inspections to be done.
- Signs that the foot is improving include:
  - Decrease in erythema
  - Pink wound
  - Reduction of swelling by comparison with the other foot
  - Wrinkles will be present in the skin of the foot where oedema has reduced
  - The skin surrounding the previously infected ulcer begins to desquamate or shed and become flaky
  - Discharge reduces
  - Smell ceases
  - Pain (if previously a problem) improves
- When there is an initial fever preoperatively, the patient's temperature is a useful indication of his progress. A steady fall in temperature is expected over the subsequent 3–4 days. If this does not occur, then uncontrolled infection should be suspected
- At operation, it is sometimes difficult to remove all infected tissue and a further operative debridement may sometimes be necessary to remove remaining necrotic tissue and control infection
- Deep wound swabs or tissue are taken twice weekly to assess the eradication of organisms.
- After surgery, the edges of the wound are debrided every 3 days and all callus, slough and non-viable tissue are removed, but it is not usually necessary to do this in theatre under anaesthetic. The wound is kept open and draining to heal from the base
- Patients will need bedrest and it is wise to give prophylactic subcutaneous heparin. Low molecular weight heparins may be used if the renal function is normal. Antithrombotic stockings should not be used on neuroischaemic feet. If they are used on neuropathic feet,

they should be folded back from the toe nails to avoid pressure on the nail sulcus
- Patients who have had toe or ray amputations need careful mobilization and rehabilitation. Too rapid mobilization can provoke Charcot's osteoarthropathy.
- For detailed descriptions of surgical procedures see Chapter 8.

Vascular control

It is important to explore the possibility of revascularization in the infected neuroischaemic foot. Improvement of perfusion will not only help to control infection, but will also promote healing of the wound if operative debridement is necessary.

Angiography

Initially, duplex angiography should be carried out to detect the presence of stenoses or occlusions which may be amenable to angioplasty or bypass. Duplex angiography is proficient at looking at the iliac, femoral and popliteal arteries, but it is sometimes difficult to obtain good views of the infrapopliteal arteries and foot arteries because of the excessive calcification in the diabetic patient. If duplex angiography is not available then MRI or CT angiography may be used to demonstrate infrapopliteal vessels and also for delineating the aortoiliac circulation.

Angioplasty

When non-invasive angiography reveals lesions that are amenable to angioplasty in the femoral and popliteal arteries, then down stream transfemoral angiography is performed followed by angioplasty. The infrapopliteal arteries are also visualized and appropriate lesions angioplastied. Angioplasty is possible at several levels of the leg arterial system to obtain straight-line flow to the foot. It is indicated for the treatment of isolated or multiple stenoses as well as short segment occlusions less than 10 cm in length in iliac, femoral and tibial arteries. Recent progress has resulted in long occlusions being satisfactorily angioplastied, either using long balloons or the technique of subintimal angioplasty, with the catheters inserted into the subintimal plane.

The aim is to improve the arterial circulation, achieve straight-line flow to the foot and bring about an increased blood supply to the site of ulceration and infection (Fig. 5.32a–c). Although the foot pulses may not be restored, there is usually a notable increase in the transcutaneous oxygen tension.

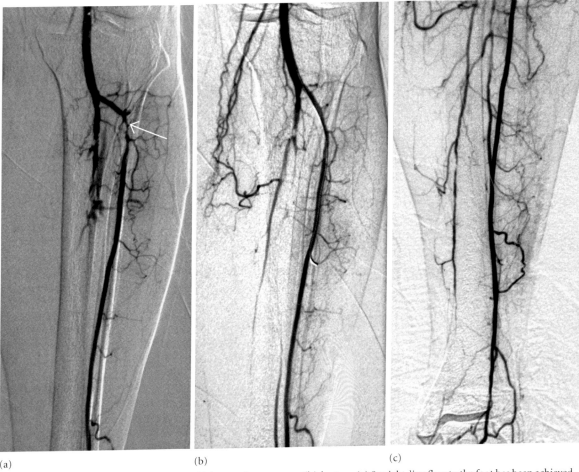

(a)   (b)   (c)

Fig. 5.32 (a) Critical stenosis of the anterior tibial artery 3 cm from its margin. (b) Angioplasty has relieved stenosis of anterior tibial artery. (c) Straight-line flow to the foot has been achieved. (Courtesy of Dr Paul Sidhu.)

Angiography and angioplasty are safe procedures with few complications so long as appropriate precautions are taken. Investigations should include:

- A recent full blood count, including a platelet count
- Blood coagulation indices
- Serum electrolytes and creatinine
- Blood grouping.

The patient should not be dehydrated. Start an insulin sliding scale together with intravenous fluids before the procedure. Dopamine is no longer used to protect kidney function but it is important to keep the patient hydrated with intravenous fluids prior to the procedure. Patients with impaired renal function should be prescribed N-acetylcysteine 600 mg bd 24 hours before the procedure and on the day of the procedure.

If the patient has previously been on warfarin then this must be stopped at least 3 days prior to the procedure and the patient changed to intravenous heparin. The heparin infusion is stopped 2 hours before the procedure. Metformin should be stopped 2 days before the procedure and restarted 2 days after the procedure. If the angiogram is required as an emergency, it may be necessary to give vitamin K to counteract the effect of the warfarin therapy.

Post-angiography, patients should be monitored closely, recording blood pressure and pulse. A rare complication is bleeding from the femoral artery injection site, which may not be immediately apparent. The pulse rate may not respond in the usual way to loss of intravascular volume because of autonomic neuropathy, therefore tachycardia may not be present. However, blood pressure will drop and an urgent blood count together with cross-matching for at least 6 pints of blood should be performed. Full resuscitation should immediately be carried out with haemodynamic monitoring. Most cases of bleeding resolve with blood replacement and tamponade themselves off spontaneously. A mass may become palpable in the lower abdomen but this may not appear until 5–6 hours after the procedure. Earlier diagnosis may be made with an ultrasound examination of the abdomen. Continued hypotension despite adequate blood replacement is an indication for surgical exploration.

Post-angioplasty it may be advisable to give heparin if a long occlusion has been treated. It is best to give unfractionated heparin intravenously. If there is any post-procedure bleeding over the subsequent few hours from the femoral artery injection site, this can be exacerbated by heparin. Unfractionated heparin can be easily stopped if given intravenously; however, low molecular weight heparin given subcutaneously is difficult to reverse and we have had one case of severe post procedure bleeding in these circumstances.

In patients with impaired renal function, serum creatinine may rise after the procedure, and should be checked after 48 hours. There may be a mild rise of serum creatinine of 50 mmol/L (0.57 mg/dL) but this falls gradually over the subsequent 10 days, but should be carefully monitored. In some cases renal impairment may be severe and renal support in the form of dialysis needed. Following angioplasty, both lower limbs should be carefully observed to detect the presence of unexpected ischaemia or emboli. Trash foot is described after angioplasty but is notably rare in our practice. The limbs should be observed for the development of a pale cold periphery which might indicate significant arterial damage either at the femoral injection site or the angioplasty site. A vascular opinion should be urgently sought if this occurs.

Arterial bypass

It is sometimes a difficult decision to balance the risk of vascular surgery in the diabetic ischaemic patient with the advantages gained by a successful arterial bypass restoring pulsatile blood flow to the foot and thereby achieving rapid healing. If angioplasty is not possible because of long arterial occlusions, bypass should be considered.

If the infection is responding to conservative treatment, with resolution of cellulitis on intravenous antibiotics, then bypass, with its inherent risks, is probably not indicated. However, if operative debridement is necessary with amputation of a toe or ray, then arterial bypass may be necessary to achieve full wound healing.

Mechanical control

Patients with extensive cellulitis should not walk. They should be on bed rest and use crutches, Zimmer frame or wheelchair for trips to the bathroom. Every step taken will spread infection.

Heels must be protected with a pillow/foam wedge under the calves to keep the patient's heels clear of the mattress when he is in bed. Special mattresses should be provided to prevent decubitus ulcers. If he slides down the bed he risks pressure lesions from the bed end.

Long periods on the operating table can lead to heel blistering and heel necrosis, and patients who go to theatre should have their heels regularly protected.

It is possible to off-load postoperative wounds in the neuropathic foot with a removable bivalved cast or windowed cast which enable wound inspection. Pressure-relieving ankle–foot orthoses (PRAFOs) are increasingly used as heel off-loaders in both classes of foot.

After operative debridement in the neuroischaemic foot, non-weightbearing is advised until the wound is healed. Patients with infected neuroischaemic feet may wear a Scotchcast boot in bed to protect the heel.

Metabolic control

It is important to make sure that there are no systemic, metabolic or nutritional disturbances to impair the response to infection and retard healing of wounds.

In severe infections, considerable metabolic decompensation may occur. Full resuscitation is urgently required with intravenous fluids and intravenous insulin sliding scale which is often necessary to achieve good blood glucose control whilst the patient is infected. This is followed by a basal-bolus regimen of three times a day short-acting insulin before meals and long-acting insulin at night. Total dose of insulin (units) = $0.5 \times$ body weight (kg), split 2/3 as bolus and 1/3 as basal.

These are complex patients. Cardiac and renal function should be assessed and any impairment should be managed carefully. Echocardiography will identify patients with left ventricular dysfunction. This is expressed as the ejection fraction and a value less than 35% increases the risk of non-cardiac surgery. Close observation and monitoring of these systems is essential to maintain correct electrolyte and fluid balance, especially postoperatively.

Neuroischaemic patients should be regularly taking statins, angiotensin-converting enzyme (ACE) inhibitors and antiplatelet agents and these should be continued if the patient is admitted to hospital. Aspirin should not be stopped before angiography or angioplasty although if the patient is taking aspirin and clopidogrel, the latter should be stopped.

High blood glucose is associated with reduced white cell function, which improves when the blood glucose is lowered.

Educational control

Patients who develop severe infection and present late may have other problems which predispose them towards neglecting infections and failing to accept care. These include:
- Drug addiction
- Psychological problems.

Drug addiction

Some of the worst neglected foot infections we have seen were in the neuropathic feet of young diabetic patients who were addicted to drugs.

CASE STUDY
Early discharge without accepting treatment by a young diabetic patient addicted to crack cocaine

A 28-year-old man with type 1 diabetes mellitus of 18 years' duration attended the Casualty department complaining of a painful foot. He was well known to the hospital and was addicted to crack cocaine. He had severe infection of the left hallux, and deep, infected ulcers over both 1st metatarsal heads (Fig. 5.33). He was admitted to the ward for intravenous antibiotics and possible surgical debridement but walked off the ward 2 hours later before treatment was started and was lost to follow-up. Three weeks later he presented again at Casualty and accepted admission. He explained that he was a crack cocaine addict and had self-discharged because he was fleeing from his dealer to whom he owed money. In the meantime he had accepted treatment from another hospital 200 miles away where he received a short course of intravenous antibiotics. Again he self-discharged when his supply of drugs ran out. Back at home he did not

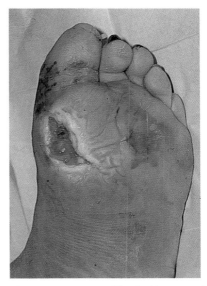

Fig. 5.33 Ulcer over 1st metatarsal head with surrounding cellulitis.

seek further treatment until he developed wet necrosis of the hallux and the pain in his foot became extremely severe.

He underwent extensive surgical debridement of the 1st ray and amputation of the hallux. The foot was slow to heal, and he frequently left the ward for periods of several hours without saying where he was going and a cast with a window over the ulcer was applied to protect his foot. Nursing staff on the ward found him a very difficult patient who would not follow advice. He discharged himself after 8 weeks, and kept two follow-up appointments in the casting clinic but was then lost to follow-up. Six months later we were told he had died after overdosing on heroin.

Key points
- Drug addiction is an enormous barrier to care. Patients are frequently non-compliant with erratic attendances. The door should always be left open to these patients
- Addicts are frequently unable to attend clinic regularly, to follow the treatment regimes suggested, to control their diabetes adequately or to attend early when problems arise
- Refusal to enter hospital and self-discharge from hospital against medical advice are also common in these very challenging patients.

Psychological problems

Concurrent psychological problems are also formidable barriers to care.

CASE STUDY
Neglected feet in a depressed man

A 45-year-old man with type 2 diabetes for 10 years and depressive illness lived alone and neglected his feet. His right foot developed ulceration over the dorsum of the 2nd toe which was complicated by cellulitis (Fig. 5.34a,b). He had peripheral neuropathy with marked clawing of the toes. He wore no socks, the ulcer was not dressed and his shoes were too tight.

Key points

- It is important for all patients and their families to understand the dangers of untreated foot infections,

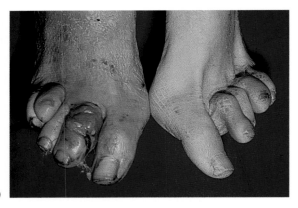

(a)

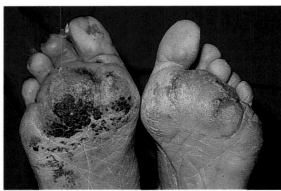

(b)

Fig. 5.34 (a) Dorsal view of both feet shows severe clawing of toes, ulceration and cellulitis. (b) Plantar view of the same pair of feet shows neglected callus and accumulated crusted exudates.

that signs and symptoms are often diminished and that it is essential to check the foot regularly to detect deterioration
- Patients with psychological problems who live alone and are socially isolated are very vulnerable
- The combined vulnerability of a high-risk diabetic foot in a patient with psychological problems can easily lead to disaster which should be preventable.

We use a question and answer sheet to educate patients as follows.

Why is foot infection a dangerous complication of diabetes?

In a diabetic foot, the usual warning signs of infection may be absent or greatly reduced, particularly if you have poorly controlled diabetes, neuropathy or poor blood supply to your feet. If you do not know you have an infection and you continue to walk then infection will be pumped through the foot with every step you take. You can become seriously ill very quickly.

Wouldn't I know there was a serious problem because my foot would hurt?

Infection in diabetic feet is not always painful, but it can quietly destroy the foot. If you wait for pain or other symptoms to develop, the foot infection may need many weeks of treatment and it may even be too late to save the foot.

How can I recognize an infection early?

Your feet should be carefully checked every day for signs of infection.

What are the signs of infection?

You should watch out for:

- Swelling of a foot or part of a foot. Compare your two feet: are they the same size?
- Colour change. Look for red patches or streaks spreading up the foot and leg, or patches of blue, purple or black near the ulcer
- Collection of fluid under the skin which may look like a clear blister, a blood blister or a blister filled with pus. These may also develop under areas of hard skin
- Pain or throbbing in the foot
- Foot develops a hot spot
- Pus or watery discharge or blood leaking from any part of the foot
- The foot smells strongly
- Your body temperature rises above 37.5°C
- Your diabetes goes out of control for no obvious reason

- You shiver and shake
- You feel very cold, or burning hot
- You feel tired, sleepy, weak or unwell with loss of appetite and 'flu'-like symptoms.

What shall I do if I can't check my own feet for these danger signs?

If it is difficult for you to see your feet clearly or to get down to your feet, then please tell the foot clinic.

Remember that symptoms that feel like flu may be due to a foot infection. Always check both your feet if you are unwell. If you call the doctor in, ask him to check your feet.

What should I do if I find a danger sign?

- Seek help the same day from your diabetic foot service or emergency department
- Do not walk on the infected foot: every step you take will pump infection through the foot and leg
- Until you get to hospital, lie with your foot up on a bed or sofa
- Do not wait until tomorrow: the worst infections are the ones which are not caught early.

Must I go at once?

Even if you have an appointment with your GP or foot clinic very soon you should never wait until then: always act the same day.

Remember that the earlier in the day that you come to clinic as an emergency, the easier it will be to sort out your problem. It is difficult to get any necessary tests and investigations performed late in the day. If you need to be admitted into hospital, and beds are in short supply, then the earlier the hunt for a bed is started the sooner your treatment can begin.

Is my foot really so important? Even if it doesn't hurt?

Please always give your foot a high priority. It may not be painful, but it is very important to start treatment as soon as possible.

What if I don't like hospital?

You may be afraid of being taken into hospital, but one thing is sure: if you delay then any hospital stay will be for much longer.

Isn't it unfair for me to get extra appointments when other people need help too and the foot service is busy?

Never delay coming to the foot clinic as an emergency because you feel it is unfair for you to receive extra appointments over and above your routine ones, or because you know the staff are very busy. Good diabetic foot services always run an emergency service in order to catch problems early. Their workload allows for emergency visits. If you do not play your part in this system and your foot is badly damaged by the delay, then the result will be extra work and trouble for everybody, especially you.

Isn't it unwise to take antibiotics for long periods?

Some patients worry about taking antibiotics for long periods. But if diabetic foot ulcers become badly infected the leg is at risk, which is why antibiotics are often prescribed earlier, and for longer periods, than for a patient who is not diabetic.

Didn't I read in the paper that antibiotics cause superbugs which are resistant?

Some patients worry because they read in the papers that taking too many antibiotics can cause germs to develop drug resistance, so that antibiotics will not work for them in the future. The most common cause of this problem is when patients do not complete a course of antibiotics. You can help prevent superbugs from emerging by never stopping your tablets without consulting your doctor. Always take your antibiotics with you wherever you go so that you do not miss a dose.

Do antibiotics cause side-effects?

Some antibiotics can cause side-effects. If you ever develop new symptoms when taking antibiotics you should rapidly contact the diabetic foot clinic and ask for advice. However, you can reduce the likelihood of problems by following precise instructions on the medication, washing down tablets with plenty of water and eating live yoghurt.

How does yoghurt help?

The reason for this is that your bowel (intestines, gut) is full of harmless microorganisms which help you to digest your food. The antibiotics kill the harmful germs in your foot, but also kill the good microorganisms in your bowel. If you eat live yoghurt you will replace the good microorganisms. Below is more information about side-effects.

Possible side-effects from antibiotics

Side-effects: what to do

- Nausea and indigestion: take tablets with lots of water and live yoghurt

If any of the following problems arise, stop the antibiotics and contact the diabetic foot service:

- Vomiting
- Diarrhoea
- Rash
- Severe itching
- Hallucinations
- Hypoglycaemia.

Except in the circumstances explained above you should never stop taking your antibiotics without checking first with the foot clinic. If you stop a course part-way through it may make the germs resistant to the antibiotic so that the antibiotic no longer works for you—or for other patients.

Remember that any other symptoms you develop may have nothing to do with the antibiotics you are taking. Always check it out with your foot clinic.

What else do I need to do if I am taking antibiotics?

Keep a precise record of all the medication you are taking and bring it with you to the foot clinic every time you come. It is very difficult for the clinic to plan your treatment when they do not know what other medication you are taking.

If you see another doctor who stops your foot clinic medication, or prescribes new medication ask him to speak to the clinic. You should also let the clinic know if any new health problems are diagnosed.

How should I look after an infected ulcer?

- Do keep your foot out of the bath or shower unless it is covered with a plastic cast protector. This protects the wound from damage, and protects other people from your infection. If infected wounds are left uncovered they are very attractive to flies, dogs and cats
- Do ensure the dressing is changed at least once a day, and the wound is washed with saline and dried carefully. Ask for help if you cannot look after the wound yourself
- If fluid strikes through the dressing so that you can see it, then it is time for the dressing to be changed
- Do not use a dressing which is designed to be left on the foot for several days. This is very dangerous for diabetic feet which lack protective pain sensation and have an infection, because the infection can spread under the area covered by the dressing and you will not know that this is happening
- Do not change the foot clinic treatment regime without consulting them first. If you have a nurse coming to your home to do the dressings and she wants to change the type of dressing used, then ask her to discuss this with the foot clinic. If your doctor changes the treatment, let the diabetic foot clinic know.

Can I use alternative medicines or folk remedies?

It is unwise to use alternative medicine, folk remedies or over-the-counter treatments for an infected diabetic foot. Always check with your foot clinic before doing this.

Is it all right to soak my foot in salty water?

If you want to do this then always check the temperature of the water first. It should be under 43°C. Use a bath thermometer to measure the temperature.

Can I put a hot poultice on my foot to draw out the infection?

No. You risk severe burns.

Anything else I should be doing?

Don't walk. Use crutches or a wheelchair if you have to move. Every step you take will spread infection along your foot. Resting your foot is essential. Every step you take will make the infection worse.

PRACTICE POINTS

- Signs and symptoms of foot infection are diminished in diabetic patients
- Microbiological investigation is essential for all infected diabetic feet
- Severe infections need intravenous antibiotic therapy and urgent assessment of the need for surgical drainage and debridement
- Infected neuroischaemic feet need vascular assessment and intervention where appropriate
- Patients with ulceration should be taught the danger signs of infection
- Without urgent treatment, severe infections will progress to necrosis.

FURTHER READING

Presentation and diagnosis

Hochman MG, Cheung Y, Brophy DP, Parker JA. Imaging of the diabetic foot. In Veves A, Giurini JM, LoGerfo FW (eds). *The Diabetic Foot*, 2nd edn. Humana Press, New Jersey, USA, 2006, pp. 227–254.

Microbiological control

British National Formulary No. 53. March 2007. BMJ Publishing Group Ltd and RPS Publishing.

Calhoun JH, Overgaard KA, Stevens CM *et al*. Diabetic foot ulcers and infections: current concepts. *Adv Skin Wound Care* 2002; **15**: 31–42.

Ulbrecht JS, Cavanagh PR, Caputo GM. Foot problems in diabetes: an overview. *Clin Infect Dis* 2004; **39** Suppl 2: S73–82.

Chantelau E, Tanudjaja T, Altenhofer F *et al.* Antibiotic treatment for uncomplicated neuropathic forefoot ulcers in diabetes: a controlled trial. *Diabetic Medicine* 1996; **13**: 156–9.

Craig JG, Amin MB, Wu K *et al.* Osteomyelitis of the diabetic foot: MR imaging—pathological correlation. *Radiology* 1997; **203**: 849–55.

Cruciani M, Lipsky BA, Mengoli C, de Lalla F. Are granulocyte colony-stimulating factors beneficial in treating diabetic foot infections? A meta-analysis. *Diabetes Care* 2005; **28**: 454–60.

Cunha BA. Antibiotic selection for diabetic foot infections: a review. *J Foot Ankle Surg* 2000; **39**: 253–7.

Edmonds M. Infection in the neuroischaemic foot. *Int J Low Extrem Wounds* 2005; **4**: 145–53.

Edmonds M, Foster A. The use of antibiotics in the diabetic foot. *Am J Surg* 2004; **187**: 25S–28S.

Edmonds ME, Foster AVM. Infections complicating diseases of the feet in renal patients. In Sweny P, Rubin R, Tolkoff-Rubin N (eds). *The Infectious Complications of Renal Disease.* Oxford University Press, Oxford, UK, 2003, **19**: 399–416.

Eneroth M, Apelqvist J, Stenstrom A. Clinical characteristics and outcome in 223 diabetic patients with deep foot infections. *Foot Ankle Int* 1997; **18**: 716–22.

Faglia E, Favales F, Aldeghi A *et al.* Adjunctive systemic hyperbaric oxygen therapy in treatment of severe prevalently ischemic diabetic foot ulcer. A randomized study. *Diabetes Care* 1996; **19**: 1338–43.

Gough A, Clapperton M, Rolando N *et al.* Randomized placebo-controlled trial of granulocyte-colony stimulating factor in diabetic foot infections. *Lancet* 1997; **350**: 855–9.

Grayson ML. Diabetic foot infections. Antimicrobial therapy. *Infect Dis Clin North Am* 1995; **9**: 143–61.

Karchmer AW. Microbiology and treatment of diabetic foot infections. In Veves A, Giurini JM, LoGerfo FW (eds). *The Diabetic Foot*, 2nd edn. Humana Press, New Jersey, USA, 2006, pp. 255–68.

Lipsky BA. Empirical therapy for diabetic foot infections: are there clinical clues to guide antibiotic selection? *Clin Microbiol Infect* 2007; **13**: 351–3.

Lipsky BA, Pecoraro RE, Larson SA *et al.* Outpatient management of uncomplicated lower-extremity infections in diabetic patients. *Arch Intern Med* 1990; **150**: 790–7.

Morrison WB, Schweitzer ME, Batte WB *et al.* Osteomyelitis of the foot: relative importance of primary and secondary MR imaging signs. *Radiology* 1998; **207**: 625–32.

Rajbhandari S, Sutton M, Davies C *et al.* Sausage toe: a reliable sign of underlying osteomyelitis. *Diabetic Medicine* 2000; **17**: 74–7.

Shank CF, Feibel JB. Osteomyelitis in the diabetic foot: diagnosis and management. *Foot Ankle Clin* 2006; **11**: 775–89.

Slater RA, Lazarovitch T, Boldur I *et al.* Swab cultures accurately identify bacterial pathogens in diabetic foot wounds not involving bone. *Diabet Med* 2004; **21**: 705–9.

Tentolouris N, Jude EB, Smirnof I *et al.* Methicillin-resistant *Staphylococcus aureus*: an increasing problem in a diabetic foot clinic. *Diabetic Medicine* 1999; **16**: 767–71.

Venkatesan P, Lawn S, Macfarlane RM *et al.* Conservative management of osteomyelitis in the feet of diabetic patients. *Diabetic Medicine* 1997; **14**: 487–90.

Wound control

Armstrong DG, Lavery LA, Sariaya M *et al.* Leukocytosis is a poor indicator of acute osteomyelitis of the foot in diabetes mellitus. *J Foot Ankle Surg* 1996; **35**: 280–3.

Grayson ML, Gibbons GW, Balogh K *et al.* Probing to bone in infected pedal ulcers: a clinical sign of osteomyelitis in diabetic patients. *JAMA* 1995; **273**: 721–3.

Lavery LA, Armstrong DG, Peters EJ, Lipsky BA. Probe to bone test for diagnosing diabetic foot osteomyelitis: reliable or relic? *Diabetes Care* 2007; **30**: 270–4.

Mumcuoglu KY, Miller J, Mumcuoglu M *et al.* Destruction of bacteria in the digestive tract of the maggot of *Lucilia sericata* (Diptera: Calliforidae). *J Med Entomol* 2001; **38**: 161–6.

Pittet D, Wyssa B, Herter-Clavell C *et al.* Outcome of diabetic foot infections treated conservatively. *Arch Intern Med* 1999; **159**: 851–6.

Vascular control

Dyet JF, Nicholson AA, Ettles DF. Vascular imaging and intervention in peripheral arteries in the diabetic patient. *Diabetes/Metabolism Res Rev* 2000; **16** (Suppl 1): S16–22.

Eagle KA, Berger PB, Calkins H *et al.* ACC/AHA Guidelines for Perioperative Cardiovascular Evaluation for Noncardiac Surgery Update. *J Am Coll Cardiol* 2002; **39**: 542–53.

Faglia E, Mantero M, Caminiti M *et al.* Extensive use of peripheral angioplasty, particularly infrapopliteal, in the treatment of ischaemic diabetic foot ulcers: clinical results of a multicentric study of 221 consecutive diabetic subjects. *J Int Med* 2002; **252**: 225–32.

Jacqueminet S, Hartemann-Neurtier A, Izzillo R *et al.* Percutaneous transluminal angioplasty in severe diabetic foot ischemia: outcomes and prognostic factors. *Diabetes Metab* 2005; **31**: 370–5.

Kay J, Chow WH, Chan TM *et al.* Acetylcysteine for prevention of acute deterioration of renal function following elective coronary angiography and intervention: a randomized controlled trial. *JAMA* 2003; **289**: 553–8.

Vraux H, Hammer F, Verhelst R *et al.* Subintimal angioplasty of tibial vessel occlusions in the treatment of critical limb ischaemia: mid-term results. *Eur J Vasc Endovasc Surg* 2000; **20**: 441–6.

Mechanical control

Knowles EA, Armstrong DG, Hayat SA *et al*. Offloading diabetic foot wounds using the scotchcast boot: a retrospective study. *Osteomy Wound Manag* 2002; **48**: 50–3.

Metabolic control

Geerlings SE, Hoepelman AI. Immune dysfunction in patients with diabetes mellitus (DM). *FEMS Immunol Med Microbiol* 1999; **26**: 259–65.

Jirkovska A, Fejfarova V, Hosova J *et al*. Impairment of polymorphonuclear leukocyte function and diabetes control in patients with diabetic foot. *Diabetes Research and Clinical Practice* 2000; **50** Suppl 1: 281–281(1).

Leibovici L, Yehezkelli Y, Porter A, *et al*. Influence of diabetes mellitus and glycaemic control on the characteristics and outcome of common infections. *Diabetic Medicine* 1996; **13**: 457–63.

Marhoffer W, Stein M, Maeser E, Federlin K. Impairment of polymorphonuclear leukocyte function and metabolic control of diabetes. *Diabetes Care* 1992; **15**: 256–60.

Sato N, Shimizu H, Suwa K *et al*. MPO activity and generation of active O_2 species in leukocytes from poorly controlled diabetic patients. *Diabetes Care* 1992; **15**: 1050–2.

Educational control

Foster A. Psychological aspects of treating the diabetic foot. *Podiatry Now* 1998; **1**: 123–6.

Malone JM, Snyder M, Anderson G *et al*. Prevention of amputation by diabetic education. *Am J Surg* 1989; **158**: 520–4.

6 Stage 5: the necrotic foot

The service of the foot
Being once gangrened is not then respected
For what before it was . . .
(Coriolanus III, i, William Shakespeare)

PRESENTATION AND DIAGNOSIS

Once the diabetic foot has developed necrosis this has very grave implications, especially in cases where the patient has a neuroischaemic foot and renal disease.

We have seen young patients with neuropathy who developed wet gangrene due to infection, undergo a minor amputation and do very well subsequently for many years. However, when the foot is neuroischaemic and develops necrosis the long-term outlook can be rather bleak, whether the necrosis be wet or dry. This is because the development of necrosis in the neuroischaemic diabetic foot is usually a marker of severe cardiovascular disease and the long-term outlook is very poor because of that underlying disease. As we have emphasized, this is particularly the case when there is a combination of neuropathy, ischaemia and renal disease. However, this situation should not be used as an excuse for therapeutic nihilism. Despite the gravity of the situation many patients can recover from the episode of necrosis and although they are sick patients, their lives can still be significantly prolonged if their feet and diabetic complications are managed well.

Many cases of necrosis can be prevented if the feet are inspected regularly and infections are detected early and treated rapidly and appropriately. It is essential for the stage 5 foot (and all stages of diabetic foot disease) to catch the foot early, diagnose it correctly, and treat it aggressively. Patients who arrive at the hospital with necrosis, even if just one toe is involved, should never be sent home from Casualty with a future outpatient appointment, but should be admitted and given urgent care by a multidis-

ciplinary team, in the clear knowledge that both the life and the limb of the patient are at risk. Necrosis is too frequently underestimated by inexperienced clinicians. The stage 5 foot should never be taken lightly or put off until another day.

Necrosis can involve skin, subcutaneous and fascial layers. In lightly pigmented skin it is easily evident but in the subcutaneous and fascial layers it is not so apparent. Furthermore, the extent of necrosis may be difficult to determine: often the blueish-black discolouration of skin is just the 'tip of an iceberg' of massive necrosis.

Other conditions may masquerade as necrosis (see Chapter 1). Purplish-black or brown discolouration of the skin also occurs after bruising and is sometimes difficult to differentiate from early necrosis associated with a history of trauma. A superficial collection of dried blood within a blister or tracking under the skin can give part of a foot a black and leathery appearance. Cyanosis of toes and feet is seen in severe cardiac and respiratory failure.

Shoe dye and the application of topical henna will result in black or brown discolouration of the skin.

Early signs of necrosis

The signs that part of a foot is becoming necrotic may be subtle in the early stages, and may mimic bruising or chilblains. A careful search should be made for early signs:

- A toe which is developing a blue or purple tinge, having been previously pink because of infection or ischaemia
- Toes which have become very pale in comparison with their fellows

A Practical Manual of Diabetic Foot Care, 2nd edition, Edmonds, Foster and Sanders.
Published 2008 Blackwell Publishing. ISBN 978-1-4051-61473

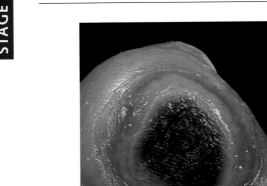

Fig. 6.1 This ulcer on the plantar surface of the hallux changed its colour from healthy pink to black over a 4-day period.

- An ulcer which has changed its colour from healthy shiny pink granulations to grey, purple or black or its texture from a smooth to a matt surface (Fig. 6.1).

Causes of necrosis

Necrosis can be due to infection, when it is usually wet, or due to occlusive macrovascular disease of the arteries of the leg, when it is usually dry. Necrosis is not, as previously thought, due to a microangiopathic arteriolar occlusive disease, or so-called small vessel disease. Health-care professionals working with diabetic foot disease should avoid using this term, which is imprecise and may lead to therapeutic nihilism.

Digital necrosis is common in patients with renal impairment, particularly those with end-stage renal failure, even though they are treated with dialysis. Patients with severe renal impairment also have a propensity to develop dry necrosis, sometimes in the presence of palpable pedal pulses and in the absence of infection. A further discussion of foot disease in the diabetic patient with renal impairment is given below.

Wet necrosis

Wet necrosis is secondary to a septic vasculitis associated with severe soft tissue infection and ulceration, and is the commonest type of necrosis in the diabetic foot. However, there is often a delay in presentation of the patient.

CASE STUDY
Puncture wound with delay in presentation of wet necrotic foot

A 38-year-old male Afro-Caribbean patient with type 2 diabetes mellitus of 2 years' known duration, and a body mass index of 31, who had been lost to follow-up after his initial diagnosis, trod on a tintack. This penetrated the sole of his shoe during his work as a school caretaker. He visited his general practitioner who prescribed a 5-day course of 250 mg amoxicillin tds. After 5 days the patient thought the foot had healed.

Two weeks later, the patient's girlfriend noted greenish discolouration of the sole of his foot and insisted that he attend the hospital Casualty department. The plantar surface of the forefoot was bulging, there was deep infection involving the 3rd, 4th and 5th web spaces and the 2nd, 3rd, 4th and 5th toes were necrotic, although this was not immediately apparent because the dorsum of the foot was heavily pigmented (Fig. 6.2a). He was admitted to hospital for intravenous antibiotics and surgical debridement, and four toes and their adjoining metatarsal heads were removed. Once the infection was controlled he insisted on returning to work. He was treated in a total-contact cast, and healed in 6 months (Fig. 6.2b). He was physically very active and his casts needed additional strengthening and very frequent replacement. On one occasion, the day after his cast had been applied, he went for a very muddy walk on Dartmoor, a national park renowned for its bogs and rocks, in his cast and returned to the clinic with the cast in tatters. He developed end-stage renal failure but continued to work and to lead an active life and while on holiday in Spain dialyzed in the local restaurant by hanging his CAPD bag from a hat stand. Two years after his admission for the foot problem he was found dead in bed from a myocardial infarction.

Key points
- Untreated infection can rapidly lead to necrosis
- Puncture wounds should be followed up very carefully as signs of infection will only become apparent when they have spread from the deep tissues to the superficial structures
- Bulging of the plantar surface indicates deep infection with collection of pus which needs drainage
- In the neuropathic foot, extensive necrosis can be successfully treated by surgical debridement with eventual complete healing
- Physically active and heavy patients need extra-strong casts.

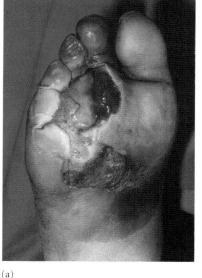 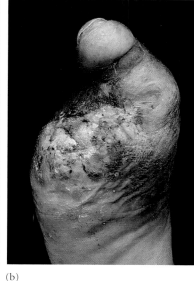

Fig. 6.2 (a) Plantar view of infection following a puncture wound which has led to wet necrosis of the forefoot requiring amputation of four toes and their adjoining metatarsal heads. (b) Full healing of the very large postsurgical tissue defect took 6 months. He wore a total-contact cast to off-load the wound.

(a)   (b)

CASE STUDY
Delay in presentation due to confusion between blood blister and wet necrosis

A 67-year-old man with type 2 diabetes which had not previously been diagnosed, developed what he took to be a blood blister on his left hallux. The lesion was not painful, he felt well, and he did not seek treatment until he noticed an unpleasant odour and went to Casualty. The toe was infected and necrotic. Pedal pulses were bounding. His vibration perception threshold was 45 volts (Fig. 6.3). He underwent amputation of the hallux and the foot healed in 4 months. Three weeks after he was discharged he re-presented at the diabetic foot clinic with a rocker-bottom Charcot foot. This was treated in a total-contact cast for 6 months and there was no progression of the deformity.

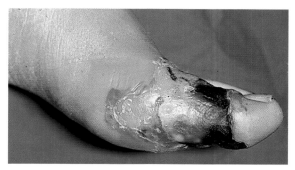

Fig. 6.3 This necrotic toe in a previously undiagnosed diabetic patient was thought by him to be a blood blister.

Key points
- Necrosis may be mistaken for blood blisters by patients and health-care professionals
- In patients with neuropathy, necrosis may not be painful
- Patients with neuropathy who undergo surgery for necrosis may develop Charcot's osteoarthropathy
- Patients with type 2 diabetes may have undiagnosed diabetes for many years and develop severe complications including neuropathy and foot ulceration by the time of diagnosis
- In wet necrosis, the tissues are grey or black, moist and often malodorous. Adjoining tissues are infected and pus may discharge from an ulcerated area between necrosis and viable tissue. There may be no clear demarcation line between necrosis and viable tissue and it may be difficult to predict exactly which areas of tissue are viable until debridement has been performed
- Once infection is established, necrosis can develop within a few hours.

CASE STUDY
Wet necrosis with rapid onset

A 73-year-old Afro-Caribbean woman with type 2 diabetes of 33 years' duration, peripheral vascular disease and a previous below-knee amputation attended the diabetic foot clinic with a 2 cm broken blister on her

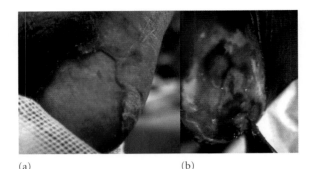

(a)   (b)

Fig. 6.4 (a) Bulla which looks clean and superficial. (b) Picture of the same foot taken 1 week later, shows an infected, necrotic heel. The patient underwent a below-knee amputation.

left heel (Fig. 6.4a). She was obese and confined to a wheelchair. She did not want to take antibiotics and said she would prefer not to have visits from the district nursing service as her daughter, with whom she lived, would look after the foot. Her daughter was carefully taught to clean and dress the foot, and advised to check it every day. We emphasized the need for immediate return to the diabetic foot clinic if any deterioration occurred. The patient returned to clinic 1 week later, for her routine appointment, with a discharging, malodorous ulcer and extensive deep necrosis (Fig. 6.4b). She was admitted to hospital and given intravenous antibiotics. She had angiography but there was severe infrapopliteal disease and no distal arterial run-off. No vascular intervention was feasible and she underwent a second below-knee amputation.

Key points
- Ischaemic foot ulcers can quickly become infected and deteriorate to wet necrosis with alarming rapidity
- Detection of deterioration was rendered more difficult because the patient had very heavily pigmented skin and did not want home nursing visits
- We encourage our patients and their families to be 'critically observant'. At the first appearance of a break in the skin, no matter how small and shallow, they are advised to seek help the same day.

Dry necrosis

Dry necrosis is hard, blackened, leathery, mummified tissue. There is usually a clear demarcation line between necrosis and viable tissue.

Dry necrosis is the result of severe ischaemia, secondary to poor tissue perfusion from atherosclerotic narrowing of the arteries of the leg, often complicated by thrombus and, occasionally, emboli.

Necrosis in the neuropathic foot

In the neuropathic foot, the first presentation of necrosis is almost invariably of wet necrosis, and this is caused when infection complicates an ulcer, leading to a septic arteritis of the digital and small arteries of the foot. The walls of these arteries are infiltrated by polymorphonuclear leucocytes leading to occlusion of the lumen by septic thrombus. This leads to the so-called 'diabetic gangrene' where a toe becomes blue and subsequently black and necrosed, while a few centimetres proximally a bounding pedal pulse can often be palpated. It is this presentation which probably gave rise to the myth of diabetic gangrene being caused by 'small vessel disease'. Sometimes the portal of entry for the infection which damages the digital arteries is on the same toe, but it may be proximal and is sometimes several centimetres away from the affected toe.

CASE STUDY
Wet necrosis in a neuropathic foot

A 28-year-old male Chinese patient, who could speak no English, had type 1 diabetes of 13 years' duration. His general practitioner referred him after he presented late with an infected plantar ulcer and patches of wet necrosis (Fig. 6.5a,b,c,d). By the time this patient reached the diabetic foot clinic, he needed a ray amputation and he was treated with amoxicillin 500 mg tds, flucloxacillin 500 mg qds, metronidazole 500 mg tds and ceftazidime 1 g tds. Infected tissue was sent from the operating theatre, and grew *Staphylococcus aureus*, *Streptococcus* group B and anaerobic streptococci. He was followed up in the foot clinic and quickly healed, but subsequently he failed to attend again.

Key points
- Untreated neuropathic ulcers which become infected lead to septic vasculitis and gangrene of the toes. This is the true 'diabetic gangrene' which can occur in the neuropathic foot with a good arterial supply
- Diabetic gangrene is preventable if infected ulcers are treated early. If intravenous antibiotics are given when the toe first takes on a blueish tinge, it is possible to prevent deterioration
- Patients who are strangers in a foreign land are very vulnerable as they may have difficulty in finding help sufficiently early.

Necrosis in the neuroischaemic foot

Both wet and dry necrosis can occur in the neuroischaemic foot.

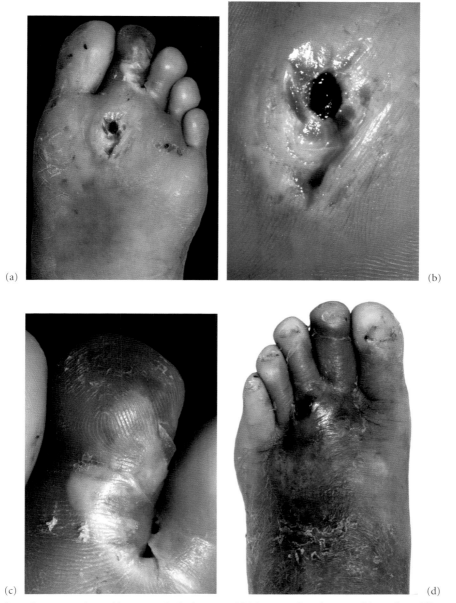

Fig. 6.5 (a) This foot of a young patient with neuropathy had developed patches of wet necrosis secondary to infected plantar ulceration. (b) Close-up view of ulcer after debridement.

(c) Wet necrosis at the apex of the 2nd toe. (d) Dorsal view to show patches of wet necrosis secondary to infection which has tracked from the plantar surface.

Wet necrosis

Wet necrosis is caused by a septic vasculitis, secondary to soft tissue infection and ulceration as in the neuropathic foot. However, in the neuroischaemic foot, reduced arterial perfusion to the foot resulting from atherosclerotic occlusive disease of the leg arteries is an important predisposing factor. When wet and infected necrosis is successfully treated with antibiotics it will desiccate and become dry necrosis.

STAGE 5

CASE STUDY
Necrosis from *Pseudomonas* infection

A 77-year-old man with type 2 diabetes of 12 years' duration developed ulceration on the lateral aspect of his right 5th metatarsal head. His feet were neuroischaemic. There was a sudden deterioration with a mild fever and spreading wet necrosis (Fig. 6.6a). A tissue sample was taken for culture which revealed a pure heavy growth of *Pseudomonas*. The patient was treated with antipseudomonal therapy in the form of ceftazidime 1 g tds and the necrosis which had previously been wet became dry and the fever resolved (Fig. 6.6b,c).

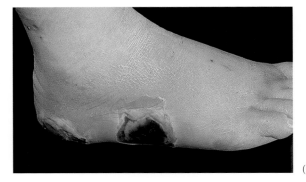

(a)

Key points
- Gram-negative organisms including *Pseudomonas*, *Citrobacter*, *Serratia* and *Klebsiella* can cause infection and necrosis in the diabetic foot
- It is important to detect such organisms by collecting a tissue specimen, if possible, or a deep ulcer swab
- Spreading necrosis in the neuroischaemic foot may be due to infection and not to increasing ischaemia and should be treated with antibiotic therapy and, if indicated, surgical debridement.

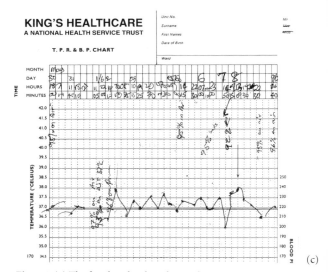

(b)

Dry necrosis
Dry necrosis is secondary to a severe reduction in arterial perfusion and occurs in three circumstances:
- Severe chronic ischaemia
- Acute ischaemia
- Emboli to the toes.

Severe chronic ischaemia
Peripheral arterial disease usually progresses slowly in the diabetic patient, but eventually a severe reduction in arterial perfusion results in vascular compromise of the skin. This is often precipitated by minor trauma, leading to a cold, blue toe which usually becomes necrotic unless the foot is revascularized. Many diabetic feet with a very low pressure index do well until the skin is breached by an injury. Inflammation and successful healing make increased vascular demands which the ischaemic foot is unable to fulfil.

Many diabetic neuroischaemic patients never complain of intermittent claudication or rest pain. If the patient has concurrent retinopathy with severe visual impairment he will frequently be unaware of ulcers or necrosis. The name 'eye–foot syndrome' has been attached to cases of middle-aged or elderly men who live alone, have undiagnosed diabetes leading to retinopathy and neuropathy, and present late with necrosis of the feet (see Pathway to amputation 3 in Chapter 7).

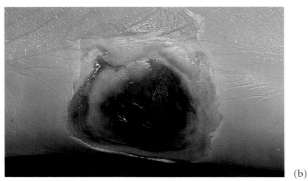

(c)

Fig. 6.6 (a) The foot has developed spreading necrosis. (b) Close-up view of the foot. (c) The patient had fever whilst the necrosis was spreading and this resolved when ceftazidime as antipseudomonal treatment was started.

Acute ischaemia
Blue discolouration leading to necrosis of the toes is also seen in acute ischaemia, which is usually caused either by thrombosis complicating an atherosclerotic narrowing

in the superficial femoral or popliteal artery or emboli from proximal atherosclerotic plaques to the femoral or popliteal arteries.

Acute ischaemia presents as a sudden onset of pain in the leg associated with pallor and coldness of the foot, quickly followed by mottling and slaty grey discolouration, and pallor of the nail beds. The diabetic patient may not experience paraesthesiae because of an existing sensory neuropathy, which also reduces the severity of ischaemic pain and may delay presentation. Some patients may complain of extreme weakness of the affected limb but not of pain.

CASE STUDY
Necrosis following acute ischaemia

A 74-year-old lady with type 2 diabetes of 32 years' duration developed acute ischaemia of her right leg (Fig. 6.7a). Postoperatively she developed blistering on the dorsum of the foot and discolouration of the tips of three toes, but the foot was well perfused and the graft was patent (Fig. 6.7b–d). She was treated conservatively with systemic antibiotics to control and eradicate infection and gentle debridement of the demarcation lines between gangrene and viable tissue. She had regular graft surveillance. After 7 months the necrotic areas autoamputated and the foot healed.

Key points

- After an episode of acute ischaemia patients may develop areas of necrosis even following successful revascularization
- Such necrosis is related to the markedly reduced perfusion during the acute ischaemic episode
- These areas of necrosis are usually dry but may become wet if they become infected
- Such necrosis can be treated conservatively
- If necrosis develops after an arterial bypass, it is important to check perfusion of the foot immediately to ensure that the graft is still patent.

Emboli to the toes

Another cause of necrosis, particularly to the toe, is the passage of emboli to the digital circulation often originating from atherosclerotic plaques in the aorta and leg arteries.

'Showers of emboli' may originate from plaques in the aortoiliac and the superficial femoral arteries. The plaques are usually irregular or ulcerated and covered with debris, particularly in the aorta. The emboli lead to cool, painful cyanotic toes and the development of areas of necrosis at the tips of the toes, which generally heal without the need for amputation (Fig. 6.8). These patients may present with palpable pedal pulses.

Emboli may also occur as a complication of invasive angiographic procedures, presenting as trash foot. Emboli may also originate from the heart. Cholesterol emboli may be related to warfarin therapy.

The initial sign of emboli may be blueish or purple discolouration which is quite well demarcated but quickly proceeds to necrosis. If it escapes infection it will dry out and mummify.

If patients with emboli have minimal or no neuropathy, the foot is extremely painful.

CASE STUDY
Emboli, minimal neuropathy and severe localized pain

A 51-year-old woman with type 2 diabetes of 7 years' duration was referred to the diabetic foot clinic by the vascular surgeon who had diagnosed peripheral embolic disease. She had very discrete areas of non-blanching blue discolouration on the tips of her right 3rd and 5th toes (Fig. 6.9). Her pressure index was 0.5 and her vibration perception threshold was 20 volts.

Angiography had shown multiple stenoses of the right superficial femoral artery and she was due for angioplasty. Aspirin and dipyridamole had been prescribed by the vascular surgeons. She had neglected toenails which were cut except for the right 3rd which she could not bear to be touched because it was so painful. She underwent angioplasty with almost immediate improvement in her pain and her pressure index rose to 0.9. The blue areas developed superficial necrosis, which healed over the next 3 months.

Key points

- Peripheral emboli present as areas of discrete blueish discolouration in one or more toes
- The origin of the emboli in this case was atherosclerotic plaques in the superficial femoral artery
- Such patients with peripheral embolic disease should receive antiplatelet therapy and vascular intervention if there is proximal arterial occlusive disease.

CASE STUDY
Trash foot after angioplasty

An 80-year-old man with type 2 diabetes of 21 years' duration had necrotic ulceration of the dorsum of the left foot. Duplex angiography revealed occlusion of the

STAGE 5

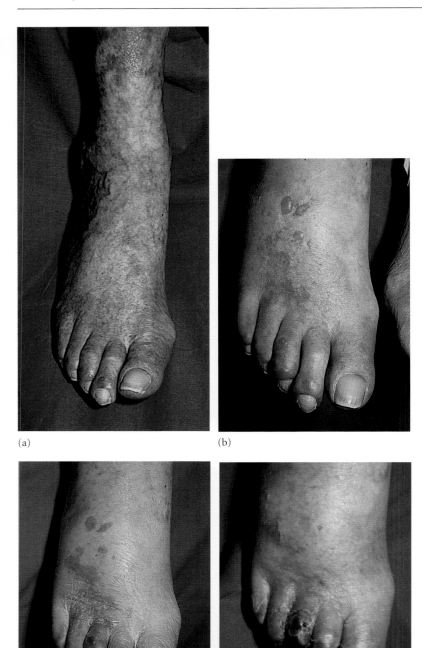

(a)

(b)

(c)

(d)

Fig. 6.7 (a) Acute ischaemia: the foot is grey, pallid and cold and needed distal bypass for limb salvage. (b) Two days after her distal bypass the foot has developed small blisters on the dorsum and the tips of the toes are discoloured. (c) Two weeks later the discoloured areas were necrotic. (d) One month after the discolouration was first noted the necrosis demarcated and stopped extending.

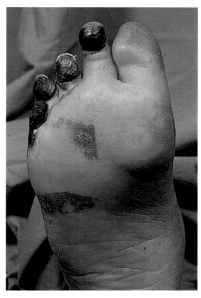

Fig. 6.8 A shower of emboli has led to necrosis of four toes.

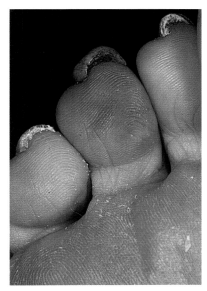

Fig. 6.9 Discrete areas of non-blanching blue discolouration on the tip of the right 3rd toe. This toe was so painful that she would not allow us to cut the nail.

superficial femoral and popliteal artery. The patient underwent subintimal angioplasty. At this procedure, it was noted that the proximal anterior tibial artery was occluded with filling into the peroneal through a collateral. The posterior tibial artery was occluded. Post-angioplasty,

embolic material passed into the distal popliteal arery. This was partly aspirated but some remained with the peroneal artery still occluded. He developed critical ischaemia and necrosis of the first to fourth toes (Fig. 6.10a). He underwent emergency embolectomy and femoral–popliteal bypass. Tissue from the necrosis grew *Klebsiella pneumoniae*. He was treated with intravenous meropenem 1 g tds and the patch of necrosis on the dorsum of the foot resolved and the digital necrosis became dry (Fig. 6.10b). However, it was complicated by further infection and thus it was decided to carry out a forefoot amputation, the femoral–popliteal bypass still being patent. The wound had nearly healed at the time of writing (Fig. 6.10c).

Key points

- Trash foot secondary to emboli may occur after angioplasty but is very rare
- It is usually treated conservatively and heparin anticoagulation may limit the damage
- In severe cases, emergency embolectomy may be required
- Necrotic toes may be amputated if the circulation is reasonable enough to expect healing of the wounds.

Necrosis and renal impairment

Patients with advanced diabetic nephropathy or end-stage renal failure have an increased propensity to develop necrosis. Most have anaemia, neuropathy (which may be aggravated by uraemia) and arterial calcification. In addition, the atherosclerotic process is accelerated. The reasons for this propensity of diabetic renal patients to develop necrosis are not entirely clear.

CASE STUDY
Necrotic finger in a renal patient

A 45-year-old man with type 1 diabetes of 30 years' duration and end-stage renal failure treated with haemodialysis, burned his finger. He had severe neuropathy of the hands as well as the feet, but no peripheral vascular disease. Despite having a bounding radial pulse, the burn became necrotic (Fig. 6.11a,b). There were no signs of infection. The necrotic area healed after 3 months.

Key points

- Necrosis is a common problem in renal diabetic patients on haemodialysis
- When necrosis develops in upper limbs there is usually no evidence of macrovascular disease or infection

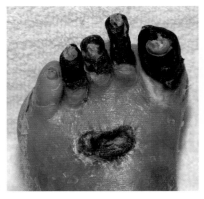

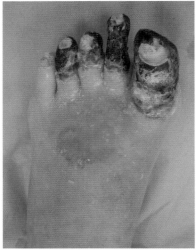

(a)

(b)

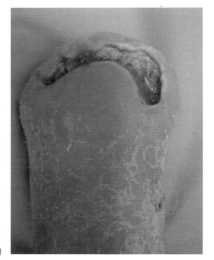

(c)

Fig. 6.10 (a) Following angioplasty, necrotic first to fourth digits with pre-existing patch of necrosis on the dorsum of foot. (b) Patch of necrosis on dorsum of foot has resolved and digital necrosis is dry. (c) Following amputation of the toes, the wound has almost healed.

- Diabetic patients on haemodialysis often have the most profound neuropathy of all patients and should be warned to check both hands and feet regularly and present early if they injure themselves
- Diabetic patients can also develop hand problems from infection of abrasions, several cases of which have been reported from Africa and labelled 'tropical hand syndrome'. In the presence of particularly severe and wide-reaching neuropathy, we have also seen neuropathic ulceration of the hands.

Necrosis can occur in the feet of diabetic renal patients with palpable pulses in the absence of severe peripheral arterial disease and in the absence of infection. An apparently small and trivial trauma such as a small split in dry skin (Fig. 6.12) or a tight nail sulcus will frequently lead to necrosis which then spreads (Fig. 6.13). Necrotic lesions often become rapidly infected in diabetic patients with renal failure.

Traumatic injuries are very common in diabetic patients in end-stage renal failure: this may be because the soft tissues of the foot are more easily damaged in end-stage renal failure, or because patients with the heavy burden of managing to cope with diabetes and renal problems become more careless about looking after their feet.

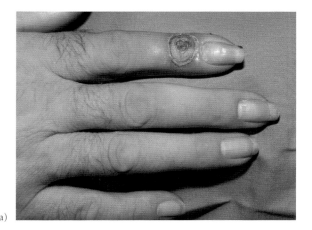

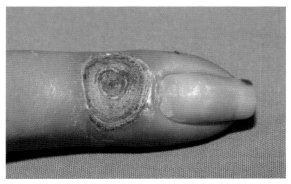

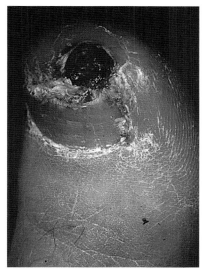

Fig. 6.13 This patch of necrosis developed on the apex of the 1st toe of a patient in end-stage renal failure treated by renal transplantation. Her pedal pulses were palpable. The patch of necrosis began as a small crack in the nail sulcus and spread very slowly to involve most of the toe, which was amputated because of severe pain. She smoked 25 cigarettes a day.

(a)

(b)

Fig. 6.11 (a) The finger of this patient on haemodialysis became necrotic after a burn. There was no infection. (b) Close-up view.

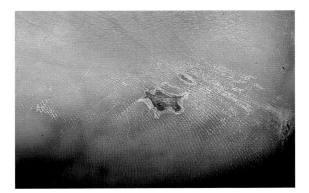

Fig. 6.12 A small split in dry skin on the border of the foot of a patient in end-stage renal failure treated with haemodialysis is becoming necrotic.

CASE STUDY
Successful treatment of infected necrotic foot in patient with renal impairment using transmetatarsal amputation and hybrid revascularization of angioplasty and distal arterial bypass

This patient presented with extensive wet necrosis of the toes in a neuroischaemic foot. She had moderate renal impairment with a serum creatinine of 194 µmol/L. She was treated with amoxicillin 500 mg tds, flucloxacillin 500 mg qds, metronidazole 500 mg tds and ceftazidime 1 g twice daily intravenously. Duplex angiography indicated superficial femoral artery, popliteal and tibial arterial disease. She underwent urgent downstream angiography which showed multiple tight stenoses in the superficial femoral and popliteal artery. A faint posterior tibial artery was seen just above the ankle, forming a plantar arch. The superficial femoral artery and popliteal artery were angioplastied. On the same day, she underwent emergency transmetatarsal amputation (Fig. 6.14a). Tissue grew *Proteus mirabilis*, *Enterococcus faecalis* and mixed anaerobes. Six days later, a popliteal to posterior tibial artery bypass was performed. The wound

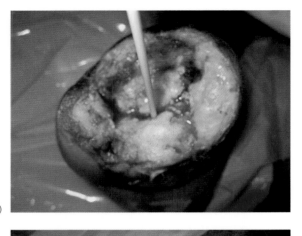

(a)

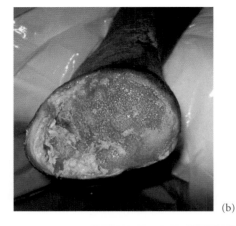

(b)

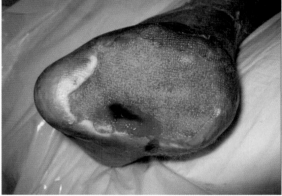

(c)

(d)

Fig. 6.14 (a) Postoperative wound with swab inserted deep into the wound. (b) Granulating wound after VAC therapy and revascularization. (c) Wound continuing to granulate and improve after further VAC therapy. (d) Wound healed after 6 months. (Courtesy of Melanie Doxford.)

responded well to vacuum-assisted closure (VAC) therapy (Fig. 6.14b,c) and eventually healed after 6 months (Fig. 6.14d).

Key points
- When ischaemic patients present with extensive wet necrosis, it is important to remove this as an emergency and then investigate the circulation
- Distal arterial bypass can be successful in patients with renal impairment
- Healing of postoperative wounds in patients with renal failure is improved with VAC therapy
- Patients who cannot be revascularized may still benefit from VAC therapy, which has improved the chances of healing postoperative wounds in diabetic patients with renal failure.

CASE STUDY
Necrosis secondary to trauma

A 60-year-old woman with type 1 diabetes of 30 years' duration and on dialysis had profoundly neuropathic feet with stenoses of the tibial arteries. She traumatized her toe and initially noted a small patch of blackened tissue which rapidly enlarged over the subsequent 10 days (Fig. 6.15). There was no overt discharge or cellulitis. She underwent successful angioplasty and her toe was allowed to auto-amputate which took 15 months.

Key points
- This foot shows typical onset of necrosis in renal failure
- Digital necrosis is often initiated by trauma, particularly in the diabetic renal foot. The reason for this is not fully

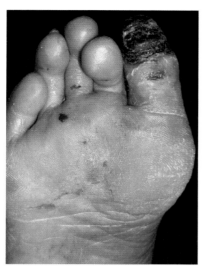

Fig. 6.15 Digital necrosis in end-stage renal failure.

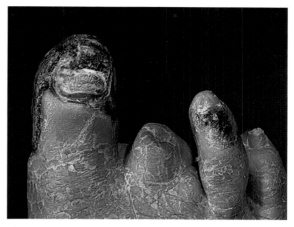

Fig. 6.16 Dry necrosis which began when the 2nd toe was pricked to obtain a blood sample. The 2nd toe has already autoamputated.

known but rheological abnormalities in microvascular flow related to the impaired renal function may contribute
· Unless full pulsatile flow and a pressure index above 1 can be achieved by revascularization, then digital amputation should be avoided
· Autoamputation is an acceptable treatment but the toe needs very close follow-up and the process may take many months.

CASE STUDY
Iatrogenic necrosis in a renal foot

A 64-year-old man with type 2 diabetes of 16 years' duration also had retinopathy, peripheral neuropathy, peripheral vascular disease and end-stage renal disease treated by renal transplantation. He had bilateral peripheral vascular disease and necrosis of the apices of the toes of his right foot, but his left foot was intact. The necrosis had started spontaneously but was slow to resolve and he was admitted for an angiogram. During the procedure he was thought to be hypoglycaemic, and a capillary blood sample was obtained by pricking his left second toe. Within 24 hours the toe turned blue and subsequently developed full-thickness necrosis which gradually spread up the foot until it affected the entire forefoot. He refused partial amputation or major amputation, and the foot was regularly debrided (Fig. 6.16). Antibiotics were administered to treat episodes of infection and the necrotic areas remained dry and eventually separated after 2 years. The

foot remained healed until he died of a myocardial infarction 6 months later.

Key points
· Blood samples should never be taken from the toes of a diabetic neuroischaemic foot
· Patients in renal failure are particularly prone to develop necrosis following an apparently trivial injury
· Once established in the toe, necrosis may spread rapidly in the forefoot.

MANAGEMENT

Whether the stage 5 foot is neuropathic or neuroischaemic it should always be regarded as a clinical emergency which should be seen by the diabetic foot service without delay and preferably the same day that it is noticed.

Patients with necrosis should not be treated solely in primary care or by health-care practitioners working alone: this is unfair both to patients and health-care professionals. Most patients will, however, need joint follow-up wound care from the community nursing team as well as the hospital.

It is important for health-care practitioners and patients to be aware that necrosis does not automatically progress to major amputation. Necrosis can often be successfully treated. However, each class of foot requires a different approach to the management of necrosis.

In the neuropathic foot, wet gangrene due to infection can be treated with intravenous antibiotics and surgical debridement.

In the neuroischaemic foot, this approach may also be used, but revascularization should be performed if feasible. If vascular intervention cannot be carried out, then surgical debridement should be avoided if possible, and intravenous antibiotics may be used to convert wet necrosis to dry necrosis.

Dry necrosis in the neuroischaemic foot can be successfully managed with revascularization of the foot and amputation of the necrotic part. If vascular intervention is impossible, some cases of dry necrosis will do well and autoamputate with conservative care alone.

Patients should be admitted immediately for urgent investigations and multidisciplinary management. It is important to achieve:
- Wound control
- Microbiological control
- Vascular control
- Mechanical control
- Metabolic control
- Educational control.

Wound control

Feet at stage 5 must always be classified as neuropathic or neuroischaemic because the treatment offered will differ according to the vascular status of the foot, and treatment decisions need to be made very quickly if the foot is to be saved.

Neuropathic foot

In the neuropathic foot, operative debridement is almost always indicated for wet gangrene. The main principle of treatment is surgical removal of the necrotic tissue, which may include toe or ray amputation (removal of toe together with part of the metatarsal) or, rarely, transmetatarsal amputation.

Although necrosis in the diabetic foot may not be associated with a definite collection of pus, the necrotic tissue still needs to be removed.

CASE STUDY
Trauma, infection, necrosis and ray amputation

A 56-year-old diabetic man with type 1 diabetes of 31 years' duration and peripheral neuropathy stubbed his left hallux when walking barefoot. He was aware that the nail was damaged but felt no pain and assumed the injury was trivial. He denied ever receiving foot care education and had not attended the diabetic foot clinic. One week later he attended Casualty with a necrotic hallux and

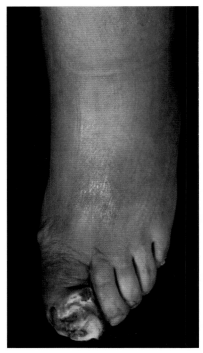

Fig. 6.17 Wet necrosis of the hallux with cellulitis spreading up the foot. There was no collection of pus but extensive sloughy tissue was present and he underwent amputation of the 1st ray.

cellulitis spreading up the foot (Fig. 6.17). Pedal pulses were bounding. Intravenous antibiotics were administered and he went to theatre within 24 hours and underwent amputation of the first ray. There was no collection of pus, but extensive sloughy tissue. The foot healed in 10 weeks.

Key points
- In the neuropathic foot, there is good arterial circulation and the treatment of choice of wet necrosis is surgical removal
- The postoperative wound in the neuropathic foot heals as long as infection is controlled
- Diabetic neuropathic patients who are ignorant of foot care are extremely vulnerable
- We give them education and frequent follow-up appointments.

Very occasionally, patients with neuropathic feet may not be suitable for or refuse operation, and the aim would then be to convert wet gangrene into dry by conservative treatment and intravenous antibiotics and allow autoamputation, where after a number of weeks or months the toe 'drops off' leaving a healed stump. Many debridements of necrotic tissue can be performed in the outpatient clinic by podiatrists. Diabetic patients do not require local anaesthetic by virtue of their neuropathy and the fact that the tissue being removed is not living and therefore insensitive.

Neuroischaemic foot

In the neuroischaemic foot, wet necrosis should also be removed when it is associated with spreading sepsis. This should be done whether pus is present or not. However, where necrosis is limited to one or two toes in the neuro-ischaemic foot we avoid surgery where possible until vascular intervention has been achieved. If angioplasty or arterial bypass is not possible, then a decision must be made either to amputate the toes in the presence of ischaemia or allow the toes, as infection is controlled, to convert to dry necrosis and autoamputate. Sometimes this decision can be a difficult one. Surgical amputation leaves a large tissue defect which, in the neuroischaemic foot, may never heal. However, a transcutaneous oxygen tension of greater than 30 mmHg on the dorsum of the foot indicates a reasonable chance of healing and postoperative VAC therapy of the wound may be useful. Autoamputation is a process which takes many months and there is always a danger that the foot may become infected if the necrotic toe is left to autoamputate.

Techniques to treat necrosis
- Outpatient sharp debridement
- Operative surgical debridement
- Facilitated autoamputation
- Larva therapy.

Outpatient debridement

The rationale for outpatient sharp debriding of necrosis is as follows:
- Removes wet necrosis, which is an excellent culture medium for microorganisms, thus rendering infection less likely (Fig. 6.18). Debridement enables inspection of the underlying tissues: are there pockets of pus, are the tissues well perfused, is there healthy granulating tissue underlying necrosis?
- Speeds healing by converting the lesion into an acute wound
- Removes a physical barrier from the edge of the wound, enabling new epithelium to grow across more easily
- The necrosis removed can be sent to the laboratory for culture and sensitivities
- Enables the true dimensions of the lesion to be seen, and in particular the depth (Fig. 6.19a,b).

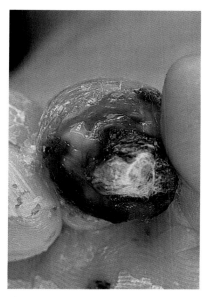

Fig. 6.18 This necrotic toe is exuding pus from along the demarcation line between necrosis and viable tissue and needs to be debrided.

The operator works from proximal to distal, away from the demarcation line, to avoid cutting into viable tissue.

Wet necrosis is grasped in forceps and gentle traction is applied so that the tissue being cut is taut, which enables greater precision (Fig. 6.20a–c).

Heaped up material along the demarcation line is removed.

When necrotic material is sent for culture the surface material is first debrided away and the tissue sample is taken from deeper areas.

Haemodialysis patients, who undergo rapid haemo-dynamic changes on dialysis, are heparinized to prevent clotting of the access graft, so ulcerated and necrotic lesions may bleed on debridement around the time of dialysis.

Operative surgical debridement (neuropathic and neuroischaemic foot)

In both the neuropathic and the neuroischaemic foot operative debridement is indicated by wet necrosis with spreading sepsis. When there is dry necrosis in the neuro-ischaemic foot, surgical debridement or amputation should be considered if the necrotic toe or any other area of necrosis is very painful, especially if the circulation is not too severely impaired, that is, a pressure index above 0.5 or a transcutaneous oxygen tension above 30 mmHg.

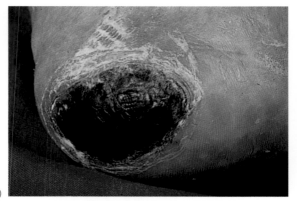
(a)

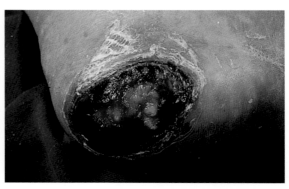
(b)

Fig. 6.19 (a) This patient has developed dry necrosis on the lateral border of the heel but the depth of the necrosis is not clear. (b) An area of necrosis has been sharp debrided to reveal the true depth of the necrosis, but viable tissue has not been injured. In this case necrosis is superficial and can be treated by regular podiatric debridement.

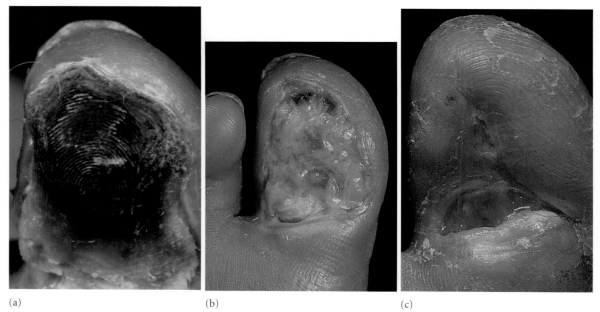
(a) (b) (c)

Fig. 6.20 (a) The proximal portion of this necrotic ulcer was wet and discharging pus. (b) The same ulcer 2 weeks later after debridement of wet necrosis. (c) Ten weeks after the first debridement the toe is healing well.

Postoperatively there may be a considerable tissue deficit with exposure of bone or tendon. Such deficits may be repaired by plastic reconstructive surgery. However, every avenue for revascularization should be explored in these patients before any surgery is contemplated.

Before surgery
The preparation and principles of operative debridement are similar to that described in stage 4. Patients will need:

- Full blood count and grouping
- Serum electrolytes and creatinine
- Blood glucose
- Liver function tests
- Chest X-ray
- ECG.

Consent should be obtained for the most extensive debridement anticipated, including digital or ray amputation.

During surgery

It is important to remove all necrotic tissue, down to bleeding tissue, as well as opening up all sinuses. Deep necrotic tissue should be sent for culture immediately. Wounds should not be sutured. A foot with a large gaping wound following extensive tissue removal may be lightly held together by winding long strips of paraffin gauze around the foot; however, the strips should be cut through to accommodate swelling and must not prevent draining of exudate.

After surgery

- At surgery all necrotic tissue should be removed but sometimes it is difficult to be sure about the viability of all tissue at the operation site
- Thus at the first postoperative dressing, the wound may still contain necrotic and sloughy tissue
- Patients are sometimes taken back to the operating theatre for the first change in dressings, where further operative debridement can be carried out if necessary.

Large, postoperative wounds following surgical debridement or ray amputation may be treated with VAC pump therapy, which is especially suitable for extensive deep wounds that have been recently debrided. It is wise to wait one day after surgery to make sure that haemostasis has been achieved before applying the VAC pump. This technique can be used to accelerate healing of such postoperative wounds in the neuropathic foot (see Chapter 5). However, the main impact of VAC therapy has been in the neuroischaemic foot and the renal foot: VAC therapy has accelerated healing of postoperative wounds in the neuroischaemic foot when applied after angioplasty or bypass, and it has great effect when applied to postoperative wounds in neuroischaemic feet which cannot be revascularized. Previously there would have been great reluctance for these feet to come to surgery because of the reduced arterial perfusion, but the VAC pump allows this process to take place because of its increased healing potential in such postoperative wounds.

CASE STUDY
Distal arterial bypass and VAC therapy in a diabetic neuroischaemic foot

A 72-year-old woman with type 2 diabetes of 32 years' duration was admitted from home where she lived with her eight cats. She had developed ulceration of the medial aspect of the foot and necrosis of the first toe. This was complicated by spreading cellulitis. Her serum creatinine was 262 μmol/L. She had had previous methicillin-resistant *Staphlyococcus aureus* (MRSA) infections of the foot.

The patient was treated with intravenous antibiotics, namely vancomycin 1 g statim, and then dosage according to serum levels, ceftazidime 1 g daily and metronidazole 500 mg tds. Tissue specimen grew MRSA and mixed anaerobes. Angiography revealed tibial disease and she underwent a popiteal to posterior tibial bypass, during which her foot was debrided. Postoperatively there was moderate slough in the wound (Fig. 6.21a) but it was decided to start VAC therapy one day postoperatively (Fig. 6.21b). This assisted in the removal of slough. The VAC dressing was changed twice a week when she also had podiatric debridement. The wound responded extremely well to this therapy (Fig. 6.21c,d).

Key points

- VAC pump therapy is now useful in accelerating healing of wounds in the neuroischaemic foot
- It is also useful in desloughing wounds which may not have been completely debrided
- VAC therapy together with bedside podiatric debridement achieves very good results in the postoperative diabetic foot wound.

Ischaemic wounds are extremely slow to heal even after revascularization, and wound care needs to continue on an outpatient basis in the diabetic foot clinic. Some feet take many months, or even years, to heal, but with patience outcomes may be surprisingly good. Even if healing is never achieved many patients prefer to live with an ulcerated foot than to undergo amputation.

Repair of tissue deficits

Debridement of necrotic lesions of the foot often leads to severe tissue deficits. Management of these soft tissue deficits is complex and skin grafts, local flaps and free tissue transfer have been used. Free tissue transfer is usually carried out for limb salvage and combined with arterial reconstruction in the ischaemic limb. Donor tissue from above the waist is usually used, particularly muscle flaps from the rectus abdominis or latissimus dorsi.

In a free tissue transfer, the arteriovenous pedicle accompanies the transferred tissue and is anastomosed to recipient vessels. A pedal or tibial vessel, which is either a bypass graft or a native revascularized artery, serves as the inflow tract for the free flap that is anastomosed using microsurgical techniques.

CASE STUDY
Toe amputation in a neuroischaemic foot

A 57-year-old man with type 2 diabetes of 6 years' duration developed a blister on his right 5th toe from a shoe

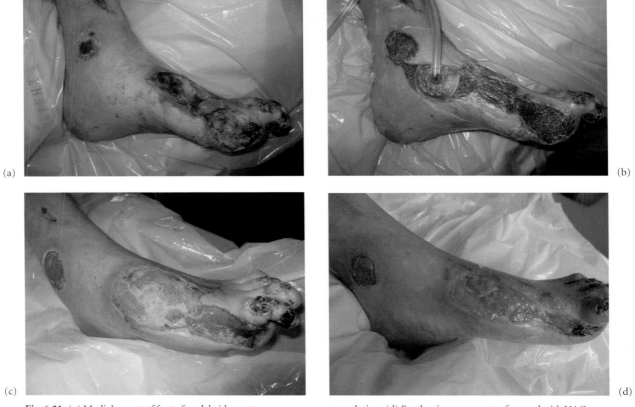

Fig. 6.21 (a) Medial aspect of foot after debridement, amputation of first toe and distal bypass. (b) Application of VAC therapy. (c) Wound improving showing evidence of granulation. (d) Further improvement of wound with VAC therapy. (Courtesy of Melanie Doxford.)

rub. After 4 days the foot became painful and discoloured and he attended Casualty. His pedal pulses were impalpable. He had wet necrosis of the 5th toe, oedema, cellulitis and lymphangitis spreading up the foot (Fig. 6.22a,b). He was admitted to hospital and given amoxicillin 500 mg tds, flucloxacillin 500 mg qds, metronidazole 500 mg tds and ceftazidime 1 g tds intravenously. He underwent angiography and angioplasty of occlusion of the anterior tibial artery and the toe was amputated. The foot healed in 8 weeks.

Key points

- In cases when the limb is not immediately threatened, and the necrosis is limited to one or two toes, it may be possible to control infection with intravenous antibiotics and proceed to urgent angiography and revascularization
- Angioplasty may improve the arterial circulation to allow healing of a toe or ray amputation
- If angioplasty is not possible then arterial bypass should be considered and the toe or ray amputation can be performed at the same time as bypass.

CASE STUDY
Large tissue deficit in a neuroischaemic foot secondary to infection needing distal arterial bypass

A 43-year-old man with type 1 diabetes of 27 years' duration, with peripheral and autonomic neuropathy, was

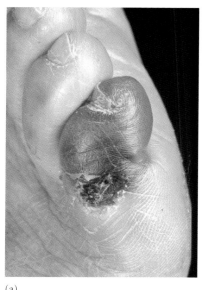
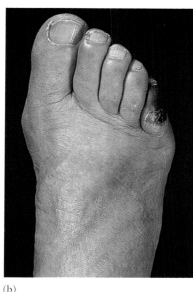

Fig. 6.22 (a) Wet necrosis of the 5th toe.
(b) Lymphangitis spreading up the same
foot.   (a)   (b)

referred with indolent neuropathic ulceration complicated by local cellulitis over the left 5th metatarsal head.
His pedal pulses were palpable. He was treated with oral
amoxicillin 500 mg tds and flucloxacillin 500 mg qds and
outpatient debridement. His deep wound swab had
grown *Staphylococcus aureus* and *Streptococcus* group G.
The cellulitis resolved and he was given a total-contact
cast. The ulcer healed after 8 weeks and he was given
bespoke shoes with cradled insoles.

Two years later he was admitted with an infected
ulcer on the plantar surface of the right heel where he
had pulled off a piece of loose skin (Fig. 6.23a). His
pedal pulses were now impalpable. He was admitted
and given intravenous vancomycin 1 g bd, ceftriaxone
1 g bd and metronidazole 500 mg tds. He had recently
had a methicillin-resistant *Staphylococcus aureus* (MRSA)
infection on the contralateral foot. Angiography showed
occlusions of the right common iliac artery and superficial femoral artery. It was planned to perform an
angioplasty of the right common iliac and right external
iliac as a crossover procedure via the left femoral artery.
However, whilst awaiting this angioplasty the patient
developed a critically ischaemic right foot. Urgent angiogram at this time showed thrombus in the right superficial
femoral artery. He underwent thrombolysis. A check
angiogram showed a patent superficial femoral artery, but
significant stenoses in the popliteal artery with a good
two-vessel run-off. He underwent a popliteal angioplasty.
Following this, transcutaneous oxygen tension was

57 mmHg on the chest and 69 mmHg on the dorsum of
the right foot. This was deemed adequate perfusion and
no further vascular intervention was attempted. The
ulceration on the right heel remained clean and VAC
therapy was applied to improve granulation.

The patient was followed up in the diabetic foot clinic
and the ulcer had almost healed after 4 months. Despite
careful education about the danger signs of deterioration
he then presented very late with chills, sweating, infection
of the heel ulcer and blue discolouration of the medial
aspect of the right foot. He had spreading cellulitis and a
2-cm area of necrosis on the medial aspect of the right
foot. Doppler waveforms were monophasic and damped.
The working diagnosis was that he had mid-foot sepsis
likely to be tracking from the ulcer and he underwent
operative surgical debridement. There was a track leading
from the heel ulcer along the extensor tendons to the mid-
foot and this was laid open. All dead and infected tissue
was excised back to bleeding tissue. Deep tissue culture
revealed MRSA and mixed anaerobes. Clinically, he was
septic and was treated with intravenous vancomycin 1 g bd,
rifampicin 600 mg bd (as an adjunctive treatment for
MRSA), metronidazole 500 mg tds and Milton irrigation
to the wound. In view of his sepsis he was also given
gentamicin 5 mg/kg daily. Angiography showed further
stenoses of the superficial femoral and popliteal artery.

Initially it was planned to carry out an angioplasty, but
it was decided that distal bypass surgery had the best
chance of restoring the pulsatile blood flow which was

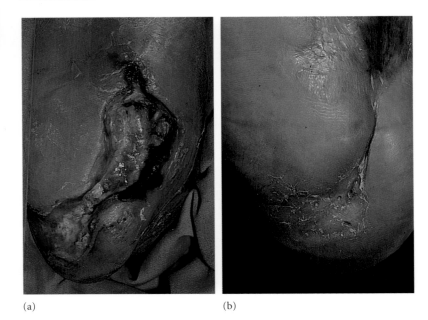

(a)   (b)

Fig 6.23 (a) Infected ulcer on plantar surface of heel. (b) The ulcer has healed following application of Apligraf.

necessary to heal his large tissue deficit. He underwent a distal bypass from the right common femoral artery to the anterior tibial artery with a reversed lower saphenous vein. The reversed lower saphenous vein was tunnelled laterally to the knee subcutaneously. There was a good quality common femoral artery and a non-calcified anterior tibial artery in mid-shin of good calibre. The bypass was successful but the plantar wound was slow to heal.

His postoperative course was stormy. He developed a fever with productive cough associated with rigors and vomiting. He was treated with vancomycin 1 g bd and meropenem 1 g tds intravenously empirically and improved. He complained of back pain and X-ray showed evidence of vertebral collapse. He had magnetic resonance imaging (MRI) of his spine as a metastatic abscess was suspected. However, the MRI showed changes consistent with a haemangioma but this did not require neurosurgical intervention. An application of Apligraf finally healed the ulcer (Fig. 6.23b).

During this admission his wife visited the hospital every day, arriving early in the afternoon and leaving late in the evening. She took a great interest in his care and learned to clean and dress the foot. She was taught the danger signs of deterioration. Subsequently he never again presented late with severe infection because his wife checked his feet every day and brought him to the diabetic foot clinic at the first sign of a break in the skin.

Key points

- Patients admitted with severe infection need intense multidisciplinary care and frequent medical and surgical review
- Surgical debridement was needed on this patient's second admission because of necrosis secondary to infection
- An arterial bypass was needed to restore pulsatile flow to heal a large tissue defect. The increase in blood flow after angioplasty may not have been sufficient
- The family of vulnerable patients should be taught to check the feet daily and respond rapidly at the first sign of a break in the skin
- Neuropathic feet eventually become neuroischaemic but this will need to be diagnosed by examination of the foot pulses at every visit
- Patients with neuroischaemic foot ulceration need long-term follow-up in a multidisciplinary diabetic foot service.

CASE STUDY
Necrotizing fasciitis in a previously neuropathic foot that had become neuroischaemic

A 67-year-old man with type 2 diabetes of 22 years' duration and a previous history of frequent neuropathic ulceration, developed fever, rigors, fatigue and malaise, and asked his general practitioner to visit him. Influenza was diagnosed and paracetamol was prescribed. The general practitioner called again, 2 days later, when the patient had not improved, and told him to continue taking paracetamol. Two days later the patient's wife became aware of an unusual odour, checked her husband's feet, and found that his hallux was purple and a large ulcer had developed on the side of his foot. Same day admission was arranged. The patient had extensive wet gangrene and necrotizing fasciitis of the plantar aspect of the foot (Fig. 6.24a,b). It was noted that the foot pulses were not palpable and Doppler studies disclosed that the patient, previously neuropathic, had become neuroischaemic.

Extensive debridement of infected soft tissue and amputation of the hallux was performed as an emergency procedure leaving him with a large tissue deficit. *Staphylococcus*

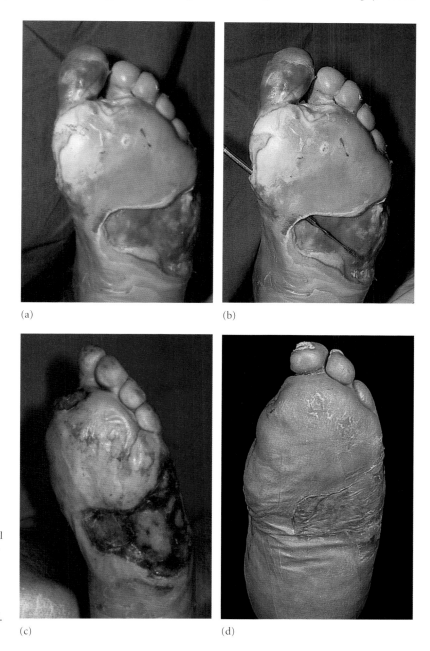

(a)   (b)

Fig. 6.24 (a) The hallux is red and purple at its tip. There is a large area of wet necrosis and sloughing of tissue on the lateral border of his foot. (b) It is possible to pass a probe from the medial to the lateral border of the foot. (c) The large tissue defect has been surgically debrided and received a split-skin graft which has taken: the hallux has been amputated. (d) The 2nd toe has also developed necrosis and autoamputated. The foot has healed.

(c)   (d)

aureus and *Pseudomonas* was grown from the tissue. He was treated with ceftazidime 1 g tds and flucloxacillin 500 mg qds. He underwent a distal arterial bypass. His postoperative progress was slow and the tissue defect was covered with a split-skin graft (Fig. 6.24c,d). After discharge he attended the diabetic foot clinic at monthly intervals for sharp debridement of callus from the skin graft.

Key points
- Diabetic foot infections may masquerade as influenza
- Patients who cancel their appointments because of 'flu-like symptoms' should have their feet checked
- Our education programme specifically warns patients that symptoms of flu may be caused by foot infections
- Soft tissue destruction in the neuroischaemic foot is usually due to infection
- Always be on the outlook for neuropathic feet that have become neuroischaemic
- Extensive tissue loss in the neuroischaemic foot should be managed ideally with an arterial bypass.

CASE STUDY
Extensive debridement of severe sepsis in a neuroischaemic foot

A 66-year-old man with type 2 diabetes of 10 years' duration went to Casualty complaining of a swollen foot with a small purple area on the medial border. His foot pulses were impalpable and his pressure index was 0.7. He was unwell with pyrexia of 39°C and had rigors. He was taken to the operating theatre for debridement. Although the area of non-viable tissue appeared to be not more than 3 cm in diameter (Fig. 6.25a), surgical debridement revealed very extensive tissue destruction involving subcutaneous tissues and bones. He underwent excision of the 1st toe, 1st metatarsal, medial cuneiform and navicular, and large areas of skin and soft tissue. Apparently healthy overlying skin covered a layer of necrosis which had tracked between skin and subcutaneous tissues like the filling of a sandwich. One week later the wound was not granulating (Fig. 6.25b). He did not want a bypass but agreed to undergo angioplasty of stenoses in his popliteal artery and tibioperoneal trunk, after which the wound granulated well (Fig. 6.25c). He was discharged after 3 months for shared care of his healing wound between community nurses and the diabetic foot clinic. However, he died of a myocardial infarct the same day.

Key points
- Surface appearances can be very deceptive: the visible area of discolouration is usually just the tip of the iceberg

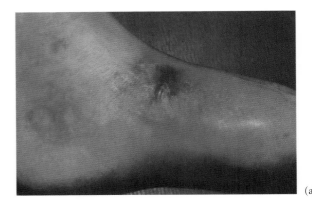

(a)

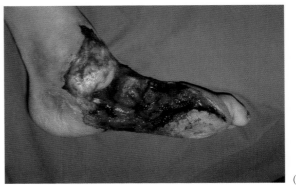

(b)

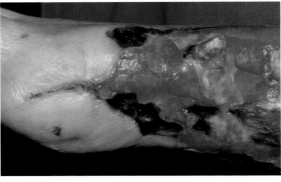

(c)

Fig. 6.25 (a) Cutaneous necrosis on the medial surface of foot indicating severe underlying tissue destruction. (b) One week postoperatively this wound is not granulating. (c) Following angioplasty the wound is granulating well 6 weeks later.

- Apparently healthy skin can cover extensive necrosis
- It is often only when surgical debridement is performed that the true extent of necrosis is understood
- If the pressure index is low and the wound is not granulating vascular intervention should be carried out

- It may take several weeks for the optimal effects of an angioplasty to take effect and granulation of the wound to take place.

Facilitated autoamputation

Careful sharp debridement is performed along the demarcation line between necrosis and viable tissue to debulk dead tissue, drain pockets of pus and prevent accumulation of debris (Fig. 6.26a,b). Scalpel and forceps are used: if necrotic material is moist then traction should be applied with the forceps to enable precise cutting with the scalpel. If tension is not applied it will be impossible to clear away the moist necrosis and the operator is in danger of cutting the patient.

If areas of the necrotic toe are moist and the necrosis is full thickness (deep to bone) then the necrotic portion may be best removed by amputating it through the interphalangeal joint distal to the demarcation line between necrosis and viable tissue. The removed necrotic apex can be sent to the laboratory for culture. Once this procedure has been performed it is easier to debride necrotic material from around the stump without damaging viable

tissue. The patient should always be warned and consulted if this procedure is to be attempted.

We remember one patient who watched with interest while his necrotic toe was amputated and asked if he could take it home. When asked why he wanted it he explained that he was meeting friends at the pub that evening and intended to drop the toe into someone's beer. The diabetic foot clinic staff confiscated the offending toe!

CASE STUDY
Autoamputation of a neuroischaemic necrotic digit

A 65-year-old man with type 2 diabetes of 12 years' duration was referred to the diabetic foot clinic with a dry necrotic 4th toe (Fig. 6.27a). He was admitted for vascular assessment but no intervention was possible so the necrosis was treated conservatively in the belief that surgical removal would leave a large defect which would be difficult to heal in an ischaemic foot. His transcutaneous oxygen tension was 25 mmHg. He was given oral anti-biotics, regular debridement along the demarcation line between gangrene and viable tissue and insulin for optimal control of his diabetes. The toes were dressed with Melolin as a non-stick dressing and pieces of gauze were placed between them to separate the gangrenous toe from its neighbours, and the community nurses visited him every day.

After 5 months the gangrenous toe autoamputated to reveal a healed stump (Fig. 6.27b).

Key points

- When it is not possible to revascularize the limb, necrotic toes may be managed conservatively by autoamputation
- We felt that the existing arterial perfusion, as reflected in the transcutaneous oxygen tension of 25 mmHg, was sufficient to allow successful autoamputation but might not enable a surgical amputation wound to heal.
- However, VAC pump therapy to postoperative amputation wounds in the ischemic foot is encouraging a trend to more digital amputations in feet that cannot be revascularized.

Larva therapy

Maggot therapy can be used to debride necrotic tissue and slough in stage 5 feet. The larvae used are those of the green bottle fly.

Medical maggots of *Lucilia sericata* (the larvae of the green bottle fly) may assist in the eradication of infection by ingesting and digesting bacteria, including MRSA, and infected, sloughy tissue. Because they feed on dead flesh and not on living flesh they are sometimes used to debride

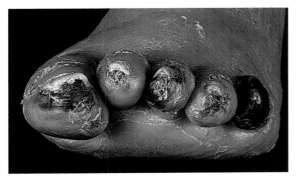

(a)

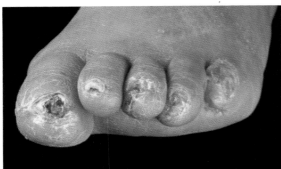

(b)

Fig. 6.26 (a) This woman with a necrotic 5th toe and necrotic apices of the 1st, 3rd and 4th toes underwent podiatric debridement. (b) The same foot 6 weeks later after regular 2-weekly debridements by the podiatrist.

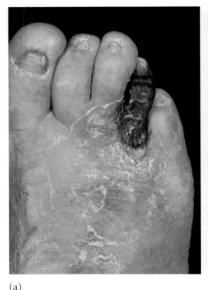
(a)

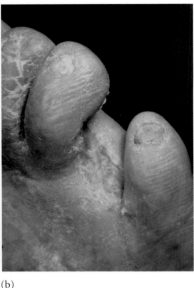
(b)

Fig. 6.27 (a) Necrotic neuroischaemic toe. (b) Autoamputation: the toe has dropped off to reveal a healed stump.

infected slough or necrotic tissue from ulcers, particularly in the neuroischaemic foot.

The maggots should be well contained within special bags provided by the 'maggot farm'. These are used to enclose the foot or part of the foot. The bag should be covered with dressings to help absorb exudate, but the maggots may drown or suffocate unless dressings are loosely applied.

Patients should be on bed rest. If the patient is allowed to walk the maggots may be crushed.

The normal skin around the wound should be masked with zinc oxide bandage to prevent the skin being affected by digestive enzymes produced by the maggots which will otherwise make it red and raw.

Copious amounts of thin discharge, which is often a rusty brown colour, and a 'fusty' smell are associated with wounds containing maggots, and patients and other members of staff should be forewarned about this.

Most patients are not bothered by the movements of the maggots within the wound, but ischaemic patients occasionally complain of increased pain during maggot therapy.

The maggots can be irrigated out of the wound on the fourth day.

- When slough is slippery and slimy, maggot debridement may be easier than sharp debridement with forceps and scalpel
- Maggots may reveal hidden depths to wounds
- Maggots can remain in the wound until they have finished feeding, but should be inspected regularly and will usually be removed on the fourth day

- Where podiatrists are unavailable, maggots may be useful for debriding infected or ischaemic wounds.

Dressing and cleaning the necrotic foot

Simple, dry, non-adherent dressings should be used. The aim is always to keep the necrosis dry and well demarcated, and to inspect the foot on a daily basis so that any new infection can be detected and treated appropriately.

It is important to separate necrotic toes from their neighbours. Dry sterile dressings are placed between the toes to keep them apart because if necrosis is in direct contact with viable tissue it can become moist, develop infection and spread to adjoining, previously healthy, tissue. Areas of the foot which are not involved with necrosis can be washed every day with warm water and mild soap, and dried carefully. Necrotic areas should be kept dry and covered with dressings.

Many chemists sell 'cast protectors' which are strong plastic bags in the shape of a leg that keep casts or bandages dry so that patients with necrosis may bathe or shower.

Necrotic toes should be kept dry.

CASE STUDY
Importance of keeping necrosis dry

A 76-year-old woman with type 2 diabetes of 7 years' duration, developed necrosis of her right 4th toe. She was

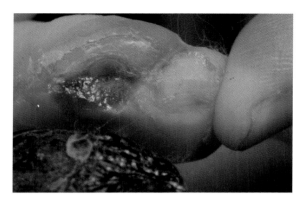

Fig. 6.28 No dressing was placed between the toes and necrosis has spread to the portion of the previously healthy toe which was in contact with the necrotic toe. A necrotic toe should always be separated from its healthy neighbours by a dry dressing placed between the toes.

neuroischaemic with a pressure index of 0.4, and no vascular intervention was possible. The necrosis was treated conservatively and her daughter was asked to keep the toe dry and to ensure that dressings were applied to separate the necrotic toe from its neighbours. However, her daughter allowed her to have a bath, and did not separate the toes with dressings. When she attended the diabetic foot clinic 1 week later, the necrosis was moist and necrosis was also present in an adjoining toe where it had been in contact with the necrotic toe (Fig. 6.28).

She was admitted to hospital and received intravenous antibiotics. The pressure index had not fallen. The necrosis became dry and well demarcated again and spread no further. Seven months later the toe separated to reveal a healed stump.

Key points
- Patients should not immerse their necrotic toes in the bath. Moistening necrosis may encourage infection
- Furthermore, if a necrotic toe is in direct contact with a viable toe, the necrotic toe may 'absorb sweat' and become moist. The area of moist necrosis is an excellent culture medium for bacteria which then spread from the necrotic toe to the adjoining toe
- If the interdigital area is macerated it is no longer a barrier to bacteria which may enter the viable toe and cause ulceration and necrosis
- Neuroischaemic feet with dry necrosis may remain at stage 5 for many months until the necrotic toe drops off to reveal a healed stump.

Microbiological control

Wet necrosis
The microbiological principles of managing wet necrosis are similar to those for the management of infection of the foot with extensive soft tissue infection or the foot with blue discolouration as described in Chapter 5. When the patient initially presents, deep wound swabs and tissue specimens are sent off for microbiology. Deep tissue taken at operative debridement must also go for culture.

Intravenous antibiotic therapy
Both neuropathic and neuroischaemic patients need parenteral therapy. They are admitted to hospital and given intravenous antibiotic therapy as follows: amoxicillin 500 mg tds, flucloxacillin 500 mg qds, metronidazole 500 mg tds and ceftazidime 1 g tds. For patients who are allergic to penicillin we substitute vancomycin 1 g bd or clindamycin 600 mg qds for amoxicillin and flucloxacillin. We use this regime because these infections are often polymicrobial. Other regimes are in use including:
- Ciprofloxacin with clindamycin
- Piperacillin/tazobactam
- Ampicillin/sulbactam
- Ticarcillin/clavulanate
- Meropenem
- Ertapenem.

Intravenous antibiotics can be replaced with oral therapy after operative debridement and when infection is controlled. On discharge from hospital, oral antibiotics are continued and reviewed regularly in the diabetic foot clinic. When the wound is granulating well and swabs are negative then the antibiotics are stopped.

It is often difficult to have all wet necrosis removed surgically. The foot may be ischaemic, and the patient may not be fit for an operation. In these circumstances we believe that it is best to leave the necrosis and convert wet necrosis to dry necrosis using antibiotics and allow it to separate. The presence of necrosis will increase the risk of infection; however, these patients are under very close surveillance and early signs of the return or spread of wet necrosis are carefully searched for.

Dry necrosis
When dry necrosis develops secondary to severe ischaemia, antibiotics should be prescribed if discharge develops, or the deep wound swab or tissue culture is positive, and continued until there is no evidence of clinical or microbiological infection.

When toes have gone from wet to dry necrosis and are allowed to autoamputate, antibiotics should only be stopped if the necrosis is dry and mummified, the foot is entirely pain free, there is no discharge exuding from the demarcation line, and swabs are negative.

In severely ischaemic feet (pressure index < 0.5) antibiotics may sometimes be continued until healing.

Daily inspection is essential. Regular deep swabs and tissue should be sent for culture and antibiotics should be restarted if the demarcation line becomes moist, the foot becomes painful, or swabs or tissue cultures grow bacteria.

Vascular control

All neuroischaemic feet that present with necrosis must have Doppler studies to confirm ischaemia. This should be followed by non-invasive investigations as described in Chapter 3.

The patient should initially have duplex angiography, which is optimal in showing stenoses or occlusions in the iliac, femoral or popliteal arteries. Tibial arteries are sometimes difficult to visualize with this technique because of excessive arterial calcification. However, if the Doppler sonograms show monophasic damped pattern at the ankle arteries this implies tibial disease. Magnetic resonance angiography may also be used to show stenoses or occlusions of the arteries of the leg, particularly in the tibial arteries (Fig. 6.29a,b).

Having diagnosed the site of disease, then revascularization can be planned.

In wet necrosis, revascularization is necessary to heal the tissue deficit after operative debridement. In dry necrosis, which occurs in the background of severe arterial disease, revascularization is necessary to maintain the viability of the limb. Revascularization can be achieved by angioplasty or bypass. However, with increasingly sophisticated techniques a hybrid procedure is often carried out which consists of initial angioplasty to one part of the circulation and then bypass to another. Thus a patient with superficial femoral artery disease as well as tibial artery disease may well undergo angioplasty above the knee to the superficial femoral artery, and then a distal bypass below the knee to achieve straight-line arterial flow. These procedures are planned in joint consultation with the interventional radiologist, vascular surgeon and diabetic foot clinic.

Angioplasty

In some patients, increased perfusion following angioplasty may be useful and this will result in an improvement in the ischaemic wound. Indeed, this is often the

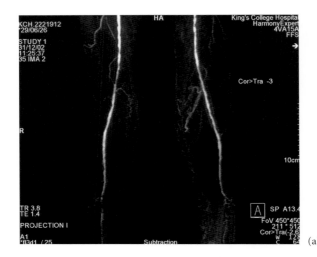

(a)

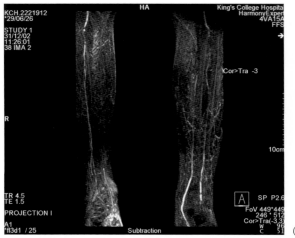

(b)

Fig. 6.29 (a) There is diffuse atheromatous disease of both superficial femoral arteries with an area of focal narrowing at the mid-level on the right. Both popliteal arteries are severely diseased. (b) On the right there is a single vessel, the anterior tibial, extending to the level of the plantar arch and it is severely diseased in the proximal aspect. There is reconstitution of posterior tibial at ankle level. On the left there is an occlusion of the tibioperoneal trunk with collaterals filling the more distal anterior and posterior tibial arteries. (Courtesy of Dr Huw Walters.)

only interventional procedure that can be performed as the patient may be too frail to undergo peripheral vascular surgery. As an alternative procedure to angioplasty, arterial stenting is now carried out. This has been fully established as a useful treatment in the iliac arteries with good long-term patency of the stent. Recently, stents have also been inserted into the superficial femoral arteries and even the tibial arteries. However, the longevity of such procedures needs to be fully established.

CASE STUDY
Stenting the superficial femoral artery

A 69-year-old woman with type 2 diabetes of 6 years' duration presented with a non-healing ulcer of the right 3rd toe. The transcutaneous oxygen on the dorsum of the right foot was 25 mmHg. Duplex angiography showed occlusion of the superficial femoral artery and this was confirmed on femoral angiography (Fig. 6.30a). The superficial femoral artery was dilated from its origin to adductor segment, but post-plasty images showed no effect. The ulceration persisted and then the artery was successfully stented. Two overlapping, subintimal 6 mm × 15 mm stents were inserted into the artery (Fig. 6.30b).

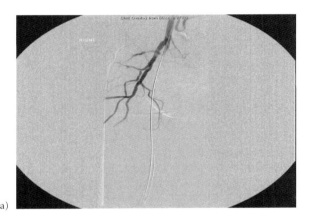

(a)

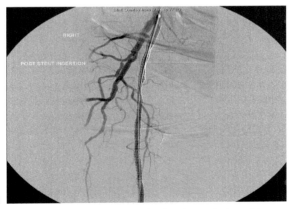

(b)

Fig. 6.30 (a) Femoral angiography showing occlusion of the superficial femoral artery. (b) Two overlapping, subintimal 6 mm × 15 mm stents inserted into the artery (Courtesy of Dr Paul Sidhu.)

It was noted that the posterior tibial artery was seen to reconstitute at the mid-calf level. This was the main artery supplying the arch of the foot. The patient then underwent popliteal to posterior tibial artery bypass.

Arterial bypass
Angioplasty rarely restores pulsatile blood flow unless a very significant localized stenosis in iliac or femoral arteries has been successfully dilated. When the limb is severely ischaemic and there is considerable tissue deficit, it is necessary to restore pulsatile blood flow. This is best achieved by arterial bypass.

Preoperative assessment
Patients will have cardiovascular disease and need preoperative assessment to maximize cardiorespiratory status. Cardiovascular risk should be carefully assessed from the history, physical examination, functional capacity and resting ECG. An estimation of low risk vs. high risk can be made from these assessments. Most patients with diabetes undergoing vascular surgery will be at high risk.

When patients are of an intermediate risk then extra preoperative tests may be needed, including echocardiography. This will identify patients with left ventricular dysfunction; a low ejection fraction (less than 35%) increases the risk of non-cardiac surgery. A useful non-invasive evaluation is perfusion nuclear imaging with thallium. Risk is increased if two or more reversible perfusion defects are present on thallium imaging. For patients with diabetes the most significant independent predictors of postoperative death are advanced age, resting ECG abnormalities and abnormalities revealed on thallium imaging.

Perioperative care
The perioperative use of β-blockers, particularly bisoprolol, is now established in patients undergoing vascular surgery. Studies using thallium reperfusion imaging as an indicator of abnormal cardiac function have shown a significant reduction in perioperative and in-hospital mortality after vascular surgery in patients randomized to bisoprolol compared with placebo. This persisted throughout the treatment period of 6 months.

Peripheral arterial disease is common in the tibial arteries, and distal bypass with autologous vein has become an established method of revascularization. A conduit is fashioned from either the femoral or popliteal artery down to a tibial artery in the lower leg, or the dorsalis pedis artery on the dorsum of the foot.

Patency rates and limb salvage rates after revascularization do not differ between diabetic patients and non-diabetic patients, and a more aggressive approach to such

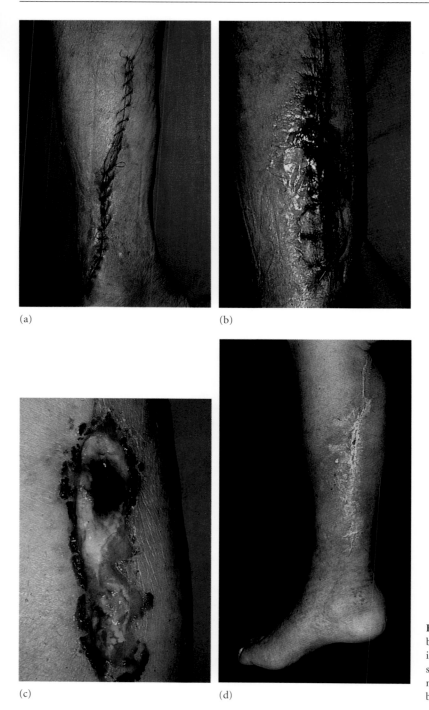

(a)

(b)

(c)

(d)

Fig. 6.31 (a) The wound has developed blueish discolouration. (b) The wound is breaking down. (c) The wound is sloughy and necrotic. (d) After 4 months, the leg is fully healed and the bypass is still working.

revascularization procedures should be promoted. Arterial bypass can be successfully carried out in patients with severe renal impairment and this should not be a contraindication.

Postoperative care

Postoperatively, the leg has wounds both where the graft has been inserted and from where the vein has been harvested. Wounds overlying the arterial graft must be kept free from infection otherwise the graft will block. Such wounds need regular cleaning and covering with dry sterile dressings, and any associated necrotic tissue which becomes bulky or moist should be gently debrided. Postoperative oedema is common and treatment with elevation is important. The patient should enter a graft surveillance programme.

CASE STUDY
Complicated leg wounds following distal bypass surgery

A 76-year-old lady with type 2 diabetes of 30 years' duration underwent a distal bypass for critical ischaemia. Three days later the proximal area of her leg wound developed blueish discolouration (Fig. 6.31a). The next day it began to break down (Fig. 6.31b) and then dehisced, revealing an area of yellow slough (Fig. 6.31c). Wide-spectrum antibiotics were prescribed. The area dried out and formed a dark brown eschar which stood proud of the area of skin. The vascular surgeon agreed that if debris accumulated in this area it should be gently debrided in the diabetic foot clinic and this was done weekly on three occasions.

When she next came to the foot diabetic clinic for her routine weekly appointment and the dressing was taken down, the eschar on the leg was seen to be gently vibrating at the same rate as the patient's pulse. The patient was taken to theatre for an emergency procedure. The artery underlying the eschar ruptured as she was being lifted onto the operating table: even though the surgeons were fully prepared there was considerable blood loss. The artery was repaired and the leg healed in 4 months (Fig. 6.31d).

Key points
- Pulsating wounds of distal bypass surgery should be referred as an emergency to the vascular surgeon
- Patients whose bypass leg wounds become infected are at great risk of losing the graft
- Outpatient debridement of leg wounds should be performed with great caution
- Leg wounds from distal bypasses should be inspected weekly until fully healed.

CASE STUDY
Septic arteritis, double ray amputation, distal bypass and skin grafting

A 71-year-old diabetic man with type 2 diabetes diagnosed when he attended Casualty with gross foot sepsis, neuropathy and peripheral vascular disease, underwent a double ray amputation for immediate limb salvage (Fig. 6.32a). This was followed by a distal arterial bypass. One week later the foot wound was debrided in the diabetic foot clinic and a split-skin graft was applied 2 days later in theatre (Fig. 6.32b) from a donor site on the patient's calf which was infiltrated with local anaesthetic through a spinal needle. He did not complain of pain from the donor site which was within the distribution of his neuropathy. On discharge he agreed to use a wheelchair but declined antibiotics and had a subsequent admission for infection which resulted in amputation of the 5th toe. The foot healed in 1 year (Fig. 6.32c).

Key points
- Infection is often responsible for tissue damage in the neuroischaemic foot and surgical debridement as an emergency may be necessary to remove necrosis
- Urgent vascular investigations should then take place to prepare for revascularization
- Wound closure may be achieved with skin grafts
- Skin grafts can be taken from within the distribution of the neuropathy to avoid general anaesthetic and postoperative pain
- Infection will destroy a skin graft and delay wound healing
- Following bypass or angioplasty, regular vascular review is essential to detect deterioration early.

Investigation of patients with emboli

When dry necrosis is secondary to emboli, a possible source should be investigated, and therefore the following investigations should be performed:
- ECG to detect atrial fibrillation or recent myocardial infarct
- Echocardiogram to detect the presence of valvular disease or thrombus in the left ventricle
- Ultrasound of abdomen to detect aortic aneurysm
- Duplex angiography of the lower limbs to detect atherosclerotic plaque in iliac or femoral arteries.

Having located the source of the emboli, appropriate treatment can be given. In general, antiplatelet therapy with aspirin is the usual treatment.

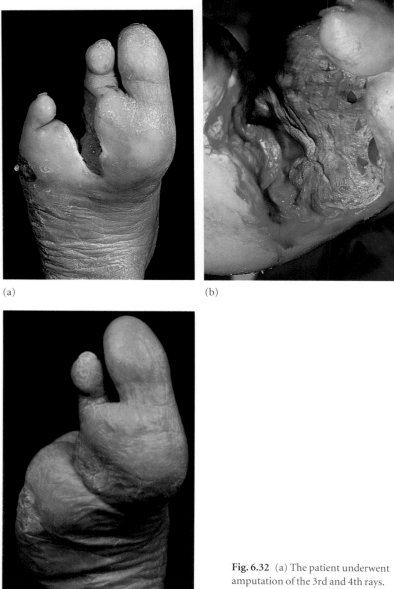

Fig. 6.32 (a) The patient underwent amputation of the 3rd and 4th rays. (b) A split-skin graft is applied to the tissue defect. (c) Foot has healed.

Mechanical control

During the peri- and postoperative period, bed rest is essential with elevation of the limb to relieve oedema and afford heel protection. Prophylaxis of deep vein thrombosis should be carried out using a low molecular weight heparin subcutaneously daily. Low molecular weight heparin is as effective and as safe as unfractionated heparin in the prevention of venous thromboembolism. However, the serum creatinine should be less than 150 μmol/L. The standard prophylactic regimen does not require monitoring.

In the neuropathic foot, non-weightbearing is advisable initially and then off-loading of the healing postoperative wound may be achieved by casting techniques.

After operative debridement in the neuroischaemic foot, especially when revascularization has not been possible, non-weightbearing is advised until the wound is healed.

If necrosis is to be treated conservatively, by autoamputation, which can take several months, then the patient needs a wide-fitting shoe to accommodate foot and dressings, or a 'Scotchcast' boot.

Patients should walk as little as possible.

Metabolic control

When patients present with necrosis, in the background of severe infection or ischaemia, they may be very ill, and will need close metabolic and haemodynamic monitoring. Considerable metabolic decompensation may occur, and full resuscitation is required with intravenous fluids and intravenous insulin sliding scale, which is often necessary to achieve good blood glucose control whilst the patient is infected or the leg severely ischaemic. High glucose levels are associated with postoperative infections in the leg as well as infections of the urinary tract and the respiratory system.

Patients will often have cardiac and renal impairment, which will need careful monitoring to optimize the regulation of fluid balance, so as to avoid hypotension from underperfusion and hypertension and peripheral oedema from overperfusion. Oedema is a potent cause of impaired wound healing. Many patients have autonomic neuropathy which may contribute to impaired blood pressure control and more frequent cardiac arrhythmias.

Nutritional impairment is denoted by a serum albumen of < 3.5 g/L and a total lymphocyte count of less than 1.5×10^9/L. A high-calorie diet should be instituted. A minimum of 1800 calories per day should be ingested to avoid the negative nitrogen balance that could accompany the depletion of protein stores.

Educational control

Gangrene can develop with alarming rapidity in the diabetic foot.

There have been cases of carers of high-risk diabetic patients being accused of neglecting their charge, when necrosis has developed rapidly and the patient has then been assessed by an inexperienced practitioner who does not realize how quickly necrosis can develop and has accused the carer of taking no action to help the patient 'who must have had gangrene for several weeks'. Health-care professionals and patients should be aware that necrosis can develop very quickly.

Fear of gangrene

Some patients and their families find necrotic feet deeply upsetting. The use of the word 'gangrene' can distress and frighten some patients. It should be explained that just because a small area of the foot has developed necrosis it does not mean that the whole foot will be destroyed or that amputation is inevitable.

The health-care practitioner should never express distaste or disgust. If he does not know the patient well, then before the foot is uncovered he should ask whether the patient has seen it. This is particularly important when the foot is first 'taken down' after surgery, because the sight of missing toes can be very upsetting and shocking.

After an amputation some patients do not want to inspect the foot at all until it is fully healed.

Patients who develop necrosis are often deeply fearful of the future. They need careful education including reassurance that much can be done to help them. Avoiding the words 'gangrene' or 'necrosis', and hiding the foot away under a dressing, can be a form of escapism which does little to address the patient's fears. We believe that practical and straightforward explanations are best.

The following educational material is in the form of commonly asked questions and answers.

If I have gangrene will I lose my leg?

Many people find gangrene a frightening word. This may be because people remember hearing about World War I and how many soldiers in the trenches developed gas gangrene which destroyed their legs and often killed them too. In fact, gangrene in the diabetic foot, although a serious problem, will not always lead to loss of the leg. In many cases the damage can be limited to loss of a small area of the skin of the foot, which will heal completely in the end leaving only a scar.

What does the word gangrene mean?

Gangrene means tissue death. There are two kinds of gangrene. One, wet gangrene, is caused by infection. The other type of gangrene, dry gangrene, is caused by a poor blood supply. When not enough blood reaches a part of the foot, the skin and flesh may die and change colour to brown or black. This is gangrene, also called necrosis.

How would I know if I was getting gangrene?

The first signs of gangrene may be that an area of the foot changes colour. It may or may not be painful. Part of the foot usually develops a blueish or purple colour.

STAGE 5

What should I do if I think I might be getting gangrene?

If you spot it early and seek treatment immediately it is often possible to treat the infection or poor blood supply and save the foot.

The worst thing you can do in these circumstances is to ignore the problem in the hope that it will go away and get better by itself. This is unlikely to happen. Go to your diabetic foot service immediately. Do not delay.

How is gangrene treated?

There are several different treatment programmes for patients with gangrene.

If the problem is due to infection, you should be admitted to hospital and given strong antibiotics through a vein in your arm. Later the black area of your foot may be taken off in the operating theatre. This will depend on how good the blood supply to your foot is. If blood flow is good then the foot should heal quickly.

If the problem is due to infection combined with a poor blood supply then you will need antibiotics but it may also be necessary and possible to improve your blood supply to the foot.

How could my blood supply be improved?

With an angioplasty. Angioplasty involves stretching a narrow blood vessel to enable more blood to pass down it.

Are there any other ways to get more blood down to the foot?

Another possibility is a bypass operation. Bypass involves attaching a new piece of blood vessel to bypass any blockage in the blood supply. If a bypass procedure is successful it may be possible to amputate the gangrenous part of your foot and achieve quick healing.

A third possibility will apply if the blood supply to your foot cannot be improved by angioplasty or bypass. Once any infection is under control the gangrenous area of your foot will dry out and drop off. This process is called autoamputation. It will take several months, and a lot of patience, before this happens.

What footwear can I wear if I have gangrene?

Until your foot is completely healed it will probably be necessary for you to wear a special shoe or cast boot to avoid any pressure on the gangrenous areas.

Will my black toe just fall off?

If your black toe becomes very loose and you are afraid of it coming off in bed, then it may be possible for the foot clinic to remove it painlessly.

Should my foot be dressed and bandaged?

Your gangrenous foot should be covered with dressings at all times. Animals and flies find gangrenous tissue very attractive.

How can I tell if my gangrenous foot is doing well?

If germs infect your gangrenous foot you will find that the black areas become wet and smell bad, and may become light grey or whiteish in colour. If this happens you should seek help from the foot clinic without delay.

Important signs that a gangrenous foot is not doing well are as follows:
- Foot becomes wet
- Foot changes colour from black or dark brown to grey
- Foot discharges fluid
- Foot swells
- Red area develops around line between gangrene and normal tissue
- Red mark spreads up leg
- Foot smells bad
- Leg or foot become more painful.

If you notice changes, go to the diabetic foot clinic at once.

What kind of dressings should be on my foot?

- You should avoid moist dressings at all costs. If gangrene becomes wet it is an excellent growth medium for bacteria and infection is likely
- Use dressings to separate black toes from their healthy neighbours, lest the problem spread from one to the other
- Avoid 'specialist' dressings and treatments like hydrocolloids, alginates, wet to dry dressings and whirlpool
- If you receive visits from a community nurse who wants to change your dressing regime, ask her to contact the diabetic foot clinic service first.

Can I bathe or shower?

Keep gangrenous toes out of the bath or shower. If gangrene becomes wet it is likely to become infected. It is possible to purchase a 'cast protector' which is a strong plastic bag shaped like a leg. You can use this to cover your foot and keep it dry while the rest of your body is bathed and showered.

How often should my foot be checked and why?

Your gangrenous foot should be checked every day for signs that it is getting worse. If this happens, talk to the diabetic foot service the same day. If it happens at a weekend then go to the Casualty department at your local hospital and ask to be seen by the diabetic team. You cannot afford to wait even one day if a gangrenous foot is going wrong: taking immediate action can save your foot.

Will I need regular appointments at the foot service?

Regular treatment is very important. When you see the podiatrist or doctor at the diabetic foot service they may use a scalpel to cut small pieces of dead tissue off your foot.

Why will they do that?

This procedure, called debridement, helps healing.

How does it help healing?

The less dead tissue there is around, the fewer germs will be on your foot. Dead tissue in direct contact with healthy tissue can cause problems, so as much dead tissue as possible will be removed when you come to clinic.

Won't it hurt?

This procedure should not be painful as the only tissue being removed is already dead. However, if it causes you discomfort you should always say so.

Why do hospitals behave as if it is their diabetes and their foot and not mine?

You may sometimes feel as if your diabetes and your foot no longer belong to you, and have passed into the possession of the eager group of people—the team of the diabetic foot clinic—who see you every time you come to clinic. Never forget—it is your foot, and you are the one who should decide what happens. You should always be told what is going to be done to you, and why, and what will happen next.

What if I don't understand what they want to do?

If you do not understand, then ask for things to be explained again. It is essential that you are aware of what is being done and take an interest. Even if you trust your foot clinic team, you should still take an interest, and try to understand why the gangrene developed, what, if anything, has gone wrong in the past and the ways that future trouble can be prevented.

What should I do if I'm away from home and my foot gets worse?

If you are away from home and your foot gives trouble you should seek treatment at the nearest hospital.

What should I do if I am admitted to another hospital or receive treatment elsewhere?

It is very important, in these circumstances, that the diabetic foot clinic is informed about what is happening. If you are under the care of less experienced people they should usually welcome input from the diabetic foot clinic.

PRACTICE POINTS

- Necrosis does not automatically lead to amputation
- Necrosis can be divided into wet necrosis and dry necrosis
- Wet necrosis in neuropathic feet needs intravenous antibiotics and surgical debridement
- Wet necrosis in neuroischaemic feet needs intravenous antibiotics, surgical debridement and vascular reconstruction
- Dry necrosis in neuroischaemic feet needs vascular reconstruction and amputation or outpatient debridement and autoamputation
- Renal patients are particularly prone to develop necrosis
- When necrosis become wet, smelly, painful or spreading then patients should seek help urgently.

FURTHER READING

Wound control

Albrektsen SB, Henriksen BM, Holstein PE. Minor amputations on the feet after revascularization for gangrene. A consecutive series of 95 limbs. *Acta Orthopaed Scand* 1997; **68**: 291–3.

Clare MP, Fitzgibbons TC, McMullen ST *et al.* Experience with the vacuum assisted closure negative pressure technique in the treatment of non-healing diabetic and dysvascular wounds. *Foot Ankle Int* 2002; **23**: 896–901.

Faglia E, Clerici G, Clerissi J *et al.* A. Early and five-year amputation and survival rate of diabetic patients with critical limb ischemia: data of a cohort study of 564 patients. *Eur J Vasc Endovasc Surg* 2006; **32**: 484–90.

Foster AV, Snowden S, Grenfell A *et al.* Reduction of gangrene and amputations in diabetic renal transplant patients: the role of a special foot clinic. *Diabetic Medicine* 1995; **12**: 632–5.

Holstein PE, Sorensen S. Limb salvage experience in a multi-disciplinary diabetic foot unit. *Diabetes Care* 1999; **22** Suppl: B97–B103.

Rayman A, Stansfield G, Woollard T *et al.* Use of larvae in the treatment of the diabetic necrotic foot. *Diabetic Foot* 1998; **1**: 7–13.

Serletti JM, Deuber MA, Guidera PM *et al.* Atherosclerosis of the lower extremity and free-tissue reconstruction for limb salvage. *Plast Reconstr Surg* 1995; **96**: 1136–44.

Sherman RA. Maggot therapy for treating diabetic foot ulcers unresponsive to conventional therapy. *Diabetes Care* 2003; **26**: 446–51.

Treiman GS, Oderich GS, Ashrafi A *et al.* Management of ischaemic heel ulcer and gangrene: an evaluation of factors associated with successful healing. *J Vasc Surg* 2000; **31**: 1110–18.

Vermassen FE, van Landuyt K. Combined vascular reconstruction and free flap transfer in diabetic arterial disease. *Diabetes Metab Res Rev* 2000; **16** Suppl 1: S33–6.

Microbiological control

Cheung AH, Wong LM. Surgical infections in patients with chronic renal failure. *Infect Dis Clin North Am* 2001; **15**: 775–96.

Edmonds ME, Foster AVM. Infections complicating diseases of the feet in renal patients. In Sweny P, Rubin R, Tolkoff-Rubin N (eds). *The Infectious Complications of Renal Disease.* Oxford University Press, Oxford, UK, 2003, **19**: 399–416.

Vascular control

Calle-Pascual AL, Duran A, Diaz A *et al.* Comparison of peripheral arterial reconstruction in diabetic and non-diabetic patients: a prospective clinic-based study. *Diabetes Res Clin Pract* 2001; **53**: 129–36.

Cohen MC, Curran PJ, L'Italien GI *et al.* Long-term prognostic value of preoperative dipyridamole thallium imaging and clinical indexes in patients with diabetes mellitus undergoing peripheral vascular surgery. *Am J Cardiol* 1999; **83**: 1038–42.

Deery HG, Sangeorzan JA. Saving the diabetic foot with special reference to the patient with chronic renal failure. *Infect Dis Clin North Am* 2001; **15**: 953–81.

Dorweiler B, Neufang A, Kreitner KF *et al.* Magnetic resonance angiography unmasks reliable target vessels for pedal bypass grafting in patients with diabetes mellitus. *J Vasc Surg* 2002; **35**: 766–72.

Dorweiler B, Neufang A, Schmiedt W, Oelert H. Pedal arterial bypass for limb salvage in patients with diabetes mellitus. *Eur J Vasc Endovasc Surg* 2002; **24**: 309–13.

Faglia E, Favales F, Morabito A. New ulceration, new major amputation, and survival rates in diabetic subjects hospitalised for foot ulceration from 1990 to 1993: a 6.5-year follow-up. *Diabetes Care* 2001; **24**: 78–83.

Fleisher LA, Eagle KA. Screening for cardiac disease in patients having noncardiac surgery. *Ann Intern Med* 1996; **124**: 767–72.

Hood DB, Weaver FA, Papanicolaou G *et al.* Cardiac evaluation of the diabetic patient prior to peripheral vascular surgery. *Ann Vasc Surg* 1996; **10**: 330–5.

Kalra M, Gloviczki P, Bower TC *et al.* Limb salvage after successful pedal bypass grafting is associated with improved long-term survival. *J Vasc Surg* 2001; **33**: 6–16.

Kaufman JL, Shah DM, Leather RP. Atheroembolism and microembolic syndromes (blue toe syndromes and disseminated atheroembolism). In Rutherford RB (ed.) *Vascular Surgery*, 4th edn. Saunders, Philadelphia, USA, 1995, pp. 669–67.

LoGerfo FW, Gibbons GW, Pomposelli FB *et al.* Trends in the care of the diabetic foot. Expanded role of arterial reconstruction. *Arch Surg* 1992; **127**: 617–21.

Morrison WB, Ledermann HP. Work-up of the diabetic foot. *Radiol Clin North Am* 2002; **40**: 1171–92.

Poldermans D, Boersma E, Bax JJ *et al.* The effect of bisoprolol on perioperative mortality and myocardial infarction in high-risk patients undergoing vascular surgery. Dutch Echocardiographic Cardiac Risk Evaluation Applying Stress Echocardiography Study Group. *N Engl J Med* 1999; **341**: 1789–94.

Pomposelli FB, Kansal N, Hamdan AD *et al.* A decade of experience with dorsalis pedis artery bypass: analysis of outcome in more than 1000 cases. *J Vasc Surg* 2003; **37**: 969–74.

Sheehan P. Introduction to diabetes: Principles of care in the surgical patient with diabetes. In Veves A, Giurini JM, LoGerfo FW (eds). *The Diabetic Foot*, 2nd edn. Humana Press, New Jersey, USA, 2006, pp. 1–38.

Treiman GS, Lawrence PF, Rockwell WB. Autogenous arterial bypass grafts: durable patency and limb salvage in patients with inframalleolar occlusive disease and end-stage renal disease. *J Vasc Surg* 2000; **32**: 13–22.

Mechanical control

Knowles EA, Armstrong DG, Hayat SA *et al.* Offloading diabetic foot wounds using the Scotchcast boot: a retrospective study. *Osteomy Wound Manag* 2002; **48**: 50–3.

Metabolic control

Deery HG. Saving the diabetic foot with special reference to the patient with chronic renal failure. *Infect Dis Clin North Am* 2001; **15**: 953–81.

Game FL, Chipchase SY, Hubbard R *et al.* Temporal association between the incidence of foot ulceration and the start of dialysis in diabetes mellitus. *Nephrol Dial Transplant* 2006; **21**: 3207–10.

Young BA, Maynard C, Reiber G, Boyko EJ. Effects of ethnicity and nephropathy on lower-extremity amputation risk among diabetic veterans. *Diabetes Care* 2003; **26**: 495–501.

Educational control

Malone JM, Snyder M, Anderson G *et al.* Prevention of amputation by diabetic education. *Am J Surg* 1989; **158**: 520–4.

Radford K, Chipchase S, Jeffcoate W. Education in the management of the foot in diabetes. In Boulton AJM, Cavanagh PR, Rayman G (eds). *The Foot in Diabetes*, 3rd edn. John Wiley & Sons, Chichester, UK, 2006, pp. 143–58.

Weinger K, Smaldone A. Psychosocial and educational implications of diabetic foot complications. In Veves A, Giurini JM, LoGerfo FW (eds). *The Diabetic Foot*, 2nd edn. Humana Press, New Jersey, USA, 2006, pp. 507–22.

7

Stage 6: the unsalvageable foot

I cannot help it now,
Unless by using means I lame the foot . . .
(Coriolanus IV, vii, William Shakespeare)

PRESENTATION AND MANAGEMENT

The stage 6 foot cannot be saved and needs a major amputation, either below, through, or above the knee. Although, as we have shown, the majority of diabetic feet can be saved and respond to good care, patients do sometimes need a major amputation either to save the patient's life from overwhelming sepsis, to control intolerable pain or to enable the patient to walk better than he can on his diseased foot.

Throughout this book we have emphasized the need for rapid access, rapid diagnosis and rapid treatment, and these are just as important at stage 6 as for the early stages.

Limbs come to amputation because they have gone down a pathway which should have been preventable. We present below six case histories which illustrate problems that frequently occur on the road to amputation.

Pathways to amputation

Pathway to amputation 1: Neglected callus destroys a neuropathic foot
- A young man with type 1 diabetes
- Denies that his diabetes is a problem
- Fails to attend the clinic regularly
- Has chronic hyperglycaemia and is depressed
- Develops retinopathy, nephropathy and neuropathy
- Denies that his feet are a problem
- Develops plantar callus which is neglected
- A neuropathic ulcer develops: it is painless and goes unreported
- Infection sets in
- Develops wet gangrene
- Presents very late, ill and toxic

- There is gas in the tissues of foot and leg
- Undergoes an above-knee amputation.

Pathway to amputation 2: Neglected injury in a neuroischaemic foot
- An elderly lady with type 2 diabetes; said to be 'mild diabetes'
- Retinopathy and neuropathy develop
- Inadequate education—patient wears slippers round house
- Drops heavy object on foot—large abrasion on right hallux
- Applies sticking plaster
- Infection develops. Patient only seeks help when infection very severe
- Feet are pulseless. Sent to hospital with necrosis
- Vascular surgeon says vascular intervention not feasible
- Has below-knee amputation
- Patient dies in postoperative period.

Pathway to amputation 3: Eye–foot syndrome
- Man with BMI ≥ 30 develops type 2 diabetes. He does not know
- Undiagnosed
- Untreated for at least 8 years. Develops retinopathy and neuropathy
- Feels tired and unwell but assumes due to age
- Lives alone, socially isolated
- Walks barefoot and cuts foot on broken glass, but unaware of this
- Develops rapidly ascending infection but only seeks help because of nausea and 'because of the smell'
- Late admission via Casualty
- Pulses not palpable
- Undergoes below-knee amputation.

A Practical Manual of Diabetic Foot Care, 2nd edition, Edmonds, Foster and Sanders.
Published 2008 Blackwell Publishing. ISBN 978-1-4051-61473

Pathway to amputation 4: Chronic ischaemia

- Elderly lady with type 2 diabetes
- Develops a 'blister' on the border of the foot
- Weekly dressings applied
- The foot does not heal. More small marginated ulcers develop
- Foot suddenly deteriorates and becomes painful
- Paracetamol prescribed. Patient told to rest
- Appointment made with hospital diabetic clinic
- Patient collapses at home. Taken to Casualty
- Gangrenous toes and severe infection with absent foot pulses
- Below-knee amputation carried out.

Pathway to amputation 5: Acute ischaemia

- Patient has type 2 diabetes
- Poorly controlled long term. Patient is a smoker
- Develops neuropathy, ischaemia, retinopathy, nephropathy
- Goes on long-haul flight
- Develops pain and numbness of right leg
- Goes to Casualty—sent home with one week's appointment for vascular clinic
- Foot and lower leg turn blue over the next 3 days
- Returns to Casualty with acute ischaemia
- Revascularization not possible
- Undergoes above-knee amputation.

Pathway to amputation 6: Mismanaged Charcot's osteoarthropathy

- Patient develops type 1 diabetes aged 8 years
- Poorly controlled
- Develops neuropathy
- Aged 25, trips and twists foot
- Develops red, hot, swollen foot and ankle
- Bandage applied. Sprain diagnosed
- Foot not painful—told it is alright to walk
- Develops unstable ankle with fracture of ankle mortice
- Develops ulcer over lateral malleolus. Infection supervenes
- Orthopaedic surgeon deems foot unsalvageable
- Below-knee amputation carried out.

Several recurring themes resonate through these case histories, including:

- Patients and health-care practitioners who underestimate the state of the foot
- Patients who wait until there is no possibility of recovery before seeking help
- Health-care practitioners who do not refer the patient on
- Long waiting times for appointments
- Lack of pain leading patients to assume that because a problem is painless it is not serious

- Ignorance about diabetes, its management and the long-term effects on the foot of poor diabetes control
- Most importantly, lack of early access to a specialized multidisciplinary team.

By the time the foot has reached stage 6 it is too late to save it: in fact, without rapid access to help, the patient with a stage 6 foot will usually die. Having reached the diabetic foot clinic it is essential that the stage 6 foot and leg are properly assessed and any necessary investigations are carried out quickly. Amputations should be performed in a humane and timely way, at the right level, with proper preparation, both physical and mental, of the patient and his family, with a view to removing the leg at the right level and achieving rapid healing. Lastly, aftercare should be excellent, with long-term follow-up, and aimed at maximizing the patient's future quality of life and ability to get out and about, enabling him to lead as full a life as possible.

Major amputation is sometimes inevitable, particularly in neuroischaemic patients. However, rehabilitation of the diabetic amputee is extremely difficult and is characterized by long stays in hospital. Major amputation, therefore, must not be taken lightly. Morbidity and mortality associated with major amputation in diabetes are very high. Within 3 years of amputation, 50% of major amputees will be dead and of the survivors, half will have lost their remaining leg. After 5 years, only 30% of major amputees with diabetes will survive. Survival of above-knee amputees is significantly less than below-knee amputees, and relative mortality is higher for females than for males. In the presence of diabetes, the risk of developing congestive cardiac failure following amputation is twice that of those who are non-diabetic. There is a need for a more aggressive approach to the management of cardiac failure and cardiovascular risk factors in those who undergo amputation and have diabetes.

Reasons for major amputation

Diabetic patients who present with extensive ulcers on their feet are sometimes offered early amputation as 'the one sure way of sorting out the problem permanently', on the basis that such an operation is likely to be inevitable at some time in the future. This approach may be useful for young, otherwise healthy, non-diabetic patients incapacitated by pain or a useless limb, whose other limb is normal. However, major amputation does not guarantee an ulcer-free existence for the diabetic patient, and non-healing ulcer alone should not normally be an indication for major amputation.

Major amputation is usually carried out for the neuro-ischaemic foot and should be rare in the neuropathic foot.

Major amputation in the neuroischaemic foot is necessary in the following circumstances when:
- Overwhelming infection has destroyed the foot and threatens the patient's life
- There is severe ischaemia with rest pain that cannot be controlled
- Extensive necrosis secondary to a major arterial occlusion has destroyed the foot.

Major amputation in a neuropathic foot should be a very rare event and necessary only when:
- Infection has irretrievably destroyed the foot
- Charcot's osteoarthropathy has destroyed the ankle joint, attempts at external stabilization have been unsuccessful and internal fixation is not possible.

CASE STUDY
Overwhelming necrosis after patient lost to follow-up

A 73-year-old man with type 2 diabetes of 25 years' duration, peripheral neuropathy, peripheral vascular disease and previous amputation of his 2nd toe for osteomyelitis, failed to attend follow-up appointments in the diabetic foot clinic. He lived alone and turned away ambulance transport, despite frequent reminders and notification of his general practitioner, who arranged weekly visits by the district nurses. His forefoot changed colour: it was initially blue and then became black but because the patient did not complain of pain no help was sought. After 5 weeks the discolouration spread up the foot. He was admitted to hospital with wet gangrene. The foot was already destroyed at presentation (Fig. 7.1). He underwent a below-knee amputation.

Key points
- Necrosis is often painless in the diabetic foot
- If dry necrosis becomes infected, wet necrosis can supervene and destroy the foot in a short time
- Regular follow-up is crucially important for high-risk diabetic patients with foot problems
- We become alarmed if high-risk patients fail to keep appointments and try to arrange for regular inspections of the feet.

CASE STUDY
Overwhelming necrosis following arterial occlusion

An 80-year-old woman with type 2 diabetes mellitus of 10 years' duration was admitted to hospital following a stroke and discharged home under the care of the

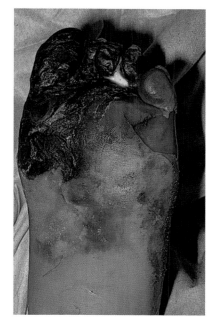

Fig. 7.1 Overwhelming necrosis: this foot was already destroyed at presentation.

general practitioner. The right foot became discoloured but she felt no pain and it was not until overwhelming necrosis of the right foot and lower limb had developed that she showed her leg to the district nurses (Fig. 7.2). When she was admitted to hospital she was moribund. She had necrosis spreading to the lower leg, which was icy cold. Clinically, this indicated a major arterial occlusion. She underwent palliative care and died shortly afterwards.

Key points
- If neuropathy is profound even occlusion of a major vessel will not be painful
- Patients who have had a stroke may have abnormal sensations and fail to complain
- Vulnerable patients in the community should have their feet checked regularly by health-care professionals.

The decision to amputate

When a major amputation is being considered the following factors should be addressed by the multidisciplinary team:
- Social factors: some practitioners believe that patients who face many weeks or months of treatment should be

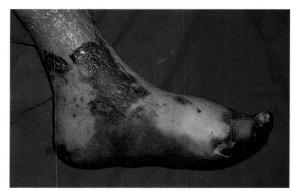

Fig. 7.2 Necrosis spreading to the leg after a major arterial occlusion.

offered a major amputation as a serious treatment option and that amputation can often be viewed very positively. Elliott Joslin felt that if life expectancy was very limited it could not be regarded as a success if the patient spent much of his remaining days in hospital to save his leg

- Emotional factors: many patients and their families react with horror to the idea of a major amputation. Depression after amputation is common
- Financial factors: diabetic foot patients may be regarded as 'expensive' patients in terms of:
    Number of bed days occupied
    Consumption of expensive antibiotics
    Costly interventions.
    However, major amputation is not cheap and involves:
    Accumulated costs of rehabilitation
    Prosthetics service
    Loss of earnings
    Costs of special services
- Functional factors: in elderly, frail diabetic patients the functional results of amputation are usually poor. Many patients do not walk again and never return to independent living.

There should be clear criteria for amputation as described above, and the decision should be made by a multidisciplinary team together with the patient and his family. Sometimes the decision is not an easy one.

CASE STUDY
Major amputation in the presence of severe comorbidity

A 78-year-old man with type 2 diabetes of 20 years' duration had had a stroke with considerable weakness of the

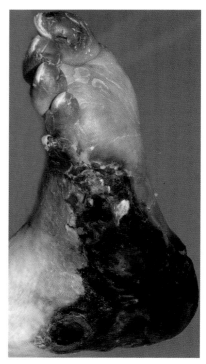

Fig. 7.3 Foot with extensive necrosis.

right arm and right leg and developed extensive necrosis of his right foot (Fig. 7.3). The decision was either to perform an amputation or embark on palliative care. The patient and his relatives wanted to 'give it a go' and he underwent a through-knee amputation. He had a stormy postoperative course complicated by pneumonia. He had tremendous problems with mobilization and died without ever going home.

Key points
- This was acute on chronic ischaemia leading to overwhelming necrosis. The patient would certainly have died without an amputation
- The decision to perform the operation was taken after long discussion with both the patient and his relatives who both favoured amputation. In these difficult cases, their opinion should be sought
- The fate of the ischaemic patient who undergoes amputation can be very disappointing but this reflects the overwhelming and widespread nature of the atherosclerotic disease.

CASE STUDY
Problems with 'the good leg'

A 39-year-old male with type 1 diabetes of 27 years' duration and end-stage renal failure treated by continuous ambulatory peritoneal dialysis had a history of bilateral neuropathic ulceration and underwent amputation of left 3rd, 4th and 5th toes. The foot healed and he was issued with an orthotic walker. The foot remained intact for most of the time, but broke down if he had to run for a bus or walked more than usual. He was desperate to wear 'normal' footwear. He was placed on the waiting list for a joint renal/pancreas transplant, but had been told that if he had ulceration the transplant could not be carried out. He had two young children and deeply resented being unable to run and walk freely and participate in sports. His orthotist referred him to the rehabilitation team who advised him to consider a below-knee amputation as he was a comparatively young man and would do well with a modern prosthesis.

When the patient discussed this proposal with the multidisciplinary diabetic foot team they perceived major amputation far less positively. They pointed out to the patient that, with a prosthetic limb, his remaining foot (with a previous history of ulceration) would be overloaded and that a major amputation could not guarantee that he would remain free from ulceration. Nonetheless he made the decision to ask for a major amputation and was put on the waiting list for an elective below-knee amputation.

One month later he attended at the diabetic foot clinic as an emergency, complaining of pain and numbness in the right foot (the 'good' foot) which had been present for several days. The foot pulses were impalpable, and the leg and foot were mottled and grey and cold from mid-calf downwards. He developed necrosis of his medial longitudinal arch and hallux that slowly extended to involve three of the lesser toes and the heel. The angiogram showed occlusion of the mid and distal popliteal artery with faint filling of the anterior tibial artery and no plantar arch was seen. The popliteal artery was angioplastied, which allowed increased flow through the popliteal artery, anterior tibial artery and some flow into the plantar vessels. He has subsequently had repeat angioplasty of the popliteal and superficial femoral arteries at 3 and 4 months after presentation, and also underwent surgical debridement of necrotic tissues. He underwent surgical amputation of the necrotic tissue and was followed up in the diabetic foot clinic (Fig. 7.4). He cancelled amputation of the left leg. Healing was protracted but the foot

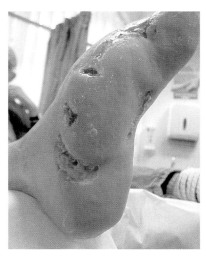

Fig. 7.4 Healing right foot.

healed after more than 2 years. Two years later he died of a stroke.

Key points
- Every foot is a precious commodity which should be preserved if at all possible because of future risks to the other foot
- The decision to undergo major amputation is particularly difficult in patients with end-stage renal failure who may be relatively young but nevertheless have considerable comorbidities
- Angioplasty can be a successful treatment for occlusion of the popliteal artery
- Angioplasty can be repeated to maintain the patency of the artery.

Choice of level of amputation

The level of amputation should be carefully considered to ensure that there is sufficient perfusion to achieve wound healing. When possible, a below-knee amputation should be carried out to conserve the knee joint and aid the fitting of a prosthesis. Preserving the knee joint lowers the energy expenditure necessary for walking. The cardiovascular cost for walking and foot plantar pressures in the opposite limb both increase in direct proportion as the amputation becomes more proximal. Postoperative mortality is higher in above-knee amputations (10–40%) than in below-knee amputations (5–20%).

The aims are:
- To keep the amputation as distal as possible
- To amputate above painful, cold, pale or discoloured tissue
- To amputate below warm, pink, well-perfused tissue.

About one-fifth of transtibial amputations and knee disarticulation amputations undergo revision surgery to proximal amputation due to healing complications.

Preoperative care

The following points should be recognized:
- Admission to hospital is always an anxious time, especially for patients fearing or facing a major amputation
- When patients are worried and anxious they may not retain information
- Information should be repeated several times and reinforced with the written word
- Patients like to feel that their limb is valuable, and that initial investigations and interventions are made in an effort to try and save the limb
- Patients want to know the reason why the leg needs to be amputated
- If patients are ill and toxic they may not comprehend what is happening
- Patients who are facing amputation should be given time to come to terms with it wherever possible
- Detailed explanations of all procedures should be given. The level of amputation should be explained and the intended site of amputation should be touched with the health-care professional's hand to demonstrate the level. The patient should be told that the wound will be covered with skin
- The effects of a general anaesthetic should be explained to the patient and family
- The stress of amputation should not be underestimated. If the operation is delayed or cancelled for any reason the patient and relatives should be informed immediately.

Physical assessment of the patient is important. Cardiorespiratory status and metabolic control should be optimized. Patients should be encouraged to cease smoking. Malnutrition increases the risk of delayed wound healing. Weight loss and diminished appetite are common and patients should be seen by the dietitian.

Antibiotic prophylaxis should be used.

Once major amputation is planned, and it is not being performed as an emergency, a lumbar epidural block with bupivicaine can be started 48 hours beforehand to relieve postoperative pain.

Perioperative care

A major amputation will put the remaining foot at great risk of ulceration.

The heel of the surviving foot should be protected on the operating table and postoperatively. One of our surgeons always wrapped several layers of thick cotton wadding (Gamgee, Robinson) around the heel of the contralateral foot to avoid pressure on the heel during the amputation.

Drains are advisable for amputations, as blood clots are a good culture medium for bacteria.

A rigid dressing applied in below-knee amputations from the end of the stump to the mid-thigh, in full extension, will reduce oedema, protect the wound and limb against trauma, and prevent knee contractures during the first three postoperative weeks.

Postoperative care

Some patients return from theatre thinking that they still have their leg as they can still 'feel' it. Without reminders they may get out of bed and try to 'stand on two feet' resulting in a fall and possible injury to the stump or the other foot.

Phantom sensation gradually decreases and may telescope so that the patient feels his foot at his thigh.

During the postoperative period, patients who have lost a limb often describe similar feelings to those described by people who have just had a chronic disease such as diabetes diagnosed, or people who have undergone a bereavement.

There may be physical sensations including:
- Fatigue
- Helplessness, muscle weakness, lack of energy
- Feeling of hollowness in stomach
- Tightness in chest and throat, and breathlessness
- Oversensitivity to noises
- Dry mouth.

Common emotional reactions include:
- Sense of unreality and light-headedness
- Feeling of observing oneself from outside
- Disbelief, confusion, hallucinations, sleep disturbance, dreams
- Preoccupation
- Sense of the presence of the lost limb
- Absent mindedness
- Sighing, crying.

Other feelings may include:
- Despair

- Sadness
- Anger and frustration
- Guilt and self-reproach
- Anxiety
- Loneliness
- Shock
- Relief.

The initial phase involves shock and disbelief, which is often followed by feelings of sadness, despair, anxiety and sometimes anger or pining. Although these feelings usually decrease as patients start to recover or adapt, individual reactions vary. It is important for patients and their families to be aware of these effects.

In the early phase, patients may feel emotionally numb, and may need help with making the simplest decisions.

Common social reactions include:

- Social withdrawal
- Avoiding reminders of the amputation.

Gradually the patient enters the recovery phase. In order to optimize recovery it is necessary for all health-care professionals to:

- Listen and give the patient time
- Acknowledge their special loss
- Acknowledge any feelings, especially negative ones such as anger, and offer reassurance that these are normal and to be expected
- Be prepared to handle the stump and encourage spouse or family to do likewise
- Be aware that some patients hate the word 'stump'
- Be aware that the first dressing change is particularly frightening. Comments about the state of the wound should be true and tactfully presented, avoiding negative facial disgust or inappropriate belittling comments
- Reassure the patient that any stump pain should settle gradually as oedema and inflammation settle and should be reduced by regularly prescribed analgesia.

The relatives of patients also need attention and sympathy. The psychological effect of amputation on the patient's relatives may be profound. We remember the wife of a major amputee who refused to have a ramp fitted to the house because she said it would spoil the look of her home. We are not sure whether she meant that ramps were unaesthetically pleasing, whether she felt there was a stigma attached to a house with a ramp, or whether she simply enjoyed being able to control their exits and their entrances. We were also unclear about the motives of another patient's wife who refused to allow him to be fitted with a prosthesis after his below-knee amputation. She said the reason was that she was afraid that he would fall over and hurt himself, but the patient himself believed that she enjoyed being in control.

Amputation wounds are often slow to heal in neuro-ischaemic patients. Infection should be treated aggressively and the vacuum-assisted closure (VAC) pump may be useful. However, if there is poor arterial perfusion to the below-knee wound it may be necessary to convert it into an above-knee amputation.

Shortly after the amputation has been performed, oedema of the stump can be a problem, and JUZO socks, which are compression stump shrinkers, provide good oedema control both in the acute stages, and long term. They are only provided after the stitches have been removed as they can otherwise drag on the wound edges and cause dehiscence. The stump is measured and the sock supplied between days 5 and 10 postamputation.

Initially, the sock is applied for 10 minutes only and the stump is then inspected for problems including colour change and breaks in the skin.

Once healed, the stump should be inspected daily for skin breakdown, which should be cleaned, dressed and off-loaded until complete healing is achieved.

Mobility aids

Before the definitive prosthesis is issued, some patients may be suitable for mobility aids.

The amputee mobility aid (AMA) is suitable for below-knee and through-knee amputees only. The stump is supported and stabilized by an inflatable bag, which also assists in reducing oedema. It is a physical and psychological boost to get the patient on his feet early. It has a knee joint.

The pneumatic postamputation mobility aid (PPAM aid) has an inflatable socket and may be used 7 days postoperatively to mobilize above-knee, through-knee and below-knee amputees. It assists in stump shrinkage, reduces pain and allows aerobic exercise to start.

The skin should always be checked before and after use of mobility aids.

When the amputation stump is slow to heal, special prostheses can be used to facilitate weightbearing and reduce pressure on the stump (Fig. 7.5).

The definitive prosthesis

The standard prosthesis contains a stump sheath worn inside a customized thermoplastic socket. This is then fitted onto a modular prosthesis. The shank of the prosthesis articulates with a prosthetic foot that is matched to the patient's physique and functional requirements.

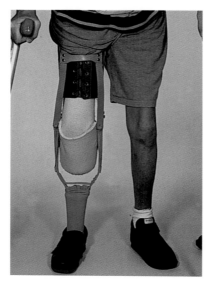

Fig. 7.5 This patient is wearing an interim prosthesis with felt cup, corset and metal shin.

Putting the definitive prosthesis on and taking it off may be difficult if hands are neuropathic and eyesight is poor, and visual inspection of the stump may be difficult. Velcro straps are useful in the patient with neuropathy and poor hand function to aid fitting and removing the prosthesis. If skin is atrophic and circulation is reduced, stasis dermatitis may be a problem, and the skin is easily injured.

Rehabilitation

The key for success in dealing with the stage 6 patient is careful follow-up. With good planning and follow-up care after a major amputation the stump will heal, but it is also important to ensure that it will remain intact. Healthcare professionals in the diabetic foot service should be aware of the presentation and management of problems with the amputated stump. Often they will be treating the remaining foot of their patients but be asked to advise on problems with the stump of the contralateral leg.

Problems with the stump include:
- Volume fluctuation
- Susceptibility to trauma
- Callus
- Ulceration
- Infection
- Ischaemia.

Volume fluctuation

It is in the early stages that the greatest changes in the stump will occur, and the size and shape of the stump can be expected to change markedly for around 1 year. During the amputee's life, his body weight and the amount he walks are likely to fluctuate, and this results in alteration of the stump volume. Cardiac and renal disease can lead to stump oedema. Fluctuating stump volume is a particular problem in diabetic amputees, and patients with neuropathic stumps may have difficulty in detecting it.

Susceptibility to trauma

Amputees are vulnerable to falls, particularly when not wearing the prosthesis, and may fracture the stump.

CASE STUDY
Fractured stump

A 62-year-old woman with type 2 diabetes of 18 years' duration underwent a right below-knee amputation after developing a deep infection of her neuropathic foot. She lived abroad and had no rehabilitation, but 4 months later she was visiting her daughter in the UK, developed neuropathic ulceration of the left hallux and was referred to the diabetic foot clinic as an emergency.

At her second visit she mentioned that she had fallen and injured her stump when transferring from a taxi to her wheelchair. She was wearing a silicone sock on her stump at the time. She felt no pain in her stump after the fall, but 3 days later she developed severe pain in the stump which kept her awake at night and was described as 'aching' and 'spasmodic'. On examination there was minimal swelling, no haematoma and no break in the skin of the stump. X-ray revealed a fracture through the tibia extending to the resected surface (Fig. 7.6). She was referred to the fracture clinic and a bivalved stump splint was applied.

Key points
- In a neuropathic stump, signs and symptoms of fracture may be minimal or delayed
- Neuropathic stumps should be X-rayed following trauma.

Callus

Patients with neuropathic stumps are prone to develop callus. If this is not debrided it will lead to ulceration (Fig. 7.7).

Ulceration

This often begins with a blister which may be caused by friction or pressure within the prosthesis socket. All tissue

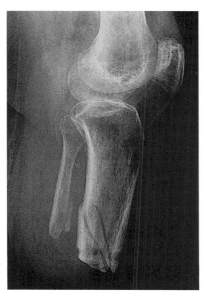

Fig. 7.6 Fracture of tibia of below-knee stump.

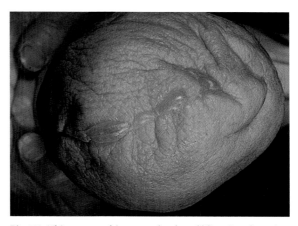

Fig. 7.8 This neuropathic stump developed blistering along the amputation scar.

Infection

There is a great risk of ulcers on the stump becoming infected, and we have seen a case of below-knee amputation being converted to above-knee amputation because of infection that occurred 4 years after the first amputation. Management is debridement, pressure relief and antibiotics.

CASE STUDY
Pain and swelling of the stump

A 65-year-old man with type 2 diabetes of 25 years' duration underwent below-knee amputation of his right leg for uncontrolled infection, which destroyed the foot and put his life at risk. He was successfully rehabilitated and walked well with a prosthesis. Three years later he was referred to the diabetic foot clinic complaining of pain and swelling of the stump in the area of the knee which made it difficult for him to use his prosthesis. There was no ulceration, but the stump was pink (Fig. 7.9a). The prosthesis socket was inspected and no areas of excessive wear were found; however, the rehabilitation team were asked to review the prosthesis. Transcutaneous oxymetry was performed to exclude ischaemia of the stump and revealed that the circulation was adequate. A diagnosis of infection was made. Broad-spectrum antibiotics were prescribed and he desisted from wearing the prosthesis, using a wheelchair and crutches instead. After 4 weeks, the redness and warmth had resolved (Fig. 7.9b) and the patient was able to wear his prosthesis again.

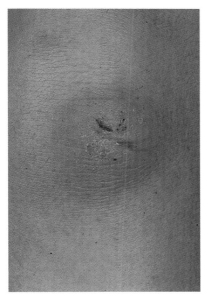

Fig. 7.7 Callus on a stump.

breakdowns should be cleaned with saline and covered with a dressing. If possible the patient should not wear his prosthesis, and should seek urgent review of the fit (Fig. 7.8).

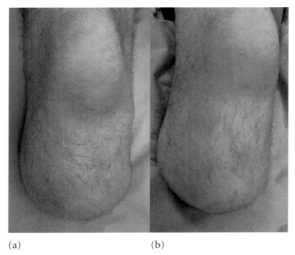

(a)   (b)

Fig. 7.9 (a) Infection in a stump presenting as pain, erythema and oedema. (b) After 1 month on antibiotics, the erythema, oedema, and pain have resolved and the patient can wear his prosthesis again.

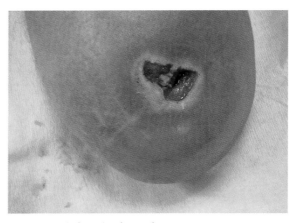

Fig. 7.10 An ischaemic, ulcerated stump.

Key points
- The diabetic foot team should be prepared to look after stumps as well as feet
- If the prosthesis is causing a problem it should be reviewed urgently by the rehabilitation team.

Ischaemia
Ischaemia can present as pain, often associated with erythema and a cold stump.

CASE STUDY
Ischaemic stump

An 84-year-old woman with type 2 diabetes of 18 years' duration underwent a below-knee amputation for extensive necrosis. She had severe cerebrovascular and cardiovascular disease and impaired renal function. She was referred to the diabetic foot clinic by the rehabilitation service as she was complaining of pain in the stump. On examination we found a cold pink stump with a painful ulcer along the old suture line (Fig. 7.10). Transcutaneous oxymetry was 15 mmHg, indicating severe ischaemia. She was seen by the vascular surgeons, and was treated conservatively with liberal analgesia and antibiotics. Her pain improved, and she died peacefully at home a few weeks later.

Key points
- Ischaemia may continue to worsen in the proximal leg after amputation and can lead to rest pain, ulceration and gangrene
- Transcutaneous oxymetry is a useful tool for assessing perfusion in the stump
- Patients attending the diabetic foot clinic may develop problems with their amputated stump and thus the multidisciplinary team should be aware of the complications that can develop and be able to commence appropriate treatment in conjunction with the local limb-fitting service.

Figure 7.11a,b shows the stump of an ischaemic below-knee amputation that has become painful and very red, and shows early signs of blistering. This was due to increasingly severe arterial disease and the patient was converted from a below-knee to an above-knee amputation.

Care of the remaining limb

After amputation, the value of the remaining limb should not be underestimated: even if the patient never walks again he will need his leg to transfer from chair to bed and lavatory, and thus maintain a little independence. It is extremely important that the patient is followed up in a multidisciplinary diabetic foot clinic. The remaining limb will need intensive prophylactic care and early treatment of ulceration and aggressive management of infection. Furthermore the development of ulceration with worsening ischaemia demands urgent vascular investigations and intervention. Intensive care of the contralateral limb has resulted in an improved outlook for this limb.

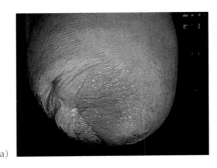

(a)

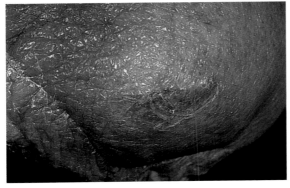

(b)

Fig. 7.11 (a) A painful red ischaemic stump. (b) Close-up view shows early signs of blistering. The patient went from a below-knee amputation to an above-knee amputation.

CASE STUDY
Gangrenous heel

A 78-year-old man with type 2 diabetes of 9 years' duration and peripheral vascular disease treated with left distal bypass presented late with infection of the left foot which resulted in overwhelming necrosis. He was ill and toxic and underwent an above-knee amputation of his necrotic left leg. Four days later a blister was noted on his right heel, which became infected and necrotic. He was given antibiotics to control infection. The necrosis dried out and became well demarcated from surrounding tissue. He underwent angiography and distal bypass to the right leg. A pressure-relieving ankle–foot orthosis (PRAFO) was issued. The foot healed in 6 months.

Key points
- Heel protection is essential for diabetic patients during the perioperative and postoperative period
- Dry necrosis of the heel can be treated by gentle debridement and does not necessarily need operative surgical debridement
- There should be close liaison between the diabetic foot service and the rehabilitation team

- The remaining foot will be at risk of overloading, and should be carefully protected during the perioperative and postoperative period. The remaining foot also needs careful attention.

Diabetic amputees should:
- Not attempt to cut their own toe nails
- Check the foot and stump every day
- Report problems immediately
- See a podiatrist regularly.

Rehabilitation physiotherapists, prosthetists, orthotists and ward staff must understand the need to avoid trauma to the remaining foot at all costs. Major amputees are among the most high-risk of all diabetic foot patients. Even with optimal foot care, foot problems occur in many major amputees, and unless they are detected early and aggressively treated by a multidisciplinary team, the outlook will be very poor.

Living with an amputation

Patients who have undergone a major amputation face the major frustrations of losing independence and being wheelchair bound. Practical help and information should always be available. Very simple advice can help with day-to-day activities, such as drink holders and trays which clamp to wheelchairs, cordless telephones and self-propelled wheelchairs if vision and manual control are adequate. Some of our amputated patients use electric wheelchairs and buggies very successfully, and one patient uses a small four-wheel drive vehicle to get into the countryside and covers very rough ground. Compact folding wheelchairs enable patients to get out by car. Manual or automatic controls for cars can enable patients to drive. Ramps and disabled lavatories foster independence.

It is important for health-care professionals to promote patient independence as far as possible. Major amputees in wheelchairs should not be moved without their permission, but should be encouraged to decide where they go and what happens to them wherever possible.

It is distressing for patients not to be offered a prosthetic limb and they may feel that it is because they have been written off, or that they do not have long to live.

CASE STUDY
Amputation for uncontrolled pain and coming to terms with limitations

An 83-year-old woman with type 2 diabetes of 14 years' duration with a previous history of stroke, who was already wheelchair bound, presented with ischaemic ulceration and severe rest pain (Fig. 7.12). She had had

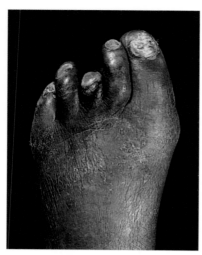

Fig. 7.12 Ischaemic ulceration in a foot with severe rest pain, which led to above-knee amputation.

transfemoral angiography and this had shown severe infrapopliteal disease with no recognizable main artery below the knee. Furthermore the arterial circulation of the foot was extremely poor with no plantar arch present. Neither angioplasty nor bypass was possible. She did not want an amputation and her ischaemic ulceration was treated conservatively. However, despite opiate analgesia it was not possible to control her pain and for this reason she underwent above-knee amputation.

Postoperatively, she was happy that she no longer had pain, and she was rehabilitated to return to her wheelchair lifestyle. She attended the diabetic foot clinic for care of the remaining foot. Three months later we noticed that she was depressed and she confided that she would have liked to have tried a prosthesis. The physiotherapists agreed to see her in the rehabilitation gym, and to let her try a pneumatic postamputation walking aid (PPAM aid) and discuss having a cosmetic prosthesis. After two sessions she came to terms with the fact that a prosthesis would not help her and declined further treatment. However, she said that she felt much happier because, as she told us, 'I was allowed to try instead of being written off'.

Key points
- Uncontrolled rest pain in the presence of unreconstructable arterial disease is an important reason for a major amputation
- Patients may resent not being offered the chance to try a prosthesis

- Help and advice on all aspects of living with an amputation are available from national organizations such as the Disabled Living Foundation in the UK and the Amputee Coalition of America.

Leaving hospital

When the time comes for the patient to leave hospital the following should be addressed:
- A wheelchair should be provided
- Wheelchair accessible accommodation should be available
- Patient is able to transfer
- Patient is managing his own programme of exercises
- Patient is medically stable
- Follow-up care has been organized.

Ideally the patient should be capable of:
- Putting on and taking off the prosthesis independently
- Walking with the prosthesis
- Moving up and down stairs
- Walking outside
- Getting on and off the floor independently.

Phantom limb, phantom pain and residual pain

Phantom limb is sensation felt at the amputated site which is not painful. Phantom pain is pain felt at the amputated site. Residual pain is stump pain felt at the site of the surgical incision.

Pain felt when wearing a prosthesis could be due to:
- Socket fitting problems
- Inappropriate prosthetic device
- Low pain threshold
- Pressure sores.

Postamputation pain is more likely if the patient has been in pain for a long time before the amputation.

Management
Treatment of phantom limb pain includes:
- Percussion therapy
- Transcutaneous electrical nerve stimulation
- Drug therapy—tricyclic antidepressants
- Ultrasound.

The aftermath of amputation: advice to health-care professionals

When catastrophes happen and patients lose a leg because of diabetic foot complications, then a storm of strong emotions, including fear and anger, is often aroused in patients and their relatives. They may seek a scapegoat—someone to blame for the amputation—as if apportioning guilt makes them feel safer because they can then deny that a similar disaster could happen to the remaining leg. Unfortunately, it is often the last person who saw or treated the foot who is blamed for the catastrophe, and the sins they are accused of may be sins of commission or sins of omission.

When patients die after an amputation, their grieving relatives may similarly look for someone to blame. If patients and practitioners do not know each other well and treatments are not explained, problems of communication are more likely to develop.

Because diabetic feet can go wrong with alarming rapidity and the triggering factors may not always be clear, practitioners are very vulnerable to criticism. We recommend the following precautions:

- Wherever possible, practitioners should not attempt to treat high-risk diabetic foot patients in isolation
- Full and careful record keeping is mandatory
- When things are going badly, patients and their families should be forewarned.

Podiatrists are particularly vulnerable to false accusations because they often work alone and patients may not understand their scope of practice. Reasons for callus removal, cutting back nails and ulcer debridement should be explained clearly. Unproven therapies should be approached with caution.

Follow-up of the patient with diabetes having had a major amputation

The long-term mortality from cardiovascular events is extremely high in these patients and many patients develop congestive cardiac failure, which needs aggressive management. Many of these patients have nephropathy, including some with end-stage renal failure who are on dialysis making them prone to peripheral oedema and electrolyte imbalance which need close attention. Cardiovascular risk factors also need marked consideration.

PRACTICE POINTS

- The main indications for amputation are severe uncontrolled pain, or major tissue deficit secondary to ischaemia or infection
- Amputees need heel protection during the perioperative and postoperative periods.

Physiotherapists, prosthetists and all members of the rehabilitation team should be aware of the vulnerability of the remaining foot:

- The stump of the diabetic amputated limb is susceptible to trauma, ulceration, infection and ischaemia, which demand urgent assessment and management
- Long-term mortality from cardiovascular events is extremely high in these patients and cardiovascular risk factors should be aggressively treated.

FURTHER READING

Adler AI, Ahroni JH, Boyko EJ, Smith DG. Lower-extremity amputation in diabetes. The independent effects of peripheral vascular disease, sensory neuropathy and foot ulcers. *Diabetes Care* 1999; **22**: 1029–35.

Anderson SP. Dysvascular amputees: what can we expect? *J Prosthet Orthot* 1995; **7**: 43–50.

Condie DN, Bowers R. Amputations and disarticulations within the foot; prosthetic management. In Smith DG, Michael JW, Bowker JH (eds). *Atlas of Amputations and Limb Deficiencies: Surgical, Prosthetic and Rehabilitation Principles.* American Academy of Orthopaedic Surgeons, Rosement, USA, 2004.

Carrington AL, Abbott CA, Griffiths J et al. A foot care program for diabetic unilateral lower-limb amputees. *Diabetes Care.* 2001; **24**: 216–21.

Cochrane H, Orsi K, Reilly P. Lower limb amputation, Part 3: Prosthetics—a 10-year literature review. *Prosthet Orthot Int* 2001; **25**: 21–8.

Davis BL, Kuznicki J, Praveen SS, Sferra JJ. Lower-extremity amputations in patients with diabetes: pre- and post-surgical decisions related to successful rehabilitation. *Diabetes Metab Res Rev* 2004; **20** Suppl 1: S45–50.

Dupre JC, Dechamps E, Pillu M, Despeyroux L. The fitting of amputated and nonamputated diabetic feet. A French experience at the Villiers-Saint-Denis Hospital. *J Am Podiatr Med Assoc* 2003; **93**: 221–8.

Ebskov LB. Relative mortality in lower limb amputees with diabetes mellitus. *Prosthet Orthot Int* 1996; **20**: 147–52.

Eneroth M. Factors affecting wound healing after major amputation for vascular disease. *Prosthet Orthot Int* 1999; **23**: 195–208.

Faglia E, Clerici G, Clerissi J. Early and five-year amputation and survival rate of diabetic patients with critical limb ischemia: data of a cohort study of 564 patients. *Eur J Vasc Endovasc Surg* 2006; **32**: 484–9.

Faglia E, Clerici G, Mantero M et al. Incidence of critical limb ischemia and amputation outcome in contralateral limb in diabetic patients hospitalized for unilateral critical limb ischemia during 1999–2003 and followed-up until 2005. *Diabetes Res Clin Pract* 2007 Feb 20. [Epub ahead of print.]

Gauthier-Gagnon C, Grise M-C, Potvin D. Predisposing factors related to prosthetic use by people with transtibial and transfemoral amputation. *J Prosthet Orthot* 1998; **10**: 99–109.

The Global Lower Extremity Amputation Study Group. Epidemiology of lower extremity amputation in centres in Europe, North America and East Asia. *Br J Surg* 2000; **87**: 328–37.

Ham R, Cotton L. *Limb Amputation—From Aetiology to Rehabilitation*. Chapman and Hall, London, UK, 1992, pp. 103–29.

Harness N, Pinzur MS. Health related quality of life in patients with dysvascular transtibial amputation. *Clin Orthop Relat Res* 2001; **383**: 204–7.

Hayden S, Evans R, McPoil TG *et al.* The effect of four prosthetic feet on reducing plantar pressures in diabetic amputees. *J Prosthet Orthot* 2000; **12**: 92–6.

Hazelgrove JF, Rogers PD. Phantom limb pain—a complication of lower extremity wound management. *Int J Low Extrem Wounds* 2002; **1**: 112–24.

Izumi Y, Satterfield K, Lee S, Harkless LB. Risk of reamputation in diabetic patients stratified by limb and level of amputation: a 10-year observation. *Diabetes Care* 2006; **29**: 566–70.

Kanade RV, van Deursen RW, Price P, Harding K. Risk of plantar ulceration in diabetic patients with single-leg amputation. *Clin Biomech* (Bristol, Avon) 2006; **21**: 306–13.

Levy SW. Stump skin problems of the amputee and the prosthetist. *Orthopädie-Technik Q* 2001; **11**: 5–7.

New JP, McDowell. D, Young RJ. Problem of amputations in patients with newly diagnosed diabetes mellitus. *Diabetic Medicine* 1998; **15**: 760–4.

Ng EK, Berbrayer MD, Hunter GA. Transtibial amputation: preoperative vascular assessment and functional outcome. *J Prosthet Orthot* 1996; **8**: 123–9.

Pecoraro RE, Reiber GE, Burgess EM. Pathways to diabetic limb amputation. Basis for prevention. *Diabetes Care* 1990; **13**: 513–21.

Reiber GE. Epidemiology of foot ulcers and amputations in the diabetic foot. In Bowker JH, Pfeifer MA (eds). *Levin and O'Neal's The Diabetic Foot*. Mosby, St Louis, USA, 2001, pp. 13–32.

Ripley DL, Ericksen JJ, Huang ME. Diabetes mellitus and functional outcome following amputation. *Arch Phys Med Rehabil* 1999; **80**: 1141.

Satterfield K. Amputation considerations and energy expenditures in the diabetic patient. *Clin Podiatr Med Surg* 2003; **20**: 793–801.

Schofield CJ, Libby G, Brennan GM *et al.* Mortality and hospitalization in patients after amputation: a comparison between patients with and without diabetes. *Diabetes Care* 2006; **29**: 2252–6.

Schoonmaker L. Rehabilitation and prosthetic intervention. Prosthetic pathways in managing the dysvascular patient. *J Prosthet Orthot* 1998; **10**: 82–4.

Smith DG. Amputation. Preoperative assessment and lower extremity surgical techniques. *Foot Ankle Clin* 2001; **6**: 271–96.

Snyder RD, Powers CM, Fontaine C, Perry J. The effect of five prosthetic feet on the gait and loading of the sound limb in dysvascular below-knee amputees. *J Rehabil Res Dev* 1995; **32**: 309–15.

Tentolouris N, Al-Sabbagh S, Walker MG *et al.* Mortality in diabetic and nondiabetic patients after amputations performed from 1990 to 1995: a 5-year follow-up study. *Diabetes Care* 2004; **27**: 1598–604.

Van Houtum WH, Lavery LA, Armstrong DG. Risk factors for above-knee amputations in diabetes mellitus. *South Med J* 1998; **91**: 643–8.

Van Ross ERE, Carlsson T. Rehabilitation of the amputee with diabetes. In Boulton AJM, Cavanagh PR, Rayman G (eds). *The Foot in Diabetes*, 4th edn. John Wiley & Sons Ltd, Chichester, UK, 2006, pp. 323–35.

Van Ross ERE. After amputation—rehabilitation of the diabetic amputee. *J Am Podiatr Med Assoc* 1997; **87**: 332–5.

Weaver FM, Burdi MD, Pinzur MS. Outpatient foot care: correlation to amputation level. *Foot Ankle Int* 1994; **15**: 498–501.

Surgical approach to the diabetic foot

For the love of God, a surgeon! Send one presently.
(Twelfth Night, *V, i, William Shakespeare*)

INTRODUCTION

In the second edition of this volume, developments in the surgery of the diabetic foot have been revisited, and in particular the surgical reconstruction of the Charcot foot is discussed.

The discovery and commercial production of insulin in the early 1920s were seminal developments in the treatment of diabetes that allowed people affected by this disease to live an almost normal life. Although insulin commuted the death sentence attributed to diabetes, it was soon recognized that it was not a cure. As people affected by this disease lived longer, they began to experience serious complications including blindness, kidney failure, heart disease, stroke and amputations. In 1934, the American diabetes specialist Elliott P. Joslin remarked that following the introduction of insulin, mortality from diabetic coma had fallen significantly from 60% to 5%. Yet deaths from diabetic gangrene had risen significantly. Joslin alleged that the reason for this complication was that physicians were not aggressive enough in their treatment of diabetes. He firmly believed that gangrene and amputations were preventable.

Diabetic gangrene is preventable in the overwhelming majority of cases . . . Hopefulness in the treatment of gangrene is possible. It comes first of all from the knowledge that the majority of the cases are needless and occur in those patients who have not been trained in the care of their feet or who have not followed training . . . prompt treatment of the infection might have prevented the gangrene.
(*Elliott P. Joslin, MD, The menace of diabetic gangrene*, N Engl J Med, *1934*)

He noted that there was almost always a history of injury to the foot that preceded the development of gangrene and led to amputation. He observed that burns and shoes were responsible for the most common injuries. Joslin's remedy was a team approach to diabetes care that emphasized patient education in foot care, dietary therapy, exercise, prompt treatment of foot infections and specialized surgical care. Joslin stressed the importance of cleanliness, daily foot inspection for early signs of trouble and preventive foot care. These recommendations are just as relevant today and are the foundation of diabetes foot care and self-management education.

Surgical management of the diabetic foot plays an integral role in the prevention and management of limb-threatening complications for people with diabetes. The objective of this chapter is to provide clinicians with a comprehensive and practical discussion of surgical management, as part of a team approach to care for patients with diabetes. It should be understood at the outset that early intervention provides the best chance of surgical cure and limb salvage. The goal is to preserve a functional plantigrade foot, and to prevent major amputation. In the words of the Roman poet Ovid, 'Stop it at the start: it's late for medicine to be prepared when disease has grown strong through long delays' (Ovid, 43BCE–18CE, *Remedia Amoris*, line 91).

For the purpose of this discussion, surgery of the diabetic foot will be stratified into three broad categories including:
- Elective surgical procedures
- Prophylactic surgical procedures
- Emergent (emergency) surgical procedures.

Elective surgical procedures

Elective surgery includes procedures that are advantageous to the patient but not urgent. For example, correction of

A Practical Manual of Diabetic Foot Care, 2nd edition, Edmonds, Foster and Sanders.
Published 2008 Blackwell Publishing. ISBN 978-1-4051-61473

a painful bunion or hammer toe in a stage 1 patient (with protective pain sensation, adequate perfusion and well-controlled diabetes) is considered elective. Yet, surgical correction of these same deformities is considered prophylactic surgery when the patient is neuropathic or neuro-ischaemic and the condition places the foot at risk for ulceration, infection and amputation. The patient's risk of developing a foot ulcer, as well as the patient's healing potential (vascular status), will determine whether a procedure is advisable or not. An important caveat is that patients must have adequate distal perfusion for surgical wounds to heal.

Elective surgery for the well-controlled, low-risk diabetic at stage 1 should be considered the same as for any other healthy patient. The surgical procedures as well as their risks and benefits are essentially the same. A discussion of these procedures is beyond the scope of this chapter, and the reader is referred to standard texts on foot surgery. Instead, the focus of this chapter is on prophylactic and emergent surgical procedures performed on the high-risk diabetic foot.

Prophylactic surgical procedures

Prophylactic surgery includes procedures which are necessary to prevent further compromise of the foot: for example, a patient with chronic recurrent ulceration beneath the hallux, who has a limitation of motion at the 1st metatarsophalangeal joint. The pathomechanical aetiology of this lesion, in an insensate patient, is hallux limitus or rigidus. Unless this condition is corrected the ulcer will never be completely resolved. Another example is the patient with a stable Charcot foot, with residual deformity, that cannot be accommodated by a shoe or brace. The deformity presents a serious and predictable risk for breakdown of the skin. We know that if this condition is not corrected, that shear stress and vertical forces on the skin will result in ulceration. Chronic, recurrent ulceration, with infection, will ultimately result in extension of the infection to bone (osteomyelitis), and amputation. Although these conditions are not immediately limb threatening, their natural history reveals that it is more likely than not that they will eventually become emergent conditions.

Emergent surgical procedures

Emergent surgery includes conditions that require immediate surgical intervention. These patients generally present to the Emergency Room/Casualty department with serious foot infections. It is important to emphasize that signs of systemic toxicity are not always present and clinical findings may be subtle. Patients may or may not be febrile and may or may not have an elevated white blood cell count; however, their diabetes is most often out of control. These patients require immediate hospitalization and work-up for infection and surgery. Depending upon the presentation, surgical treatment may include: incision and drainage of pus, exploration of wounds, debridement of necrotic soft tissue and bone, revascularization and local amputation of the foot. The urgency and aggressiveness of surgical care is determined by the nature of the presentation and by the clinician's familiarity with the diabetic foot. Limb-threatening conditions in seriously ill patients require immediate medical and surgical triage.

PRINCIPLES OF SURGICAL MANAGEMENT

A team approach to the medical care of patients with diabetes is necessary for successful surgical management. Prior to surgical intervention, patients require thorough preoperative medical assessment and aggressive management of their diabetes and comorbid conditions. Prompt attention must be directed to cardiovascular, renal, peripheral vascular and infectious disease issues. There is also a need to assess the patient's nutritional status and requirements for help from the dietitian. Wounds will not heal without adequate nutrition, nor will they heal with insufficient distal perfusion. Clinicians should be well trained to recognize emergency diabetic foot problems, and to distinguish immediately between limb-threatening and non-limb-threatening presentations. Successful surgical intervention demands timely drainage of infection and debridement of necrotic, bacteria-laden tissues. The risk of tissue loss and amputation is increased with inadequate antibiotic coverage and long delays in providing surgical care. It is important to emphasize that antibiotics alone are not sufficient for the management of most diabetic foot infections. Infected wounds must be incised and dependent drainage established. Postoperatively, patients must be followed closely with lifetime surveillance in the diabetic foot clinic. Appropriate footwear and preventive services are required.

Principles of surgical management include:

- Prompt detection and intervention
- Preoperative medical work-up and clearance for surgery

- Medical management of diabetes and comorbid conditions
- Targeted antibiotic coverage of infection
- Vascular work-up
- Consultations:
  Foot and ankle surgeon
  Infectious disease specialist
  Vascular surgeon
  Diabetologist
  Prosthetist/orthotist
  Physiotherapist
- Wound care and dressings
- Postsurgical surveillance
- Podiatric care, footwear and orthoses.

GOALS OF DIABETIC FOOT SURGERY

- Establish dependent drainage
- Remove bacteria-laden necrotic soft tissues
- Remove infected/necrotic bone
- Correct deformity
- Reduce risk of ulceration or amputation
- Restore stability and alignment
- Preserve function
- Achieve a cosmetically acceptable result
- Prevent major amputation of the leg.

SURGICAL PROCEDURES

Incision and drainage

Incision and drainage is the basic tenet of treatment for nearly all infections of the diabetic foot. Streptococcal cellulitis is an exception to this rule. Initial drainage of an abscess can be performed in the emergency department or at the bedside, under local field block or regional ankle block anaesthesia (Fig. 8.1a,b). Drainage means opening up all collections of pus (abscesses), with gentle probing of the superficial and deep tissues for sinus tracts. If present, sinus tracts need to be laid open. Bacteria-laden necrotic tissues are debrided and dependent drainage is established. Sometimes amputation of a toe(s) or ray(s) may be necessary to establish drainage; however, this is best done in the operating theatre. In severe limb-threatening situations, guillotine amputation of the foot may be necessary to stem systemic toxicity. It is important to emphasize that medical treatment of infection, solely with antibiotics, is insufficient to resolve the majority of diabetic foot infections. In the simplest and most common scenario, surgical debridement of ulcers is the main-

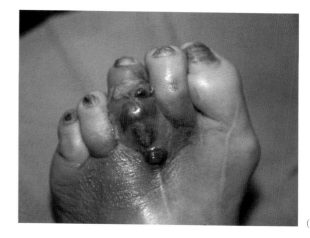

(a)

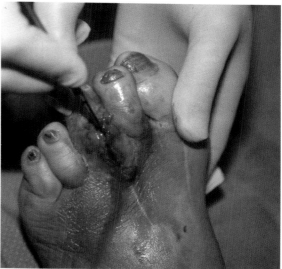

(b)

Fig. 8.1 (a) Abscess on 3rd toe with cellulitis, left foot. (b) Incision and drainage of the abscess, at the bedside.

stay of treatment. Salvage of the diabetic foot may require aggressive debridement and revascularization.

Gas in the soft tissues is a serious finding requiring an immediate trip to the operating theatre for open drainage of all infected spaces, and intravenous broad-spectrum antibiotics. This presentation is characterized clinically by crepitus, a crackling sensation noted on palpation of the affected soft tissues. This finding is confirmed on radiographic examination of the foot. Gas formation by infecting bacteria is common in diabetic foot infections, and is caused by both clostridial and non-clostridial organisms.

One or more incisions may be necessary. Whenever possible, incisions should be directed longitudinally on the foot, so as to avoid the neurovascular structures. It is important to inspect the foot for involvement of the deep compartments, as well as to look for infection that tracks along fascial planes and tendon sheaths. Several trips to the operating theatre may be required. It is incumbent upon the surgeon to plan the incisions with regard to foot function and ultimate surgical repair.

CASE STUDY
Infection

A 53-year-old man with a history of schizophrenia, poorly controlled type 2 diabetes of 9 years' duration and a dense peripheral neuropathy with sensory loss extending above the ankle, had developed his own unique method for sensory testing. He used a lit cigarette to establish the level of sensory loss on his lower legs and had several circular scars and burns in various stages of healing. He was followed for routine care in the diabetic foot clinic, for treatment of an intractable plantar keratosis beneath his right 5th metatarsal head. Having missed his last scheduled appointment, the patient finally returned to clinic with the chief complaint of pain in his right foot that had started 2 weeks before.

Physical examination revealed swelling, cellulitis and increased skin temperature of the forefoot with an abscess overlying the 5th metatarsophalangeal joint (Fig. 8.2a). Inspection of the plantar aspect of the foot revealed a thick callus, with haemorrhage, beneath the 5th metatarsal head. The 5th toe appeared blueish-black. Laboratory studies revealed an elevated white blood cell (WBC) count of 17,000/µL, and elevated fasting serum glucose 203 mg/dL (11.3 mmol/L). Radiographic evaluation revealed subluxation of the 5th metatarsophalangeal joint. The patient was admitted to the hospital for surgical management and intravenous antibiotics. At the bedside, the abscess was incised and drained, revealing a purulent-sanguineous discharge (Fig. 8.2b). Using a sterile probe, the dorsal wound was found to communicate with the plantar aspect of the joint, and exited through the bottom of the foot. Wound cultures revealed a single organism, *Staphylococcus aureus*, sensitive to penicillinase-resistant penicillins. Five days following hospital admission, the patient's WBC count was 12,600/µL, dry gangrene had clearly demarcated at the base of the 5th toe, and the cellulitis and swelling had subsided. Fifth ray amputation was advised; however, the patient did not immediately consent to surgery. The surgical management will be continued

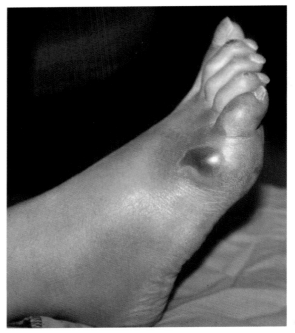

(a)

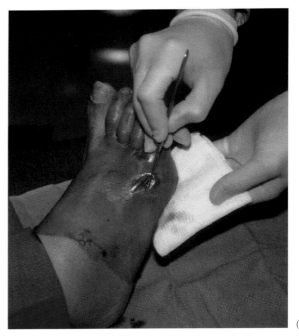

(b)

Fig. 8.2 (a) Abscess with cellulitis, right foot. Tense bulla overlying the 5th metatarsophalangeal joint. (b) Incision and drainage, at the bedside.

later in the section covering amputations and 5th ray resections.

CASE STUDY
Limb-threatening deep plantar space infection

A 69-year-old Afro-American man with type 2 diabetes of 22 years' duration and peripheral vascular disease, presented to the diabetic foot clinic with a limb-threatening deep plantar space infection of his left foot. Physical examination revealed an erythematous, swollen foot with fluctuance in the medial arch. There was a full-thickness ulcer noted beneath the 1st metatarsal head, with pus present in the wound. The ulcer probed to bone. He was febrile with an elevated WBC count and elevated serum glucose 400 mg/dL (22.2 mmol/L). The patient was admitted to hospital, and preoperative laboratory testing, chest X-ray, electrocardiogram and medical consultation were obtained. Empiric intravenous antibiotic therapy was initiated and the patient was taken to the operating theatre the same evening for extensive incision and drainage of his foot. The incision extended from the 1st metatarsal head to his ankle (Fig. 8.3).

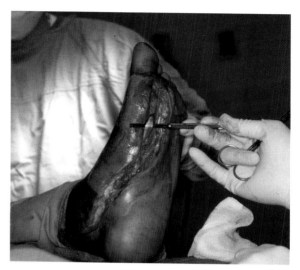

Fig. 8.3 Deep plantar space infection, left foot. Incision and drainage performed in the operating room. The flexor hallucis longus tendon is visible in the wound.

CASE STUDY
Complicated (severe) wound infection accompanied by systemic toxicity and metabolic instability

An unemployed 56-year-old Afro-American man with type 1 diabetes of 13 years' duration had a past medical history remarkable for polysubstance abuse, hepatitis C, dysthymic disorder as well as diabetic peripheral sensory neuropathy. He presented to the Emergency department with a chief complaint of intermittent fevers, chills and pain in his left foot (pain scale 9/10). The condition of his foot began 3 weeks earlier with ulceration at the site of a callus on the bottom of his big toe and on the ball of his foot. The ulcers became infected 2 weeks prior to his presentation and he began to experience increased pain in his foot within the last week. He was febrile, 103.2 °F (39.6°C) and tachycardic at 106/minute. Blood pressure was 138/93 mmHg. Examination of the left foot revealed a full-thickness ulcer beneath the hallux with purulent, foul-smelling, brownish-red drainage (Fig. 8.4a). A second full-thickness ulcer was present beneath the second metatarsal head. The ulcers did not probe to bone. The left foot and ankle were oedematous with cellulitis extending to the medial arch and on to the dorsum of the foot. Palpation of the arch resulted in increased drainage

from the wound. The foot was hot. Pedal pulses were palpable. Radiographs revealed gas in the soft tissues along the medial side of the foot. Laboratory studies revealed a markedly elevated WBC count 20,300/μL with 92.4% granulocytes, erythrocyte sedimentation rate was 37 mm/h, and serum glucose was 373 mg/dL (20.7 mmol/L). Blood and wound cultures were performed and the patient was admitted directly to the Acute Medicine Service. The patient was empirically started on IV ampicillin/sulbactam. Podiatric surgical consultation was requested and the patient was taken to the operating room the following morning for amputation of his great toe, incision and drainage, and wound debridement (Fig. 8.4b). Surgery was performed under regional ankle block anesthesia with monitored anesthesia care. On the morning of surgery the patient's WBC count had increased to 23,800/μL with 64% granulocytes. Blood culture was positive for viridans streptococci (alpha haemolytic). Wound cultures were positive for viridans streptococci, *Streptococcus* group G (beta haemolytic), methicillin-sensitive *Staphylococcus aureus* and *Escherichia coli*. On the day following surgery the patient's WBC count decreased to 11,300/μL. Within the next few days his blood sugars normalized. The patient was taken back to the operating room for wound debridement and revision of his surgical wound.

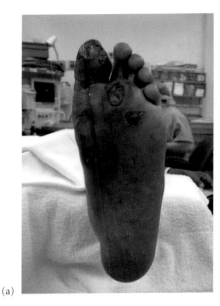

(a)

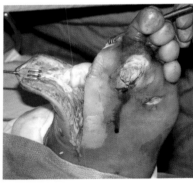

(b)

Fig. 8.4 (a) Severe wound infection in left foot accompanied by systemic toxicity and metabolic instability. Pus is seen exuding from the hallux. (b) Intraoperative photograph following amputation of the hallux, incision and drainage, and wound debridement. Infection tracked along the long flexor tendon into the medial plantar space. The first metatarsal head is visible in the wound.

Key points

- Seek prompt surgical consultation.
  The mainstay of therapy for moderate to severe diabetic foot infections is *timely and aggressive surgical intervention*, including incision and drainage, debridement of infected or necrotic tissues and limited resections of bone or amputations. This approach may diminish the need for more extensive amputation of the foot or leg

- Determine severity of the infection and select an empirical antibiotic regimen based on the severity and likely aetiological agents. Initial antibiotic therapy should be broad, providing coverage for aerobic gram-positive cocci, gram-negative rods and anaerobes. Therapy should be targeted to culture and susceptibility results
- Stabilize the patient prior to transfer to the operating room
- Ensure that blood glucose levels are adequately controlled.

Hammer toe correction

Patients with diabetes often develop one or more digital contractures. Flexion contracture of the toes develops as a result of biomechanical imbalance between the long flexor and extensor tendons to the toe. The intrinsic muscles of the foot, the interossei and lumbricales, function to stabilize the toes on the weightbearing surface. Weakness of these muscles, secondary to motor neuropathy, results in the development of hammer toes and, in some cases, claw toes.

Hammer toe

A hammer toe is characterized by hyperextension of the toe at the metatarsophalangeal joint, and flexion contracture of the toe at the proximal interphalangeal joint. The resulting deformity, like a swan's neck, results in retrograde force on the metatarsal head, causing increased plantar pressure, metatarsalgia, callus formation and eventually ulceration. Friction and pressure caused by the shoe on a prominent proximal interphalangeal joint results in the development of a corn and, eventually, an ulcer. Pressure at the tip of the flexed toe may result in a distal corn and eventually an ulcer (Fig. 8.5a).

Claw toes

Claw toes are characterized by flexion contracture at both the proximal interphalangeal joint and distal interphalangeal joint. Claw toes are often associated with cavus (high arched) feet (Fig. 8.5b).

Mallet toe

Mallet toe is a digital deformity characterized by flexion at the distal joint. Risk of ulceration is associated with each of these three digital deformities, at the tips of the toes and over the prominent interphalangeal joints.

Surgical correction of digital deformities may be indicated in high-risk patients with loss of protective sensation. Surgical intervention becomes a more pressing issue once the patient has developed ulceration and/or

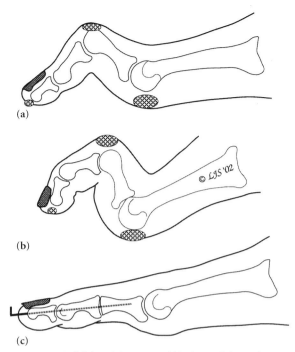

Fig. 8.5 Digital deformities. Areas of friction and elevated pressure are identified beneath the metatarsal head, over the prominent proximal interphalangeal joint, and at the tip of the toe. (a) Hammer toe. (b) Claw toe. (c) Surgical correction of hammer toe deformity with proximal interphalangeal joint arthroplasty and internal fixation with a Kirschner wire.

infection. Chronic, recurrent plantar ulceration beneath a metatarsal head may require correction of the digital deformity to relieve pressure beneath the metatarsal head (Fig. 8.5c).

Proximal interphalangeal joint arthroplasty

Proximal interphalangeal joint arthroplasty is indicated for correction of rigidly contracted hammer toes with or without ulceration at the tip of the toe, or over the prominent proximal interphalangeal joint (Fig. 8.6a).

Technique

The procedure is performed in the operating theatre under local anaesthesia and sedation, with an ankle tourniquet for haemostasis. If an ulcer or corn is present over the proximal interphalangeal joint, it is excised, using two converging semi-elliptical incisions. The incisions are carried down to the subcutaneous tissue and the

ulcer is excised. The extensor tendon is exposed (Fig. 8.6b) and transected at the level of the interphalangeal joint. The tendon is retracted proximally, exposing the head and neck of the proximal phalanx. The medial and lateral collateral ligaments are freed using a Beaver No. 64 mini-blade or scalpel with a No. 15 blade. The head of the proximal phalanx is then transected at the surgical neck using double action bone-cutting forceps or a power saw (Fig. 8.6c). The bone is examined for evidence of osteomyelitis which, if present, would dictate removal of additional bone. The extensor tendon is then repaired with absorbable sutures at the level of the proximal interphalangeal joint. If there is evidence of extension of the toe at the metatarsophalangeal joint, then the extensor tendon can be lengthened or transected, followed by a dorsal transverse metatarsophalangeal capsulotomy. A McGlamry elevator is helpful to release adhesions of the plantar structures. If the metatarsophalangeal joint contracture has not been corrected, then partial metatarsal head resection may be required. In the presence of infection the wound should be packed open, with a return to the operating theatre for delayed primary closure within a week. For clean wounds, the skin is closed with 5–0 nylon simple interrupted sutures (Fig. 8.6d). The use of a 0.45 Kirschner wire, placed across the joint, is optional. When used to maintain the corrected position of the toe, the wire is placed in a retrograde fashion, from the proximal interphalangeal joint, out through the tip of the toe. It is then driven back into the proximal phalanx. It is wise to reserve the use of internal fixation for clean, elective cases.

Dressings and postoperative care

Dressings consist of non-adherent fine mesh gauze (petrolatum, 3% Xeroform or Adaptic) and a dry sterile gauze bandage with the toe splinted in its corrected position. A surgical shoe is dispensed and the patient is able to ambulate as tolerated. The first postoperative dressing change is within 1 week. Sutures are removed in 10–14 days, and if a Kirschner wire was used it is removed at 3 weeks. The patient is able to return to a roomy shoe with a broad toe box after 3–6 weeks, as oedema resolves.

CASE STUDY
Rigid hammer toe deformity

A 64-year-old man, a retired pilot, with type 2 diabetes of 16 years' duration, was followed regularly in the diabetic foot clinic for treatment of a rigid hammer toe deformity of his right 2nd toe, with recurrent ulceration over the proximal interphalangeal joint. The patient underwent an

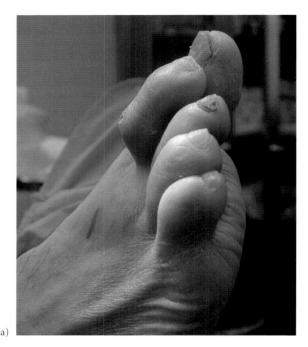

(a)

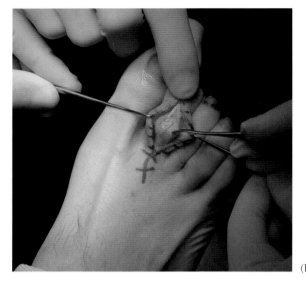

(b)

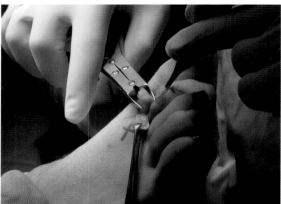

(c)

(d)

Fig. 8.6 Surgical correction of hammer toe deformity.
(a) Preoperative appearance of a rigid hammer toe, 2nd toe, right foot. Notice the very prominent deformity at the proximal interphalangeal joint. (b) The extensor digitorum longus tendon and joint capsule are identified overlying the proximal interphalangeal joint. (c) Removal of the head of the proximal phalanx with double action bone-cutting forceps.
(d) Immediate postoperative appearance.

elective proximal interphalangeal joint arthroplasty, with lengthening of the extensor hallucis longus tendon and dorsal capsulotomy of the metatarsophalangeal joint. A Kirschner wire was not used in this case, and the toe was splinted in its corrected alignment. The postoperative course was uncomplicated.

Mallet toe correction—distal interphalangeal joint arthroplasty

Mallet toe correction is indicated for lesions that develop at the tip of the toe. In the presence of mallet toe deformity the tip of the toe is traumatized with every step that the patient takes. The initial lesion is a callus, which eventually progresses to a preulcerative lesion (haemorrhage within the callus) and then to a full thickness ulcer that may probe to bone.

Technique

The procedure is performed in the operating theatre under local anaesthesia, with a Penrose drain applied as a tourniquet at the base of the toe. No tourniquet is used if there is a question of vascular compromise. Two semi-elliptical incisions are made in a transverse manner over the distal interphalangeal joint of the toe. The incisions are carried down through the skin, the extensor tendon and joint capsule, and these structures are removed. The interphalangeal joint is identified and the collateral ligaments are severed using a Beaver No. 64 mini-blade. The blade is kept close to bone at all times. The distal aspect of the middle phalanx is transected with a power saw or with bone-cutting forceps. It may be necessary to release the long flexor tendon, and this can be done through the same dorsal incision. The deformity is reduced and the dorsal capsule and skin are repaired in the usual fashion. In the absence of ulceration or infection, the corrected position of the toe is maintained by placing a 0.45 Kirschner wire across the joint in a retrograde manner, as described for hammer toe correction.

Dressings and postoperative care

Same as for hammer toe correction.

Hallux limitus/rigidus with plantar ulceration of the hallux

Limited joint mobility of the 1st metatarsophalangeal joint, with decreased range of dorsiflexion, results in elevated plantar pressure beneath the hallux. Repetitive moderate stress on the skin is observed clinically by the formation of a callus beneath (or plantar medial to) the hallux interphalangeal joint (Fig. 8.7). Haemorrhage within the callus represents a preulcerative condition that requires regular debridement and footwear modification. The natural history for hallux interphalangeal joint lesions is for the preulcerative condition to progress to a full-thickness ulcer and eventually to amputation. Correlation between elevated plantar pressure and a lesion beneath the hallux can be demonstrated qualitatively using a Harris footprint mat, or quantified using an electronic gait platform or in-shoe measuring device. Location of the peak plantar pressure corresponds with the location of the callus or ulcer. All too often, the initial

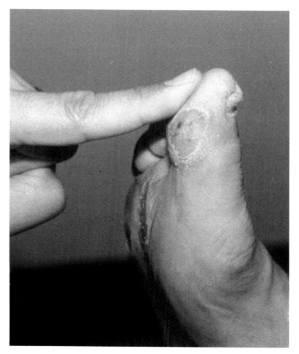

Fig. 8.7 Hallux limitus. There is a callus with preulcerative changes on the plantar medial aspect of the great toe.

treatment for this condition focuses on the wound and totally ignores the pathomechanical aetiology of the ulcer. Although local wound care and off-loading of the foot may result in healing of the ulcer, this outcome is short-lived. The ulcer inevitably recurs and becomes a chronic non-healing wound. The obvious risk, for a diabetic patient, is wound infection, extension of infection to bone and eventual amputation of the hallux.

Surgical treatment for hallux interphalangeal joint ulcers is directed at increasing the dorsiflexory range of motion of the hallux. Some authors advocate hallux interphalangeal joint arthroplasty and report an overall success rate of 91%, with only minor complications. Most authors, however, advocate a procedure to increase dorsiflectory range of motion at the level of the 1st metatarsophalangeal joint. Keller arthroplasty is the procedure most often cited for surgical correction of recalcitrant interphalangeal joint ulceration of the hallux in adults. Downs reported successful results of this procedure in a series of patients ranging in age from 30 to 65 years. Postoperatively, all ulcers healed promptly with no recurrence at follow-up after 2–5 years. Dannels reported similar results in a series of Native American Indians with diabetes, with an age range of 39–58 years.

Keller resectional arthroplasty of the 1st metatarsophalangeal joint

Technique

This procedure can be performed under regional ankle block anaesthesia, with an ankle tourniquet. A dorsal longitudinal incision is made over the 1st metatarsophalangeal joint just medial to the extensor hallucis longus tendon. The incision starts at the neck of the proximal phalanx and extends ~2 cm proximal to the metatarsal head. Skin hooks are used to retract the skin edges, small bleeders are clamped and electrocoagulated, and the incision is then carried deep through the capsule down to bone. Subperiosteal dissection is carried out over the proximal phalanx. The joint capsule is reflected, allowing direct visualization of the metatarsophalangeal joint. The collateral ligaments are cut using a Beaver No. 64 mini-blade or No. 15 blade and the proximal one-quarter to one-third of the proximal phalanx is transected, perpendicular to the long axis of the phalanx, with a power saw (Fig. 8.8,

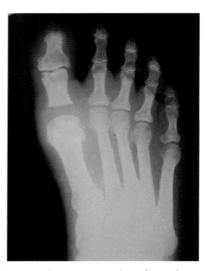

Fig. 8.9 Postoperative anteroposterior radiograph reveals resection of the proximal one-third of the phalangeal base of the hallux.

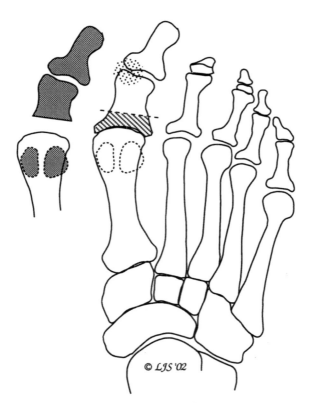

Fig. 8.8 Keller resectional arthroplasty of the 1st metatarsophalangeal joint, before and after removal of the proximal one-third of the base of the proximal phalanx.

Fig. 8.9). The most difficult part of this procedure is removing the phalangeal base. The bone is grasped with a bone clamp and the intrinsic muscle attachments, for the flexor hallucis brevis and the adductor hallucis, are carefully freed using a Beaver No. 64 mini-blade. Care must be taken to avoid cutting the flexor hallucis longus tendon. The wound is irrigated with normal sterile saline and a piece of Gelfoam sponge (haemostatic absorbable gelatin) is placed in the void created by removal of the phalangeal base. The joint capsule is closed with 3–0 absorbable sutures in a simple interrupted fashion. If possible, the capsule should be purse stringed, interposing soft tissue between the metatarsal head and the phalangeal base. The skin is closed with a 4–0 absorbable suture in a running subcuticular fashion and Steri-Strips are placed across the incision. The use of one or two Kirschner wires to maintain the hallux position is at the surgeon's discretion. I have not found it necessary to use Kirschner wires, and prefer splinting, with early passive range of motion exercises to maintain hallux dorsiflexion.

Dressings and postoperative care

Dressings consist of non-adherent fine mesh gauze (petrolatum, 3% Xeroform or Adaptic), and a fluffy dry sterile compression gauze bandage, with the hallux splinted in its corrected position. A surgical shoe is dispensed. The patient is instructed to rest at home, remain non-weightbearing and to elevate his feet for 48 hours. He is then allowed partial weightbearing in a surgical shoe with crutches or a walker. The first postoperative dressing change is within 1 week. Dressings are changed weekly for 3–4 weeks postoperatively. Sutures are removed in 14–21 days, and the patient is allowed to return to a roomy shoe with a broad toe box in 3–6 weeks.

Advantages
- Performed under local anaesthesia with minimal risk
- Minimally debilitating
- Increases range of motion at the metatarsophalangeal joint
- Decompresses the hallux interphalangeal joint ulcer and allows for rapid healing
- Patients may begin protected weightbearing immediately.

Disadvantages
- Reduction in plantar flexion strength of the great toe
- Loss of toe purchase
- Weakness during the toe-off phase of gait
- Shortening of the great toe.

Complications
- Postoperative infection
- Development of lesser metatarsalgia
- Cock-up deformity of the hallux
- Digital fracture(s)
- Charcot's osteoarthropathy (rarely).

CASE STUDY
Hallux limitus

A 46-year-old man with type 2 diabetes of 12 years' duration, documented peripheral neuropathy with loss of protective sensation and history of a chronic non-healing ulcer on the plantar medial aspect of his right hallux interphalangeal joint, had limited joint mobility in the 1st metatarsophalangeal joint, with approximately 10° of hallux dorsiflexion (Fig. 8.10). Quantitative plantar pressure measurements revealed markedly elevated peak plantar pressure, 95 N/cm^2, beneath the great toe (Fig. 8.11). The maximum peak pressure corresponded to the precise location of his ulcer. Radiographs revealed no evidence of osteomyelitis. Conservative treatment consisted of local wound care, total-contact casting, a walking brace and extra-depth shoes with total-contact orthoses. Over a period of several months the ulcer showed some improvement with off-loading; however, it never completely healed. The ulcer became infected on two occasions with *Staphylococcus aureus*. The infections resolved promptly with oral antibiotics.

It became clear that the ulcer would not heal without surgical intervention, and that the patient was at high risk for future infections and amputation of his hallux. Keller resectional arthroplasty of the 1st metatarsophalangeal

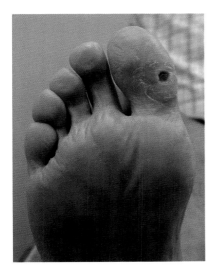

Fig. 8.10 A 46-year-old man with hallux limitus and a chronic ulcer beneath the hallux interphalangeal joint, right foot.

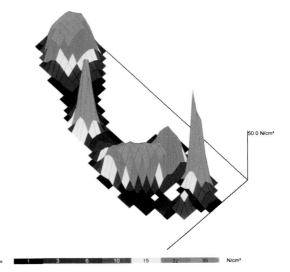

Fig. 8.11 EMED three-dimensional display of peak plantar pressures beneath the right foot. The peak pressure beneath the hallux was 95 N/cm^2.

joint was proposed as a salvage procedure and the patient consented. Within 4 weeks following the procedure, the hallux ulcer was completely healed. A complication occurred on postoperative day 18, with development of pain and swelling at the base of the right 2nd toe. The patient indicated that his foot began to hurt as he was walking to his car. X-rays revealed a non-displaced fracture of the proximal phalangeal base of the 2nd toe. The 2nd and 3rd toes were splinted, the patient was placed in a walking brace, and the foot healed without further complications.

Sesamoidectomy

Sesamoidectomy is indicated for the treatment of a discrete intractable lesion, beneath the 1st metatarsal head, that fails to heal or remain healed with a conservative approach to treatment (local wound care, total-contact casting or attempts to off-load the forefoot with orthoses and custom footwear). Sesamoidectomy is also indicated for the curative treatment of osteomyelitis of the sesamoid bone. This procedure is appropriate for the treatment of neuropathic patients with evidence of increased plantar pressure beneath the 1st metatarsal head. Weightbearing radiographs taken with a radio-opaque open circle marker placed over the ulcer will confirm the relationship between an enlarged or arthritic sesamoid bone and the plantar lesion. There may also be evidence of a plantar flexed 1st metatarsal associated with a cavus foot deformity. Excision of the tibial sesamoid, fibular sesamoid or both sesamoids may be indicated.

Technique

Surgical approach to the tibial sesamoid can be either medial or plantar. A low medial longitudinal incision is centred over the 1st metatarsophalangeal joint between the dorsal and plantar cutaneous nerves to the hallux. This incision is deepened to the level of the joint capsule and the capsule is incised in the same plane. The tibial (medial) sesamoid is visualized within the joint capsule beneath the metatarsal head. The capsule is grasped with a clamp and the sesamoid is shelled out with a Beaver No. 64 mini-blade or No. 15 scalpel blade. The fibular (lateral) sesamoid is more difficult to reach through a medial incision, and may be more accessible from a dorsal longitudinal approach, over the first webspace. This is a reasonable approach if the sesamoid is located in the intermetatarsal space.

A plantar approach is indicated for excision of the ulcer, and allows for direct visualization of both sesamoid bones.

Dressings and postoperative care

The decision to close the wound primarily or to pack it open will vary with each case. Infected or contaminated wounds should be packed open, and either allowed to heal by secondary intention or brought back to the operating theatre for delayed wound closure. Dressings consist of a dry sterile compression gauze bandage with the hallux splinted in its proper alignment. The patient is instructed to rest at home, remain non-weightbearing and elevate his feet for 48 hours. If the wound was packed open, the dressing is changed on the first or second postoperative day. If possible, arrangements should be made for a visiting nurse to perform the necessary daily dressing changes. The patient is then allowed limited protected weightbearing in a walking brace. The first postoperative visit is scheduled within 1 week with weekly visits scheduled until the wound is healed. Once healed, the patient will require therapeutic shoes and insoles.

Advantages
- The procedure is performed under local anaesthesia with minimal risk
- Surgical simplicity
- Low morbidity.

Disadvantages
- Possibility of developing a hallux hammer toe or hallux abducto valgus deformity.

Complications
- Infection, wound dehiscence and hallux hammer toe.

CASE STUDY
Removal of sesamoids

A 69-year-old man with type 2 diabetes of 22 years' duration and peripheral neuropathy had a history of chronic full-thickness ulceration beneath his left 1st metatarsal head. The ulcer did not probe to bone (Fig. 8.12). Radiographs revealed a hypertrophic tibial sesamoid (Fig. 8.13). Conservative treatment was employed for 4 months with no improvement in his condition. The patient was offered the option of surgical treatment and he consented. In this case, the plantar ulcer was excised and both medial and lateral sesamoids were removed (Fig. 8.14a,b). The wound was packed open and allowed to heal by secondary intention.

Lesser metatarsal osteotomy

Dorsiflexory metatarsal osteotomies are performed for the treatment of lesser metatarsalgia, most often for

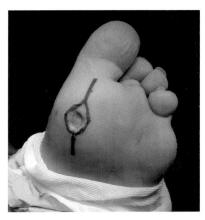

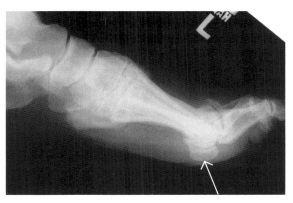

Fig. 8.12 Preoperative appearance of a chronic ulcer beneath the tibial (medial) sesamoid, left foot.

Fig. 8.13 Lateral radiograph of the left foot, reveals a hypertrophic tibial sesamoid. The ulcer was located beneath the sesamoid.

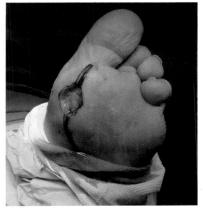

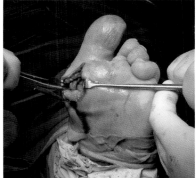

Fig. 8.14 Sesamoidectomy. (a) Intraoperative photograph, the ulcer has been excised. (b) The hypertrophic tibial (medial) sesamoid has been grasped with a bone clamp and is being removed from the wound.

(a)

(b)

intractable plantar keratoses (IPKs), when non-surgical methods have failed. These procedures are controversial and are often plagued by postoperative complications such as transfer lesions, non-union or malunion, and floating toes. Infection and screw failure have also been reported. Caution should be exercised when considering these procedures for neuropathic individuals. Metatarsal osteotomy is not advised in the presence of infection or full-thickness ulceration beneath the metatarsal head.

Fig. 8.15 illustrates a chronic IPK with preulcerative haemorrhage within the callus and a long 2nd metatarsal. This is an appropriate indication for lesser metatarsal osteotomy. Multiple lesser metatarsal osteotomies have been described to include transverse, oblique and closing wedge procedures. Two of the more popular distal procedures are the vertical chevron metatarsal osteotomy and the Weil shortening osteotomy. Both procedures require internal fixation.

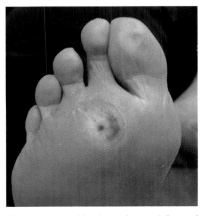

Fig. 8.15 Chronic intractable plantar keratosis beneath the 2nd metatarsal head. The callus has been debrided, revealing preulcerative haemorrhage within the skin. This is an indication for lesser metatarsal osteotomy.

The Weil osteotomy

The Weil shortening osteotomy is a distal lesser metatarsal procedure, designed to shorten one or more of the central metatarsals (2nd, 3rd and sometimes the 4th) without elevating or depressing the metatarsal head. The head moves proximal to the existing plantar callus, and decompresses the metatarsophalangeal joint. The procedure should be reserved for cases that fail conservative treatment, and only used in cases where the affected metatarsals are comparatively long. Complications are similar to those associated with other metatarsal osteotomies.

Technique

The procedure is performed in the operating theatre under local anaesthesia with an ankle tourniquet. A dorsal longitudinal incision is made over the metatarsophalangeal joint and then deepened to the joint capsule. The capsule is dissected between the extensor digitorum longus and the extensor digitorum brevis. The capsule is reflected, allowing for release of the collateral ligaments. Two small Hohmann retractors are inserted under the metatarsal neck to provide sufficient exposure to the metatarsal head. The toe is plantar flexed and the osteotomy is performed with a long, thin sagittal saw blade. The osteotomy cut begins at the distal dorsal edge of the articular cartilage and is directed proximally, oblique to the metatarsal shaft, and as parallel as possible to the sole of the foot. The distal fragment is displaced proximally, 3–5 mm, and fixed with a single self-drilling, self-tapping partially threaded 2.0 mm screw. The screw is directed from dorsal-proximal to plantar-distal. The bone peak is then resected with a rongeur and smoothed with a burr (Fig. 8.16a–c). The joint capsule is closed with 3–0 absorbable (Dexon or Vicryl) sutures and the skin is closed with 4–0 absorbable subcuticular sutures, or nylon simple interrupted sutures.

Dressings and postoperative care

Standard dressings are utilized. The patient is allowed to ambulate with crutches and partial weightbearing, in a surgical shoe. Sutures are removed in 10–14 days and patients can return to their normal footwear in 2–4 weeks, as dictated by the clinical course.

Advantages

- Simple and reliable procedure
- Stability of the osteotomy with a large area of bone to bone contact
- Pressure relief beneath the metatarsal head
- Helpful for reduction of dorsally dislocated metatarsophalangeal joints

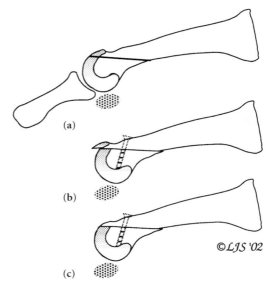

Fig. 8.16 The Weil lesser metatarsal shortening osteotomy. (a) The lesser toe is plantarflexed, and the oblique osteotomy cut begins at the distal dorsal edge of the articular cartilage. (b) Proximal displacement of the metatarsal head, approximately 3–5 mm. Note that the head of the metatarsal is now proximal to the plantar callus. Fixation is with a single 2.0 mm screw. (c) Resection and smoothing of the bone peak.

- Pressure relief beneath the metatarsal head
- Early return to weightbearing.

Complications

- Transfer lesions
- Recurrent symptomatic plantar keratosis
- Infection
- Floating and stiff toes.

Metatarsal head resection

Resection of a single metatarsal head is indicated for one of the following reasons, when non-surgical methods fail to achieve the desired result:

- For removal of infected bone, in the case of chronic osteomyelitis
- For decompression of a plantar ulcer, as an alternative to metatarsal osteotomy, to facilitate wound healing
- For deformity of the 5th metatarsal with painful callus on the plantar or lateral aspect of the metatarsal head.

Resection of the metatarsal head can be performed through a dorsal incision over the metatarsophalangeal joint, or in the presence of a deep plantar ulcer, the ulcer

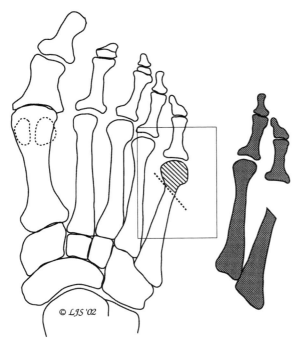

Fig. 8.17 Technique for 5th metatarsal head resection. Before and after removal of the metatarsal head. Note that the osteotomy is angled in an oblique manner at the surgical neck of the metatarsal.

and the metatarsal head can both be excised through a plantar approach.

Fifth metatarsal head resection (Fig. 8.17)

This procedure is well suited for older sedentary individuals, and for patients with osteopaenia or osteomyelitis of the metatarsal head, where a transpositional osteotomy is not appropriate. Although transfer lesions (callus or ulcer) have been reported to occur beneath adjacent metatarsal heads, following metatarsal head resections, this is not a frequent problem with 5th metatarsal head resections.

Technique

Fifth metatarsal head resection is performed under local anaesthesia with IV sedation. An ankle tourniquet is used for haemostasis. A 4 cm dorsal longitudinal incision is made over the 5th metatarsophalangeal joint and shaft, just lateral to the extensor digitorum longus tendon. The incision is carried down to fascia, the skin edges are retracted, and the incision is then continued through joint capsule and deep to the periosteum. The joint is visualized, collateral ligaments are cut with a Beaver mini-blade,

and the metatarsal is cut in an oblique manner, at the surgical neck, from distal-medial to proximal-lateral. The metatarsal head is removed, and the wound is irrigated. Gelfoam is placed in the void, and the capsule is closed with 3–0 absorbable sutures in a simple interrupted fashion. The skin is closed with 4–0 nylon sutures, in a simple interrupted and horizontal mattress fashion. Drains are generally not necessary.

Dressings and postoperative care

Dressings consist of non-adherent fine mesh gauze (petrolatum, 3% Xeroform or Adaptic), and a fluffy dry sterile compression gauze bandage. A surgical shoe is dispensed. The patient is instructed to rest at home, remain non-weightbearing and to elevate his feet for 48 hours. He is then allowed partial weightbearing in a surgical shoe with crutches or a walker. The first postoperative dressing change is scheduled within 1 week. Dressings are changed weekly for 3–4 weeks postoperatively. Sutures are removed in 14–21 days, and the patient is allowed to return to a roomy shoe with a broad toe box in 3–4 weeks.

Advantages

- Can be performed under local anaesthesia with minimal risk
- Simple procedure
- Can be used for osteomyelitis
- Can be closed primarily
- Rapid return to weightbearing
- Limited disability, and rapid recovery.

Disadvantages

- Possibility of a transfer lesion (callus or ulcer).

Complications

- Postoperative infection
- Delayed healing
- Regrowth of the transected metatarsal with recurrence of the lesion.

CASE STUDY
Fifth metatarsal head resection

An 80-year-old active man with peripheral neuropathy and loss of protective sensation presented to clinic with a prominent, painful tailor's bunion that could not be satisfactorily accommodated by footwear. The patient had a 5th metatarsal head resection performed 2 years earlier, for correction of a similar condition affecting his right

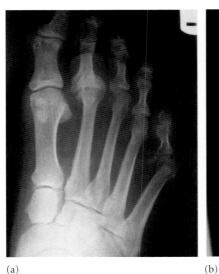
(a)

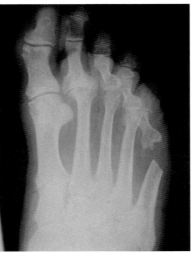
(b)

Fig. 8.18 (a) Preoperative anteroposterior radiograph reveals deformity of the right 5th metatarsophalangeal joint with lateral bowing and prominence of the 5th metatarsal head. (b) Postoperative anteroposterior radiograph reveals resection of the 5th metatarsal head.

foot. He was very satisfied with the results and returned for surgical correction of his left foot. The surgical procedure and postoperative course were uneventful. The surgical outcome was excellent (Fig. 8.18a,b).

Achilles tendon lengthening

Increased pressure on the plantar aspect of the forefoot has been shown to be associated with limited joint mobility and with equinus deformity of the ankle. In the presence of peripheral neuropathy, elevated pressure beneath one or more metatarsal heads can result in the development of ulceration. Ankle equinus may also contribute to the development of Charcot's osteoarthropathy with collapse of the mid-foot or avulsion fracture of the posterior process of the calcaneus. Armstrong and coworkers, at the University of Texas Health Science Centre at San Antonio, reported on a study to determine the degree to which pressure on the plantar aspect of the forefoot is reduced following percutaneous lengthening of the Achilles tendon in high-risk subjects with diabetes. They demonstrated that peak plantar forefoot pressures were reduced by approximately 27% following percutaneous Achilles tendon lengthening. These authors suggest that lengthening of the Achilles tendon, in high-risk patients with diabetes, may decrease the likelihood of ulceration and may increase the efficacy of pressure-reduction modalities such as casts or braces. In fact, this procedure facilitates the healing of recalcitrant forefoot plantar ulcers.

CASE STUDY
Percutaneous lengthening of Achilles tendon

A 55-year-old Afro-American man with poorly controlled type 2 diabetes ($HbA_{1c} = 10.6\%$) of 8 years' duration, and dense peripheral neuropathy was seen regularly in the diabetic foot clinic for treatment of a chronic non-healing full-thickness ulcer located beneath the 2nd and 3rd metatarsal heads of his left foot. The ulcer did not probe to bone. Treatment consisted of wound debridement, total-contact casting, walking brace and a variety of topical wound healing agents.

Diagnostic studies
- Serial X-rays were negative for osteomyelitis; however, they revealed a long 3rd metatarsal
- MRI was unremarkable
- Non-invasive vascular studies were normal with evidence of strong pedal pulses
- EMED plantar pressure measurements revealed markedly elevated peak plantar pressure, 117 N/cm^2, located beneath the 2nd to 3rd metatarsal heads, right foot
- Arthrometric evaluation revealed ankle joint dorsiflexion was $-6°$ with the knee extended, $-2°$ with the knee flexed on the right ankle.

The proposed treatment for this patient was a percutaneous lengthening of the right Achilles tendon, by triple hemisection, under local anaesthesia. The patient consented to this minimally invasive procedure. Within 3–4 weeks the plantar ulcer was completely healed and has remained healed for the past 3 years. Peak pressure at the site of ulcer was significantly reduced to 42 N/cm^2. The surgical technique is described below.

Percutaneous Achilles tendon lengthening—triple hemisection

Technique

This procedure is indicated for correction of mild to moderate gastrocnemius-soleus ankle equinus. Three hemisections of the tendon are performed, two medial and one lateral. The distance between the hemisections is determined by the overall size of the tendon and the amount of lengthening desired. An alternative procedure, attributed to Hoke, incorporates two posterior and one anterior hemisections of the Achilles tendon, and is performed in the frontal plane through a medial approach.

The patient is placed in a prone position on the operating room table. Local anaesthesia is infiltrated just above the Achilles tendon on the back of the leg. A tourniquet is not required for this procedure. The surgeon stands at the end of the operating table facing the foot, which hangs over the end of the table. The plantar surface of the foot is placed against the abdomen of the surgeon and gently dorsiflexed while palpating the Achilles tendon. A skin marker is used to define the borders of the tendon, from its insertion into the calcaneus, to its proximal myotendinous junction. The proposed cuts in the tendon are drawn on the skin, as shown in Fig. 8.19a. These marks help the surgeon to remember the direction of the cuts. The distal cut is made 1.0–2.5 cm superior to the tendon's insertion into the calcaneal tuberosity. A Beaver No. 64 mini-blade is introduced through the skin and tendon in a perpendicular manner, bisecting the tendon. The tendon is then lifted away from the leg, and the blade turned medially. Hemisection of the tendon is accomplished by gently working the blade against the tendon until its fibres are completely cut. When satisfactorily performed a gap can be palpated in the tendon. Avoid forcefully pushing the blade against the tendon as this may result in tenotomy, with rapid loss of resistance, followed by uncontrolled movement of the blade and subsequent laceration of the skin or the surgeon's finger. This procedure is repeated in the opposite direction, 2.5–4.0 cm more proximally, and then again 2.5–4.0 cm more proximal to the second cut. The foot is then firmly dorsiflexed to an angle greater than 90°, generally 5° above neutral (Fig. 8.19b). Overcorrection should be avoided, as this may lead to rupture of the tendon or a calcaneus deformity. The stab wounds are generally so small that they do not require sutures. However, if desired, a single interrupted 5–0 nylon suture can be used.

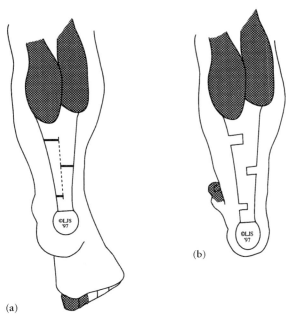

Fig. 8.19 (a) Percutaneous lengthening of the Achilles tendon—triple hemisection. Proposed cuts in tendon. From Sanders (1997) with permission from Elsevier Science. (b) Dorsiflexion of foot after triple hemisection.

Dressings and postoperative care

Dressings consist of non-adherent fine mesh gauze (petrolatum, 3% Xeroform or Adaptic), and dry sterile gauze dressing. A well-padded plaster splint is applied to immobilize the foot and ankle, and to maintain the ankle in approximately 5° of dorsiflexion. At the first dressing change, the patient is placed in either a short-leg walking cast or a walking brace for 6 weeks. The decision to cast or brace should be determined on an individual basis, based upon the surgeon's assessment of patient compliance.

Advantages

- Simple to perform
- Minimally invasive procedure
- Effective for relieving elevated forefoot plantar pressures.

Disadvantages

- Over lengthening of the tendon can result in a calcaneus gait.

Complications

- Tendon rupture
- Infection
- Development of a plantar heel ulcer

• In cases with moderate to severe shortening of the Achilles tendon, open lengthening of the tendon may be necessary.

Partial calcanectomy

Partial calcanectomy is indicated for the surgical management of large non-healing wounds located over the heel, with or without osteomyelitis. These wounds are typically chronic decubitus ulcers located on the posterior aspect of the heel, or neuropathic ulcers on the plantar surface of the heel. Regardless of the aetiology, heel ulcers are often unresponsive to conservative therapy and are frustrating to treat. Partial calcanectomy is a viable alternative to below-knee amputation for these patients, provided that they have adequate distal perfusion. The procedure eradicates infection and achieves wound closure and limb preservation. Patients who are ambulatory before surgery are generally able to resume the same level of function postoperatively. Smith and coworkers proposed the following preoperative criteria for performing a partial calcanectomy:
• Ankle–brachial index > 0.45
• Transcutaneous oxygen tension ($TcPo_2$) > 28 mmHg
• Serum albumin > 3.0 g/dL
• Total lymphocyte count of more than 1500.

Advantages
• Simple procedure
• Low morbidity
• Rapid convalescence
• Good functional results.

Disadvantages
• None. This is a salvage procedure.

Complications
• Infection
• Delayed healing
• Failure to heal.

CASE STUDY
Partial calcanectomy

A 59-year-old Caucasian man with type 2 diabetes of 7 years' duration and history of multiple foot surgeries for the treatment of infected neuropathic plantar ulcers underwent a successful transmetatarsal amputation of his right foot, 2 years earlier. He had recently been treated for a full-thickness ulcer beneath his 4th metatarsal head.

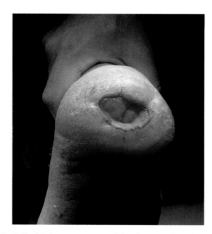

Fig. 8.20 Full-thickness neuropathic ulcer on the plantar aspect of the right heel, with osteomyelitis of the calcaneus.

This lesion was unresponsive to conservative care, and an Achilles tendon lengthening procedure was performed. The forefoot ulcer healed quickly following the tendon lengthening; however, the patient went on to rupture his tendon and developed a calcaneus gait. The result of elevated pressure beneath his heel was the development of a chronic full-thickness ulcer, approximately 3.0 × 2.0 cm (Fig. 8.20). Although the patient had adequate distal perfusion, the ulcer failed to heal with conservative therapy; total-contact casting, local wound care and antibiotics. Osteomyelitis was suspected. Partial calcanectomy, a salvage procedure, was offered to the patient as an alternative to below-knee amputation and he consented to the operation.

Technique
The procedure is performed under spinal anaesthesia using a thigh tourniquet for haemostasis. The patient is placed in a prone position on the operating theatre table. Two converging semi-elliptical incisions are made surrounding the ulcer. The incisions are carried deep to bone, and the ulcer is completely excised. The incision is extended proximally, to expose the posterior aspect of the calcaneus, and deepened to the fascia overlying the Achilles tendon (Fig. 8.21). A No. 15 blade is used to transect the tendon at its insertion on the posterior tubercle of the heel. The tendon is dissected free, grasped with an Allis clamp and reflected out of the wound. Dissection is then directed close to bone, exposing the body of the calcaneus. In the case cited above, the posterior aspect of the heel was resected, using a sagittal saw, in a plane entering the

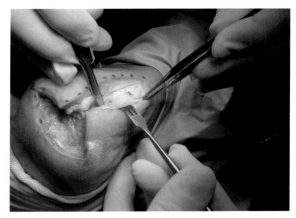

Fig. 8.21 The heel ulcer has been excised and the incision extends proximally over the Achilles tendon.

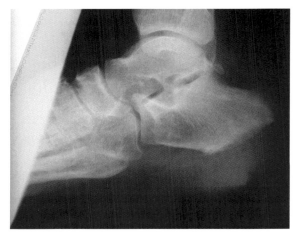

Fig. 8.22 Partial calcanectomy of the right foot. Postoperative lateral radiograph of the same patient shown in Figs 8.20 and 8.21.

posterior superior aspect of the calcaneus and exiting plantarly at the insertion of the plantar fascia. Inspection of the residual calcaneus revealed healthy cancellous bone. The wound was thoroughly irrigated using 2 L of normal sterile saline solution containing an antibiotic. Three drill holes were then made in the posterosuperior aspect of the calcaneus, for reattachment of the Achilles tendon, using 0 Ethibond non-absorbable sutures. A tube low suction (TLS) drain was inserted, exiting through the lateral aspect of the heel. The deep tissues were closed with 2–0 absorbable sutures. The skin was closed using a combination of 3–0 nylon vertical and horizontal mattress sutures, and simple interrupted sutures. (*Caution*—infected wounds should be packed open and allowed to heal by secondary intention, or brought back to the operating theatre for delayed wound closure.) Figure 8.22 is the postoperative lateral radiograph, which reveals the amount of bone that was removed.

Dressings and postoperative care

Dressings consist of non-adherent fine mesh gauze (petrolatum, 3% Xeroform or Adaptic), placed on the suture line, a bulky gauze fluff dressing and additional padding for protection of the heel and lateral border of the foot. Dressings are held in place by gauze bandage. A well-padded plaster splint is applied to immobilize the foot and ankle. Drains are generally removed after 48 hours. Moderate bleeding from the cut cancellous bone is to be expected, especially over the first 12–24 hours, and dressings may need to be reinforced with additional absorbent material. After 7 days, a well-padded short-leg non-weightbearing cast is applied. The cast is changed at 2-week intervals for inspection of the wounds. Sutures are left in place for 3–4 weeks. Once the skin is healed, the patient is placed in a walking brace for 4 weeks and is then allowed to ambulate in a therapeutic shoe with an ankle–foot orthosis (AFO).

AMPUTATIONS OF THE FOOT

Amputations of the foot can be divided into emergent and non-emergent procedures. Non-emergency amputations allow some flexibility in the creation of skin flaps, selection of level and wound closure. These cases generally include neuropathic feet that are structurally or functionally impaired, with satisfactory circulation and controlled infection. They are characterized by moderate to severe forefoot deformities with associated chronic non-healing wounds that are recalcitrant to conservative medical and surgical management. In some cases, the presenting deformities are the residuals of prior infection, tissue necrosis and chronic non-healing wounds.

Emergent amputations include those performed for gangrene, severe soft tissue infection, osteomyelitis, peripheral vascular disease, tumours or trauma. The main consideration in determining the level of amputation in these cases is the extent of healthy tissue. When infection is the primary issue, an open or guillotine amputation may be necessary. In most cases, adequacy of blood supply to the foot ultimately determines the level at which successful amputation can be performed. Although non-invasive laboratory methods have been proposed for evaluating wound healing potential, clinical experience and judgement are most often relied upon.

Preoperative physical examination should include a quantitative assessment of ankle joint dorsiflexion. Contracture of the Achilles tendon is generally more apparent prior to amputation of the forefoot, and suggests the need for tendon lengthening at the time of amputation. The procedure is performed as necessary, in the presence of equinus or excessive spasticity. In many cases equinovarus deformity is a complication of Lisfranc and Chopart amputations. A longitudinal open procedure or percutaneous approach can be utilized according to the surgeon's preference.

Wound healing criteria for amputation surgery

Measurements of TcPo$_2$ are useful to accurately predict the presence of critical vascular disease and the success of major or minor amputations. TcPo$_2$ levels ≥ 30 mmHg bode well for healing of a forefoot amputation, and are more accurate predictors than a palpable pedal pulse. TcPo$_2$ levels < 30 mmHg indicate significant vascular disease and foreshadow wound healing failure and amputation. These patients require well-timed vascular surgery consultation, arteriography and revascularization.

Toe pressures, measured by photoplethysmography, are helpful to predict the healing potential of primary forefoot amputations. In a retrospective study of 136 amputations, Vitti and coworkers observed that healing occurred in all diabetics with preoperative toe pressures > 68 mmHg. Other preoperative criteria for wound healing include: an ankle–brachial index > 0.50, serum albumin > 3.0 g/dL, serum protein > 6.0 g/dL and total lymphocyte count > 1500. Patients should be medically stable, with diabetes and infection under control.

It is important to note that the preoperative wound healing criteria listed above are only guidelines. The most important factors are individualized patient assessment and clinical experience.

Selection of anaesthesia

Amputations at the level of the forefoot or mid-foot can be performed safely under regional ankle block anaesthesia, or if desired under spinal or epidural anaesthesia. In a series of consecutive transmetatarsal or midfoot amputations performed by the author, an ankle block was administered in 83% of the cases. Patients receiving regional ankle block anaesthesia with intravenous

sedation tolerate surgery well, with minimal anaesthesia risk.

Digital amputations

Digital amputation is indicated in the presence of fixed digital deformity, osteomyelitis, septic arthritis or recurrent ulcers over the interphalangeal joint or distal aspect of the toe. Neuroischaemic patients may present with severe necrotic ulceration of the distal third of the toe. In yet another scenario, patients undergoing invasive cardiovascular procedures may develop a shower of cholesterol emboli to their toes, with resultant gangrenous changes involving the tips of their toes.

A common clinical scenario is the neuropathic patient, with a hammer toe deformity, who presents with a superficial ulcer over the proximal interphalangeal joint of the 2nd or 3rd toe. This may have started as a 'simple' corn. Local wound care is initiated; however, the ulcer is refractory to treatment. The toe becomes infected, very swollen (sausage-like), and shortly thereafter the head of the proximal phalanx is visible in the wound. There is little recourse but to amputate the entire toe.

In some cases, when the lesion is limited to the distal portion of the toe, a terminal amputation can be performed at the distal joint. Amputation of a single lesser toe generally causes very little disability. However, amputation of the great toe with its metatarsal head alters weightbearing and increases the vulnerability of the remaining toes.

When performing digital amputations the surgeon can be creative with skin closure. Medial and lateral skin flaps are most often employed because they protect the neurovascular structures on either side of the toe. However, dorsal and plantar flaps are also acceptable. The length of the flaps can also vary, with one flap being longer than the other. This is an important consideration for wound closure, when there has been skin loss due to infection or necrosis.

Partial digital amputation of the hallux

Distal amputation of the hallux, sometimes referred to as a terminal Syme's amputation, is indicated for lesions of the distal toe or nail bed, e.g. osteomyelitis of the distal phalangeal tuft, ulceration of the nail bed or tumour. The procedure employs either resection of the tuft of the distal phalanx or disarticulation of the toe at the interphalangeal joint. This procedure preserves acceptable length and function of the hallux. A similar surgical approach can be modified for the lesser toes.

Technique

The procedure for amputation through the hallux inter-phalangeal joint is performed in the operating theatre under local anaesthesia and sedation, with a Penrose drain applied as a tourniquet around the base of the great toe. A long plantar and short dorsal skin flap is fashioned. The transverse dorsal skin incision is made, proximal to the posterior nail fold, at the level of the interphalangeal joint. The incision extends from medial to lateral and is then directed distally around the end of the toe, to form a long plantar flap. The toe is disarticulated at the interpha-langeal joint and all tissues are excised (nail plate, nail bed, nail matrix and distal phalanx). A long plantar flap is fash-ioned (trimmed to fit), and sutured without tension to the short dorsal flap with 4–0 nylon simple interrupted sutures. If the toe is infected at the time of surgery, the wound should be left open or very loosely approximated. The patient can then be brought back to the operating theatre for delayed wound closure when the infection is resolved.

Dressings and postoperative care

Dressings consist of non-adherent fine mesh gauze (petrolatum, 3% Xeroform or Adaptic), and a fluffy dry sterile compression gauze bandage. A surgical shoe is dis-pensed. The patient is instructed to rest at home, remain non-weightbearing and to elevate his feet for 48 hours. He is then allowed partial weightbearing in a surgical shoe with crutches or a walker. The first postoperative dressing change is scheduled within 1 week. Dressings are changed weekly for 3–4 weeks postoperatively. Sutures are removed

in 14–21 days, and the patient is allowed to return to his regular footwear as soon as the operative site is completely healed and swelling has subsided.

Amputation of the lesser toes can be performed by a transphalangeal approach or by disarticulating the toe at the metatarsophalangeal joint. Some authors have sug-gested leaving a 'button' of proximal phalanx intact over the metatarsal head. However, there is a need for caution. The residual portion of the proximal phalanx can cause discomfort and become a future site of ulceration. I have found that transphalangeal amputations often result in dorsiflexion of the residual phalangeal stump, with irrita-tion of the skin over the prominent bone. For this reason I disarticulate the toe at the metatarsophalangeal joint.

Hallux amputation (Fig. 8.23a,b)

Amputation of the great toe invariably results in biome-chanical dysfunction of the foot. The degree to which this occurs depends upon whether or not a portion of the 1st metatarsal has also been removed. The loss of propulsive function is not detrimental to neuropathic patients who already have an apropulsive gait. Of greater concern, however, are the following postoperative sequelae:

- Compensatory flexion contracture of the 2nd toe
- Ulceration at the tip of the 2nd toe
- Lesser metatarsalgia
- Pathological fractures
- Ulceration beneath the 1st or 2nd metatarsal heads (Fig. 8.24).

These complications may eventually result in a more proximal amputation.

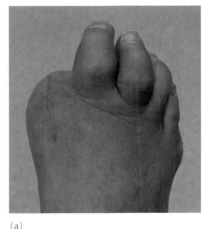
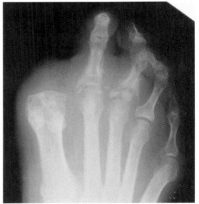

Fig. 8.23 Hallux amputation in a neuropathic patient. (a) Clinical appearance 5 months following disarticulation of the hallux at the metatarsophalangeal joint, with medial and lateral skin flaps for closure. There is moderate to severe swelling of the 2nd and 3rd toes. (b) Anteroposterior radiograph reveals pathological fractures of the proximal phalanges of the 2nd and 3rd toes.

(a)

(b)

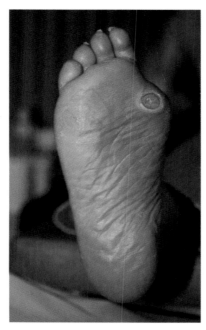

Fig. 8.24 A full-thickness neuropathic plantar ulcer developed beneath the 1st metatarsal, as a complication of amputation of the hallux with resection of the 1st metatarsal head.

Technique

Caution—amputation of the hallux is deceptively simple. Surgeons often find that, once the hallux is amputated, they are unable to close the surgical wound without removing the metatarsal head and a portion of the shaft. This will always occur when using a racquet incision encircling the base of the great toe. The dilemma is how to prevent this from happening. The approach, when feasible, should be to develop a long medial or lateral skin flap that will allow for closure over the disarticulated 1st metatarsal head.

Ray amputations

A ray resection consists of excision of a toe and its corresponding metatarsal. The most frequent complication of a ray resection is transfer ulceration. The overall success rate for ray amputations is low; however, there is reasonable success with resection of a central ray (2nd or 3rd), or 5th ray. Amputation of the hallux and 1st metatarsal frequently results in imbalance of the medial column of the foot with a poor functional outcome. Therefore, it is very important to preserve 1st metatarsal shaft length whenever possible.

Amputation of the 5th ray alone is indicated when infection and necrosis involve the 5th toe and/or the skin over the metatarsophalangeal joint. This can develop in neuroischaemic patients from unremitting pressure, caused by a tight shoe or bandage, over the lateral aspect of the 5th metatarsal head. In neuropathic individuals, repetitive moderate stress on the skin beneath a prominent 5th metatarsal head will eventually result in callus formation, ulceration and infection. The primary objective of this procedure is to achieve adequate resection of the infected or necrotic tissues, in order to create a wound that can be closed without tension. The configuration of the skin incision is determined by the extent of the infected necrotic tissues to be excised. Whenever possible, the 5th metatarsal base should be preserved together with its muscle attachments for the peroneus brevis and tertius. This is important for the prevention of varus deformity of the foot. Varus deformity occurs when inversion of the foot is left unopposed. Following ray resection, part or all of the incision may be left open, with the patient returning to the operating theatre for delayed primary closure. Ray resections are sometimes performed as an initial incision and drainage procedure to control infection prior to a more definitive amputation.

CASE STUDY
Ray resection to control infection with delayed primary closure

A 53-year-old man with poorly controlled type 2 diabetes of 9 years' duration was admitted to hospital with the provisional diagnosis of cellulitis of the right foot and infected abscess of the 5th metatarsophalangeal joint. Initial surgical treatment was incision and drainage of the abscess. Dry gangrene demarcated at the base of his 5th toe (Fig. 8.25). Although the patient initially refused

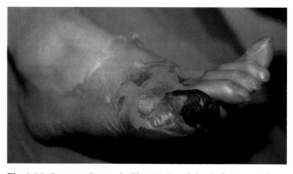

Fig. 8.25 Same patient as in Fig. 8.2. Resolving infection with dry gangrene demarcated at the base of the right 5th toe.

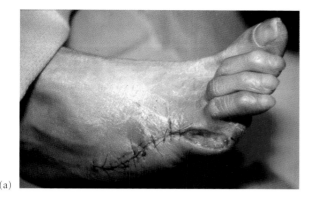

(a)

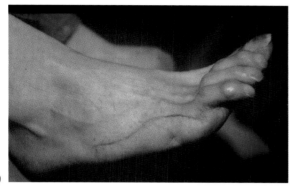

(b)

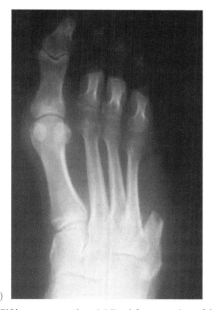

(c)

Fig. 8.26 Fifth ray amputation. (a) Partial amputation of the right 5th ray. The distal portion of the wound was left open. (b) Appearance of the right foot healed after delayed wound closure. (c) Anteroposterior radiograph reveals resection of the distal two-thirds of the 5th metatarsal.

further surgical treatment, he eventually changed his mind and consented to surgery. He was taken to the operating theatre where, under regional ankle block anaesthesia and sedation, his right 5th toe was amputated together with the distal two-thirds of the 5th metatarsal. The proximal portion of the wound was closed with 3–0 nylon simple interrupted sutures, and the distal portion was packed open. One week later, the patient returned to the operating room for delayed primary closure of the wound (Fig. 8.26a–c).

Technique

The 5th ray is amputated through a dorsolateral approach, with a racquet incision encircling the 5th toe. The toe is disarticulated at the metatarsophalangeal joint, and all necrotic tissues are excised. The incision is then extended proximally, in a curvilinear fashion over the 5th metatarsal shaft, to the level of the base. Dissection is kept close to the bone. The soft tissues are retracted using blunt Senn retractors. The exact amount of bone to be removed is determined, at the time of surgery, by how well the skin edges can be approximated without tension. Removing more bone may facilitate closure of the wound. The 5th metatarsal shaft is cut in an oblique manner, using a sagittal saw, from distal-medial to proximal-lateral. The reason for this angled cut is to avoid a bony prominence that could cause pressure on the skin. The wound is then thoroughly irrigated with normal sterile saline solution using a pulsed irrigation system. The decision to close the wound or to pack it open is based upon the appearance of the wound and the results of reliable wound cultures.

CASE STUDY
Transfer ulceration following 5th ray resection

A 55-year-old Caucasian man with type 2 diabetes of 5 years' duration and symptomatic peripheral sensory neuropathy with loss of protective sensation presented to the Emergency department with a 2-day history of intermittent fever chills and cellulitis of his left foot. He was admitted to the Acute Medicine Service, and was empirically started on intravenous ampicillin/sulbactam. Past medical history revealed a 2-year history of recurrent ulceration, infection and osteomyelitis of his left 5th metatarsal, for which he underwent partial 5th ray amputation approximately 1 year earlier at another hospital. The patient subsequently developed a callus beneath his 4th metatarsal head and this progressed to a blister and then to a full-thickness ulcer. He experienced recurrent bouts of ascending cellulitis of his foot and leg over the past 6 months. On admission the patient was afebrile, pulse 91, respiration 20, BP 169/94 mmHg. The patient weighed 142 kg and was 175 cm tall, his BMI was 43. Examination of the left foot revealed erythema of the foot with a forefoot varus deformity. There was a callus beneath the 4th metatarsal head and 'blister' overlying the lateral aspect of the 4th metatarsal head. Debridement revealed a full-thickness ulcer, 10 mm × 8 mm, which did not probe to bone. The base of the ulcer contained beefy red granulation tissue (Fig. 8.27a). A small amount of serosanguinous drainage was present. Debridement of the plantar callus revealed a second more superficial ulcer.

Wound culture was reported as *Staphylococcus aureus*, MRSA. Blood culture was negative. Radiographs (Fig. 8.27b) and MRI were negative for osteomyelitis. Local wound care, intravenous and oral antibiotics (trimethoprim-sulfamethoxazole), total-contact casts, removable cast walker, custom made footwear and orthotics resulted in improvement; however, the ulcers failed to heal completely. After 7 months of conservative management the veteran underwent a successful transmetatarsal amputation. The left foot remains well healed with no new ulcers or infections (Fig. 8.27c).

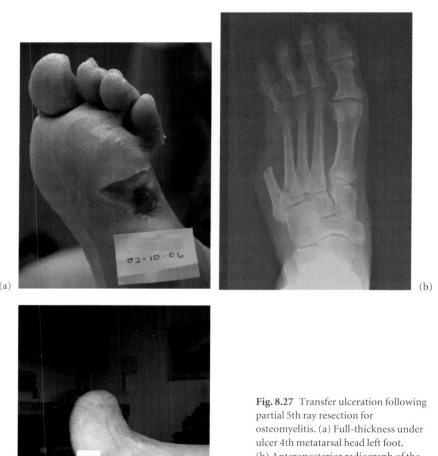

(a)

(b)

(c)

Fig. 8.27 Transfer ulceration following partial 5th ray resection for osteomyelitis. (a) Full-thickness under ulcer 4th metatarsal head left foot. (b) Anteroposterior radiograph of the left foot demonstrates partial amputation of the 5th ray. There is no evidence of osteomyelitis. (c) Conservative management failed to resolve the ulcer and after 7 months a successful transmetatarsal amputation was performed.

Key points
- The most frequent complication of ray resection is transfer ulceration
- Overall success rate of ray amputations is low
- Resection of more than one ray generally results in failure
- Evaluate the patient, the wound, the infection and foot structure
- Varus deformity of the forefoot contributes to increased pressure on the lateral border of the foot. In this case, we were unable to mitigate the pressure over a prominent 4th metatarsal head in a morbidly obese individual with peripheral sensory neuropathy.

Transmetatarsal and mid-foot amputations

Amputations through the forefoot and mid-foot include the transmetatarsal, Lisfranc and Chopart amputations. The Lisfranc amputation is performed at the tarsometatarsal joints and the Chopart amputation is performed at the mid-tarsal joints (Fig. 8.28). Mid-foot amputations frequently develop equinovarus deformity, which requires Achilles tendon lengthening or tenotomy. When preoperative criteria are met, healing occurs in > 80% of transmetatarsal and mid-foot amputations.

Transmetatarsal amputation
Indications
The indications and technique for performing a transmetatarsal amputation have changed very little since McKittrick and Warren initially described them in the 1940s and 1950s. They proposed three basic criteria, and I have added a fourth:
- Gangrene of one or more toes, without entering on to the foot
- Stabilized infection or open wound involving the distal portion of the foot
- An infected lesion in a neuropathic foot
- Moderate to severe forefoot deformity.
Careful preoperative preparation is necessary with drainage of infection, culture-directed antibiotics and daily wound care. Successful amputation requires attention to detail, careful planning of skin flaps, atraumatic operative technique and, whenever possible, primary closure of the wound. The use of an ankle or thigh tourniquet is desirable; however, this is at the discretion of the surgeon. Relative contraindications to the use of a tourniquet include ischaemia or recent lower extremity revascularization. A bloodless field enables the surgeon to work more efficiently and saves operating time. However, prior to closing the wound, the tourniquet must be released and all bleeders ligated or coagulated. Meticulous haemostasis is required to prevent blood loss and haematoma formation. If ankle equinus is noted, it should be corrected at the same time as the transmetatarsal amputation.

Technique
The patient is placed in a supine position with the foot and lower half of the leg prepped and draped in the usual manner. Bony landmarks are identified for the 1st and 5th metatarsal heads and bases. The desired level of bone resection is determined, e.g. mid-shaft level, and then using a skin marker a line is drawn across the dorsum of the foot from mid-shaft of the 1st metatarsal to mid-shaft of the 5th metatarsal. Lines are then extended distally, along the 1st and 5th metatarsal shafts, to the bases of the hallux and 5th toe, and then curved across the plantar skin just proximal to the sulcus of the toes. This approach will create a short dorsal and long plantar flap.

Starting anteromedially at the 1st metatarsal shaft, the knife is held perpendicular to the skin and an incision is made through the skin, across the dorsum of the foot, ending at the previously determined level on the 5th metatarsal shaft. The dorsal incision is deepened to expose the long extensor tendons. Vessels are identified, ligated or electrocoagulated. The incision is then carried down to bone. Prior to transection of the metatarsals, an osteotome or key elevator is directed distally away from the dorsal skin incision, to reflect the soft tissues and periosteum. The dorsal flap should not be undermined.

Incisions are then carried distally toward the toes and then across the plantar aspect of the foot, developing a

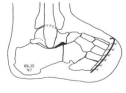
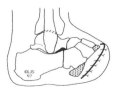
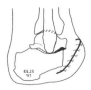

Fig. 8.28 Transmetatarsal and mid-foot amputations. Three levels of amputation. From Sanders (1997) with permission from Elsevier Science.

Transmetatarsal   Lisfranc   Chopart

long, thick myocutaneous flap. The plantar flap is re-tracted using rake retractors. It is important to keep the dissection close to the metatarsal shafts, thereby creating a thick viable plantar flap. The plantar flap is reflected proximally to the intended level of bone resection. The metatarsal bones are then cut transversely, with a power saw, at the level of the dorsal skin flap. The cuts are angled slightly from dorsal-distal to plantar-proximal. The 1st and 5th metatarsals are bevelled medially and laterally to prevent focal points of pressure. The distal foot is grasped securely with a small bone clamp, and then removed by sharp dissection.

The plantar flap is inspected, and debrided as neces-sary. Exposed flexor tendons should be grasped without tension and excised. Antibiotic solution is used to irrigate the wound. The plantar flap is then brought up over the resected metatarsals and approximated with the dorsal flap. If the plantar flap is too long, redundant skin should be remodelled. The flap should be carefully marked with a skin marker and excess skin removed. Accurate trimming of the skin is accomplished by placing several Allis tissue forceps on the edge of the skin to be excised. The surgical assistant holds the forceps with gentle tension, and a fresh blade is used to trim the excess skin. Placing a malleable retractor beneath the plantar flap, while it rests on the dorsum of the foot, provides a firm supporting surface to cut on.

The tourniquet is deflated prior to wound closure, and bleeders are ligated or coagulated. Some oozing of blood from the transected bone marrow and from muscle is to be expected. The skin flaps are approximated without ten-sion and secured with a few simple interrupted, subcuta-neous 3–0 absorbable sutures. A TLS drain is placed in the wound, exiting the skin on the dorsolateral aspect of the foot. Skin flaps are carefully positioned and secured with 4–0 nylon sutures in a simple interrupted fashion, or with stainless steel staples. The technique for performing a transmetatarsal amputation is illustrated in Fig. 8.29a–f.

Dressings and postoperative care

Dressings consist of non-adherent fine mesh gauze (petrolatum, 3% Xeroform or Adaptic), placed on the suture line, wide gauze sponges (4 × 8 s, with a long dorsal and plantar tail, secured around the stump) and padding for protection of the heel and lateral border of the foot. Dressings are held in place by gauze bandage. A well-padded plaster splint is applied to immobilize the foot and ankle. Drains are generally left in place for 48 hours. Normal sterile saline moist-to-dry dressings are applied when there is persistent drainage from the wound or

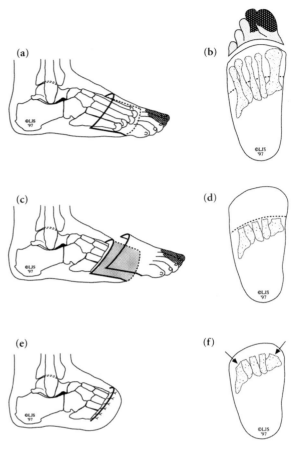

Fig. 8.29 Technique for performing a transmetatarsal amputation. (a) Incision with creation of a long plantar flap. (b) Plantar view. The plantar incision is made just proximal to the sulcus of the toes. The dotted line represents the dorsal skin incision and its relationship to the metatarsal shafts. (c) Removal of the forefoot, leaving a thick myocutaneous plantar flap. (d) Resection of the metatarsals. (e, f) The plantar flap has been remodelled, approximated with the dorsal skin flap and sutured in place. The lateral view depicts how the metatarsals have been cut, from dorsal-distal to plantar-proximal. The plantar view (arrows) illustrates how the cuts are bevelled on the 1st and 5th metatarsal stumps. From Sanders (1997) with permission from Elsevier Science.

when portions of the wound remain open. Sutures are removed after 14–21 days, and the patient is then placed in a short-leg removeable cast walker, non-weightbearing, for an additional 3–4 weeks. The patient is then transi-tioned to full weightbearing, in therapeutic high quarter depth inlay footwear. Shoe modifications include a stump filler and stiffened outer sole.

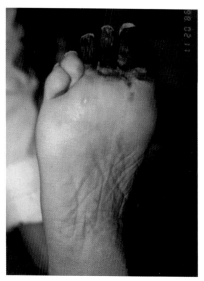

Fig. 8.30 Dry gangrene of the hallux, 2nd and 3rd toes. From Sanders (1997) with permission from Elsevier Science.

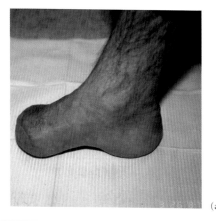

(a)

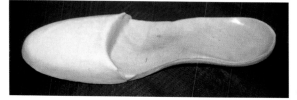

(b)

Fig. 8.31 Transmetatarsal amputation. (a) Postoperative appearance of the foot. (b) Custom-made orthosis, for use in extra-depth shoes.

CASE STUDY
Transmetatarsal amputation

A 56-year-old man with type 1 diabetes and schizophrenia was referred to the diabetic foot clinic for dry gangrene of his hallux, 2nd and 3rd toes (Fig. 8.30). The patient was new to our clinic, having been transferred from another hospital. The patient's medical history was quite remarkable: he had recently been very ill, in ketoacidosis, with a blood sugar level > 1200 mg/dL (66.7 mmol/L). The gangrenous changes in his toes developed during this episode, and appeared to be related to a shower of emboli to his toes. Pedal pulses were present and Doppler studies were otherwise normal. He underwent a successful transmetatarsal amputation with an unremarkable postoperative course (Fig. 8.31a). A custom-made orthosis with a stump filler was provided for the patient for use in extra-depth therapeutic shoes (Fig. 8.31b). The patient is very satisfied with the results of his amputation and ambulates normally without a limp. This transmetatarsal amputation has been durable with no further complications for more than 15 years.

CASE STUDY
Transmetatarsal amputation with long laterally based plantar flap

A 66-year-old man with type 2 diabetes of 30 years' dura-

tion and severe occlusive peripheral vascular disease had a chronic non-healing ulcer affecting his right great toe. The ulcer became infected and the patient developed dry gangrene of the hallux with cellulitis of the foot. The gangrenous right hallux was amputated, and 3 days later the patient underwent a right femoral to dorsalis pedis bypass graft. The amputation site remained dry and necrotic (Fig. 8.32a) with no evidence of healthy granulation tissue. We believed that the wound would not heal, and 1 week later, the patient was brought back to the operating room for a definitive transmetatarsal amputation (Fig. 8.32b,c). The procedure was performed under spinal anaesthesia, without a tourniquet.

This was a challenging case that stretched the indications and limits for a transmetatarsal amputation. The success of a transmetatarsal amputation depends upon the presence of healthy plantar skin, for the creation of a plantar flap. In this case, gangrene and tissue loss extended on to the plantar skin, effectively narrowing the plantar flap. Preparing the flap in a normal manner would have left a large uncovered defect on the medial aspect of the amputation stump. To remedy this, we developed a long laterally based plantar flap, which was rotated medially to cover the wound. The operation was successful and the

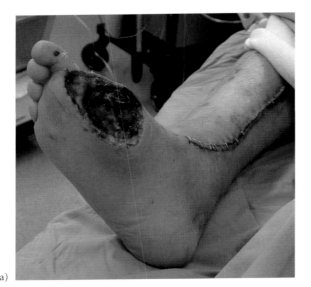

(a)

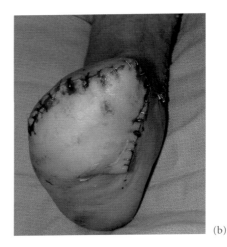

(b)

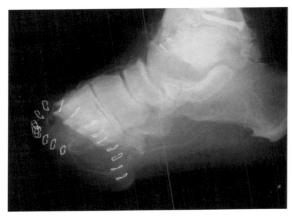

(c)

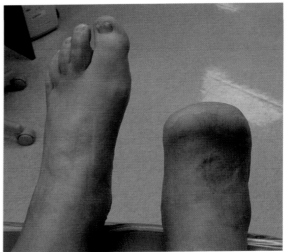

(d)

Fig. 8.32 Transmetatarsal amputation. (a) Preoperative appearance of the right foot with a large necrotic wound at the site of a failed hallux amputation. (b) The plantar flap has been rotated medially to achieve closure of the surgical wound.

(c) Lateral radiograph reveals the level of amputation. Notice the angled cuts of the metatarsals. Stainless steel staples were used to close the wound. (d) Healed transmetatarsal amputation right foot.

patient has a functional, durable foot that has remained lesion free for the past 5 years (Fig. 8.32d).

Transmetatarsal amputation with excision of plantar ulcer

Chronic non-healing neuropathic plantar ulceration is often associated with the complications of soft tissue infection and osteomyelitis. Cases that are refractory to conservative care may benefit from a modified transmetatarsal amputation with excision of a triangular wedge of skin from the plantar flap. I have also employed this

technique, in the absence of a plantar ulcer, to remodel excessively broad plantar flaps, thereby avoiding redundant skin and unsightly dog-ears.

Technique

Following a standard transmetatarsal amputation procedure, the plantar flap is revised as illustrated in Fig. 8.33a–e. The ulcer is completely enclosed in a triangle with its apex located proximally. Several Allis tissue forceps are applied to the distal flap and the wedge of skin is excised. It should be emphasized that the Allis clamps are

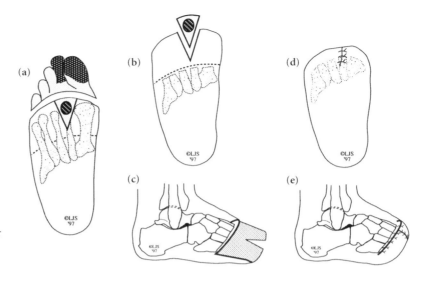

Fig. 8.33 Technique for modified transmetatarsal amputation with excision of a plantar ulcer. (a) A triangular wedge is drawn on the skin, enclosing the plantar ulcer. (b) The forefoot has been amputated and the triangular wedge of skin has been excised. (c) Plantar flap prior to approximation of the two segments of skin. (d) Plantar flap has been repaired with simple interrupted sutures. (e) Completed repair with approximation of the dorsal and plantar skin flaps. From Sanders (1997) with permission from Elsevier Science.

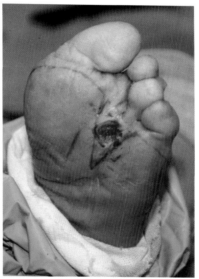
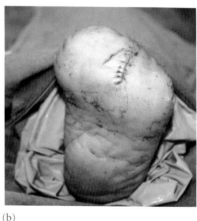

Fig. 8.34 Transmetatarsal amputation with excision of plantar ulcer. (a) Intraoperative view of the right foot, with the skin marked for excision of the plantar ulcer and creation of the plantar flap. (b) Completed transmetatarsal amputation with repair of the plantar flap. From Sanders (1997) with permission from Elsevier Science

(a) (b)

only applied to skin that is to be excised. A wide malleable retractor, placed beneath the flap, provides a firm supporting surface for the excision. The two segments of the plantar flap are then approximated with absorbable simple interrupted sutures placed within the wound, and 4–0 nylon in the skin. The dorsal and plantar flaps are closed, over a TLS drain, in the usual manner (Fig. 8.34a,b). Dressings, posterior splint and cast are applied as for a basic transmetatarsal amputation.

Open transmetatarsal amputation

Extensive forefoot infection or gangrene that extends on to the plantar skin may preclude a standard forefoot or mid-foot amputation. In these cases, an open or guillotine amputation performed at the mid-metatarsal level may be required. Guillotine amputations have a major disadvantage, in that they require extensive revision. A better alternative is to fashion flaps in the usual manner but to leave the wound open, with the intent to perform a delayed primary closure. The main disadvantage of open procedures is the prolonged length of time for healing, and the need for frequent dressing changes and debridement. Ideally, the wound will form a healthy granulation tissue base that can support a split-thickness skin graft or healing by secondary intention.

Amputations through the mid-foot

Lisfranc and Chopart amputations are frequently complicated by the development of equinus deformity. Equinovarus deformity is associated with Lisfranc disarticulation. Amputation at the tarsometatarsal joints appears to be the most proximal level that allows for satisfactory function of the foot. For surgery to work at this level, care must be taken to preserve the base of the 5th metatarsal with its tendinous attachments, for eversion of the foot. The Achilles tendon should be lengthened, as necessary.

Chopart's mid-tarsal joint amputation has the advantage of producing less limb shortening than a Syme's procedure because the talus and calcaneus are retained. However, complications are commonly reported with the Chopart amputation. Severe equinus deformity develops due to loss of the tibialis anterior, long extensor and peroneal tendons, with resultant failure to balance the force of the triceps surae. The resulting foot is short with a very small weightbearing surface, and is at increased risk of further breakdown. Some authors advise reattachment of the tibialis anterior to the talus to prevent equinus deformity of the hindfoot. However, long-term results demonstrate inevitable development of equinus deformity, even with tenotomy of the Achilles tendon.

Modified Lisfranc amputation

Modifications of the Lisfranc amputation include preservation of the 5th metatarsal base, and the 2nd metatarsal base, in its intercuneiform mortise.

Technique

The patient is placed in a supine position with the foot and lower half of the leg prepared and draped in the usual manner. This procedure is performed in a manner similar to the transmetatarsal amputation, with the development of a longer plantar flap and short dorsal flap. The dorsal skin incision is made just distal to the 1st metatarsocuneiform joint and carried across the dorsum of the foot, ending just distal to the 5th metatarsal base. Occasionally it may be necessary to develop a longer dorsal flap to compensate for devitalized plantar skin. The medial and lateral incisions are carried distally along the metatarsal shafts to the necks of the metatarsals and then curved plantarly across the ball of the foot. The plantar flap is developed to the intended level of disarticulation.

The 1st metatarsal base is disarticulated from the medial cuneiform. Using a power saw, and working from medial to lateral, the 2nd metatarsal is transected at the level of the 1st and 3rd cuneiforms, leaving its base intact in the intercuneiform mortise. The 3rd and 4th metatarsals are then disarticulated, followed by transection of the 5th metatarsal, just distal to its base. Although the 5th metatarsal base will leave a prominence of bone, this generally does not cause a problem. Wound closure is performed in the same manner as described above for a transmetatarsal amputation. Dressings and postoperative care are also the same. High-top shoes or chukka boots with a stump filler and mild rocker sole are well suited for this level of mid-foot amputation.

CASE STUDY
Lisfranc amputation

A 50-year-old man with a history of iv drug abuse and type 2 diabetes underwent amputation of his right 2nd toe and was referred to us for surgical management of his infected right foot. Examination revealed several draining ulcers and sinus tracts, extending from the site of his amputated 2nd toe, to beneath the 2nd and 3rd metatarsal heads and into the central plantar space (Fig. 8.35a,b). Radiographs revealed osteolytic changes in the 2nd and 3rd metatarsals consistent with osteomyelitis. The patient was given the options of a partial foot amputation or below-knee amputation, and he chose to preserve his leg. He was taken to the operating theatre where under spinal anaesthesia and ankle tourniquet, he underwent a Lisfranc amputation of his right foot. The technical difficulty in this case was related to the poor condition of the plantar skin. We were unable to fashion a healthy long plantar flap. Closure was accomplished by creating a slightly longer dorsal flap (Fig. 8.35c). The surgical wound healed satisfactorily (Fig. 8.35d). The Achilles tendon was not lengthened in this case, and a mild equinovarus deformity developed. The right foot held up well, for approximately 9 years, until the patient developed a new ulcer and recurrent infections. He unfortunately went on to a below-knee amputation.

Chopart amputation
Technique

The incision for a Chopart amputation starts medially, at the level just proximal to the navicular tuberosity and extends over the dorsum of the foot to a point midway between the 5th metatarsal base and the lateral malleolus.

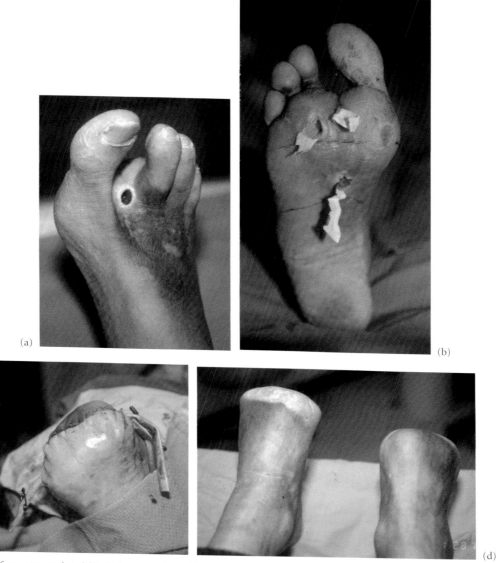

(a)

(b)

(c)

(d)

Fig. 8.35 Lisfranc amputation. (a) Initial presentation with a non-healing wound at the site of prior amputation of the 2nd toe, right foot. (b) Multiple draining plantar ulcers with sinus tracts. (c) Completed repair with a long dorsal flap and short plantar flap. (d) Healed Lisfranc amputation right foot, compared with transmetatarsal amputation of the left foot. Part (d) from Sanders (1997) with permission from Elsevier Science.

Medial and lateral incisions are then carried distally, over the 1st and 5th metatarsal shafts. At mid-shaft, the incision is curved down across the sole to fashion a plantar flap. The plantar flap is developed in a careful manner, using rakes for retraction, to the level of the mid-tarsal joint. The ligaments around the talonavicular and calcaneocuboid joints are divided. A suture is placed in the end of the tendon of the tibialis anterior. Soft tissue attachments are sharply dissected free from the foot, and it is disarticulated from the rearfoot. A drill hole is made in the talus for attachment of the tibialis anterior. The plantar flap is trimmed to size. Tourniquet is released and bleeders ligated or electrocoagulated. The skin flaps are then approximated, over a drain. The Achilles tendon is tenotomized. Standard dressings and splints are applied as for a transmetatarsal amputation.

Early consultation with an orthotist/prosthetist is advised for fabrication of an appropriate AFO or prosthesis.

CASE STUDY
Chopart's amputation

A 54-year-old man with type 2 diabetes of 17 years' duration and Charcot's arthropathy had chronic ulceration beneath the calcaneocuboid joint of his left foot. He also had nephropathy, peripheral vascular disease, retinopathy, neuropathy, congestive heart failure, hypertension and cardiovascular disease. He presented to the Emergency department with fever, rigors and a grossly infected left foot. Radiographs and clinical examination confirmed gas in the soft tissues on the dorsum of his foot, and over the 1st metatarsal to the level of the medial cuneiform. On admission his serum glucose was 398 mg/dL (22.1 mmol/L), WBC count was 18,300/μL, with 96% granulocytes. The patient was diagnosed with gas gangrene, a limb-threatening infection, and was emergently taken to the operating room for a guillotine amputation of his forefoot, under general anaesthesia. The surgical wound was left open. Intraoperative wound cultures revealed anaerobic Gram-positive cocci, *Peptostreptococcus magnus* and *Peptostreptococcus asaccharolyticus*. Blood cultures also grew *Peptostreptococcus magnus*. In consultation with the infectious disease specialist, he was placed on intravenous piperacillin/tazobactam and clindamycin. Daily dressing changes were performed, until the wound was clean and free from infection. The patient was given the options of a Chopart's amputation, to salvage a portion of his foot, or a below-knee amputation. He was opposed to losing his leg and chose the first option.

The patient returned to the operating theatre where under spinal anaesthesia, and a thigh tourniquet, he underwent a Chopart's amputation of his left foot. In an effort to prevent the development of ankle equinus, the tibialis anterior and extensor digitorum longus tendons were attached to the residual neck of the talus. In addition, the Achilles tendon was tenotomized. A small split-thickness skin graft was applied to the wound for coverage. The operative sites were bandaged and the foot was placed in a well-padded posterior splint. The patient was seen by an orthotist/prosthetist who provided a temporary clamshell total-contact cast.

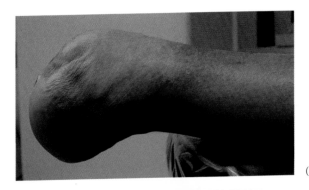

(a)

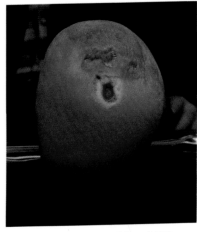

(b)

Fig. 8.36 (a) Chopart's amputation left foot. (b) Plantar ulcer.

In spite of our efforts to prevent the development of ankle equinus, this occurred, and was complicated by the development of recurrent ulceration. (Fig. 8.36a,b).

Outcomes of transmetatarsal and mid-foot amputations

Of the three levels of amputation discussed in this chapter, the transmetatarsal amputation is the most successful with respect to functional outcomes, patient satisfaction and long-term results. Transmetatarsal amputation preserves foot function, is cosmetically acceptable, does not require a prosthesis and enables fitting with commercially available footwear. Amputations performed at the tarsometatarsal and mid-tarsal joint levels frequently result in deformity and difficulty fitting shoes. Limb salvage can be achieved, with functional outcomes, by the motivated patient and knowledgeable surgeon with the use of these procedures.

SURGICAL MANAGEMENT OF THE CHARCOT FOOT

Most authors agree that non-operative treatment is the standard for the majority of patients with Charcot's osteoarthropathy of the foot and ankle. However, surgical intervention is indicated when deformity is severe, the foot/ankle is unstable or weightbearing is difficult. Careful patient selection and timing of operative treatment are critical considerations for successful outcomes. Unstable joints and deformities that predispose to shearing stress and ulceration can be corrected, but only after the acute inflammatory phase (stage of development) has subsided. Operative intervention during the acute phase of Charcot's joint disease may contribute to further destruction and is ill advised.

Indications and criteria

Instability, deformity, chronic ulceration and progressive joint destruction, despite rest and immobilization, are the primary indications for surgical intervention in diabetic individuals with Charcot's joint disease.

The patient's age, physical condition, compliance and comorbidities must also be considered in the surgical decision-making process. The benefits of surgery must be weighed carefully against the possible risks and complications. A simple ostectomy or limited arthrodesis may be all that is required. Relative contraindications to surgical management of the Charcot foot include infection, ischaemia, active bone disease, poorly controlled diabetes mellitus, a medically unstable patient and a history of poor compliance.

Criteria for surgical intervention
- Foot/ankle deformity
- Instability
- Ulceration
- Adequate circulation
- Medically stable
- Infection controlled.

Surgical procedures for the Charcot foot

Ostectomy

The most commonly employed procedure for the treatment of chronic neuropathic ulceration involves excision of bony prominences through either a plantar, medial or lateral approach. Decompression of the ulcer may be sufficient to prevent recurrence even when there is resid-

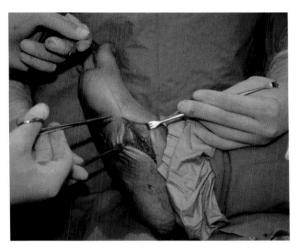

Fig. 8.37 Medial approach for ostectomy of the medial cuneiform.

ual deformity of the foot. Excision of the ulcer, resection of underlying bony prominence, with primary or secondary closure of the wound, is a reasonable method of treatment associated with minimal morbidity.

Technique
The surgical approach to ostectomy can be direct or indirect, and is determined by the location of deformity and condition of the skin. Bone can be resected through a plantar approach; however, it is easier to do this through either a medial (Fig. 8.37) or lateral (Fig. 8.38a,b) approach. Excision of the ulcer with resection of bone provides a quick fix for chronic plantar ulceration; however, recurrence is common.

CASE STUDY
Percutaneous lengthening of Achilles tendon with ostectomy of cuboid

A 63-year-old man with type 2 diabetes of 12 years' duration presented to the diabetic foot clinic with a chief complaint of pain, redness and swelling of his left foot. This condition began 1 week earlier with sudden onset and with no history of injury. Physical examination revealed instability of the mid-foot, ankle equinus, bounding pedal pulses, absent deep tendon reflexes at the ankle and loss of protective sensation. He was unable to perceive the Semmes–Weinstein 6.10 (90 g) monofilament. Radiographs revealed fracture dislocation of the tarsometatarsal joints (Lisfranc's

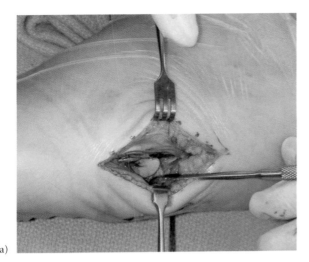

(a)

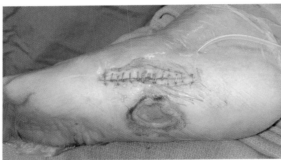

(b)

Fig. 8.38 Lateral approach for ostectomy of the cuboid. (a) Incision on the lateral border of the left foot. The articular surface of the cuboid is visible in the wound. (b) A large plantar ulcer is seen below the incision.

joint). The patient was afebrile with no elevation in his WBC count. His diabetes was very poorly controlled as evidenced by a markedly elevated HbA$_{1c}$ of 12.2%. Initial treatment consisted of a well-padded compression dressing and elevation of the limb. The patient was then immobilized in a non-weightbearing cast, which was changed every 3 weeks for 2.5 months. During a cast change, at 12 weeks postimmobilization, an ulcer was noted at the apex of his collapsed mid-foot (rocker-bottom deformity). Radiographs revealed that the ulcer was located directly beneath the cuboid, which was plantarly displaced. The surgical treatment for this patient included percutaneous lengthening of the Achilles tendon, with ostectomy of the cuboid performed through a lateral approach. Intraoperative and postoperative photographs illustrate the surgical approach (Fig. 8.38a,b). His postoperative course

was uncomplicated and his plantar ulcer healed well. He was seen by an orthotist who provided custommoulded shoes and a patella tendon bearing (PTB) orthosis (Fig. 8.39a,b). Ulceration recurred when the patient stopped wearing his custom shoes and PTB orthosis.

CASE STUDY
Charcot foot with cellulitis, full-thickness plantar ulceration and abscess. Collapse of the medial arch with deformity of the medial cuneiform

A 64-year-old Caucasian man with poorly controlled type 2 diabetes of 8 years' duration and a 5-year history of neurogenic arthropathy of his left foot presented to the diabetic foot clinic with an acute infection of his left foot. He stated that over the last few days he had experienced increased pain, redness and swelling of his left foot accompanied by fever and chills. At presentation his vital signs were: temperature 38.2°C, pulse 90, respiration 18, BP 136/84 mmHg. WBC count was elevated at 17,300/μL with 85.5% granulocytes. Serum glucose was 253 mg/dL (14 mmol/L). The foot was erythematous, swollen and hot. The medial arch of the left foot was collapsed, with prominent bony deformity. A full-thickness ulcer was present beneath the apex of the medial cuneiform. The ulcer did not probe to bone. A purulent exudate was present. Cellulitis extended approximately 8 cm around the ulcer (Fig. 8.40a). Infection appeared to involve the medial and central plantar spaces. Pedal pulses were palpable. Neurological exam revealed a dense peripheral neuropathy with loss of protective sensation, absent vibratory sensation below the malleoli and absent deep tendon reflexes at the ankle. Wound and blood cultures were performed. The patient was admitted to the Acute Medicine Service and he was empirically started on intravenous piperacillin/tazobactam. Radiographs revealed chronic neuropathic changes of the foot characterized by collapse of the mid-foot with sclerosis of the tarsal bones, lateral displacement of metatarsals 2 through 5, and medial subluxation of the first cuneiform with bony fragmentation. There was soft tissue swelling and air in the medial and plantar soft tissues. An incidental finding was the presence of a broken needle in the plantar soft tissues between the 2nd and 3rd metatarsals (Fig. 8.40b). Podiatric surgical consultation was requested and on the second day following hospital admission the patient was taken to the operating room for incision and drainage (I & D) with wound debridement. An oblique incision was made across the bottom of the foot, from proximal medial

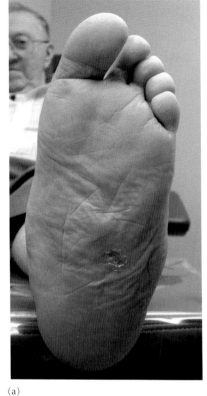

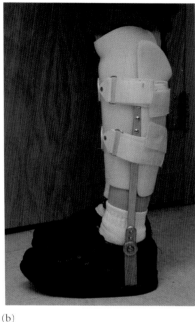

Fig. 8.39 The same patient as in Fig. 8.38a,b. (a) The foot is well healed. (b) Patella tendon bearing brace with custom-moulded shoes and rocker soles.

(a)

(b)

to distal lateral, exposing the medial and central plantar spaces. A portion of the medial band of the plantar fascia was found to be necrotic and was excised. Deep wound cultures were performed. The wound was irrigated with 1 L of normal sterile saline containing 1 g of cefazolin, and packed open. Blood cultures were reported as no growth. The initial wound culture grew out *Pseudomonas aeruginosa*, *Enterobacter cloacae*, viridans streptococci and MRSA. The intraoperative wound culture grew only MRSA. Vancomycin was added to the piperacillin/tazobactam. Initial wound care consisted of moist-to-dry normal sterile saline dressings. An Indium-111 bone scan was negative for osteomyelitis. Vacuum-assisted closure (VAC) was then employed to promote granulation tissue formation and wound healing. This therapy resulted in the formation of exuberant granulation tissue (Fig. 8.40c). Although this might have normally provided a healthy bed for a split-thickness skin graft (STSG), deformity of the foot precluded this option. A STSG could not withstand the abnormally high plantar pressures associated with the pathomechanics of this Charcot foot. The

option of conservative surgical reconstruction was discussed with the patient and he consented to have this performed. He returned to the operating room, 6 weeks after I & D, for ostectomy of the medial cuneiform under general anaesthesia. The wound was debrided and exuberant granulation tissue was excised. The prominent medial cuneiform was resected medially and plantarly, through a separate incision, thereby reducing the deformity. A portion of the medial cuneiform was preserved so as to maintain stability of the medial column of the foot (Fig. 8.40c,d). The wounds were closed primarily over a closed suction drain, and the patient was immobilized in a multipodus boot. Postoperative care consisted of non-weightbearing in a removable cast walker for 14 weeks, transitioning to gradual weightbearing in custom footwear (Fig. 8.40e).

Key points

- Seek prompt surgical consultation
- The mainstay of therapy for moderate to severe diabetic foot infections is *timely and aggressive surgical intervention*, including incision and drainage, debridement

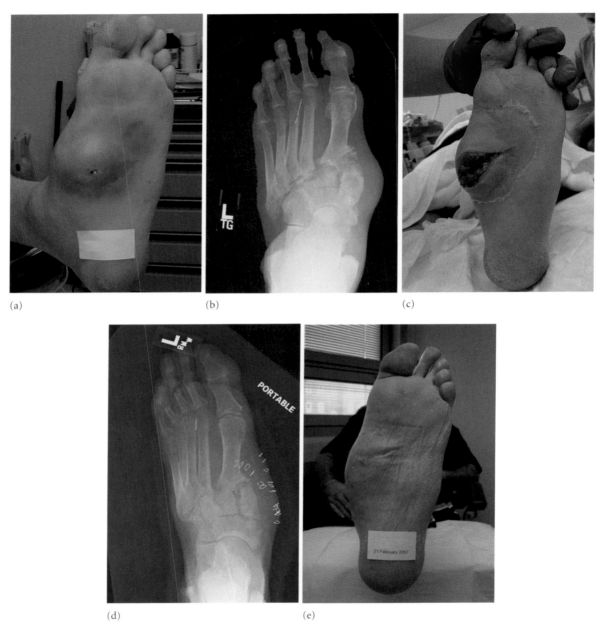

(a)   (b)   (c)

(d)   (e)

Fig. 8.40 A 64-year-old man with poorly controlled type 2 diabetes and neurogenic arthropathy presents with an acute infection of his left foot. (a) Cellulitis of the left foot with collapse of the medial arch. A full-thickness ulcer is seen beneath the apex of the medial cuneiform. (b) Anteroposterior radiograph of the left foot demonstrates soft tissue swelling with chronic neuropathic changes characterized by collapse of the mid-foot with sclerosis of the tarsal bones, lateral displacement of the metatarsal bones, and medial subluxation of the medial cuneiform with bony fragmentation. A sewing needle is seen in the plantar soft tissues between the 2nd and 3rd metatarsals. (c) Appearance of the left foot after 6 weeks of intravenous antibiotics (vancomycin). There is rigid deformity of the mid-foot with exuberant granulation tissue in the wound. (d) Anteroposterior radiograph, following the patient's return to the operating room for exostectomy and excision of the chronic wound with primary closure. (e) Postoperative appearance of the left foot 3 months following surgery. The skin is well healed; however, there is residual deformity of the foot that predisposes the patient to future ulceration. Close surveillance is required.

of infected or necrotic tissues and limited resections of bone

- Surgical correction of underlying foot deformities associated with recalcitrant ulceration and infection should be considered
- Infection must be adequately treated prior to exostectomy
- Removal of a foreign body (needle), that has been identified as an incidental radiographic finding, deep in the foot of an asymptomatic patient, is not required.

Arthrodesis

Mid-foot and hindfoot arthrodesis of neuropathic joints should be considered salvage procedures, as they are technically demanding and frequently associated with complications. Recent reports have been encouraging with respect to satisfactory outcomes of these procedures as an alternative to amputation of the limb. However, there is still a need for caution, as surgical complication rates remain high. Stabilization of the medial column of the foot is crucial to the success of mid-foot arthrodesis.

Factors leading to successful arthrodesis include the preoperative condition of the foot, control of infection, operative technique and postoperative management. In general, no patient should be considered for surgery until the acute arthropathy has subsided. The precise timing for this has not been quantified. Regardless of which joints are fused, basic surgical techniques remain the same.

Technique for successful arthrodesis
- Thorough removal of all cartilage and detritus
- Careful removal of sclerotic bone down to healthy bleeding bone
- Meticulous fashioning of congruent bone surfaces for apposition
- Rigid fixation of bone.

Modern surgical techniques for internal and external fixation have greatly increased the chances for successful outcomes. Of equal importance is the necessity for prolonged postoperative immobilization, often two to three times longer than that required for a patient without neuropathic bone disease. Patients must remain non-weightbearing, and require physiotherapy and rehabilitation, with a gradual return to protected weightbearing.

The following case is a striking example of acute Charcot's arthropathy, with fracture dislocation of the mid-foot, that required realignment arthrodesis with fusion of the medial column of the foot.

CASE STUDY
Open reduction and rigid internal fixation of mid-foot fracture-dislocations

A 53-year-old Caucasian man, a janitorial worker, with type 2 diabetes of 6 years' duration, presented to the diabetic foot clinic with the chief complaint of sudden and unexpected swelling of his left foot. There was no history of injury, ankle sprain, tripping or falling. Physical examination revealed moderate to severe redness, swelling and elevated skin temperature, approximately 4°C, of the left foot and ankle. Swelling extended up the leg to the knee. The medial column of the foot was unstable. Pedal pulses were present and there were no breaks in the skin. The patient had a dense peripheral neuropathy with loss of protective sensation, absent deep tendon reflexes at the ankle and elevated vibratory perception threshold > 45. The patient's body mass index was 35 kg/m^2. Laboratory data revealed an elevated HbA$_{1c}$ = 8.0%, mild anaemia, and normal WBC count. Radiographs revealed fracture-dislocation of Lisfranc's joint, with medial dislocation of the 1st metatarsal, and fracture dislocation of the 2nd metatarsocuneiform joint. In addition, there were dorsally displaced fractures of the 2nd, 3rd and 4th metatarsal heads (Fig. 8.41a,b).

He was initially placed in a well-padded Jones compression dressing and admitted to the medical centre for bedrest and elevation of his left lower extremity. Within 1 week, the swelling began to subside and he was placed in a short-leg non-weightbearing cast. The cast was changed 2 weeks later. Interim evaluation at day 21 revealed resolution of the swelling, redness and elevated skin temperature. The medial column of the foot (1st ray) remained unstable. At this time the process was considered to be subacute, and surgical intervention was advised. The following criteria for surgical intervention were met:
- Foot deformity/instability
- Adequate circulation
- Medically stable
- No evidence of infection.

The patient underwent successful open reduction and rigid internal fixation of his mid-foot fracture-dislocations, under spinal anaesthesia, using a thigh tourniquet for haemostasis.

Technique
An 8 cm linear incision was made over the medial aspect of the 1st metatarsal and medial cuneiform. The incision was carried deep to bone and all soft tissues were reflected from the cuneiform and metatarsal, revealing complete

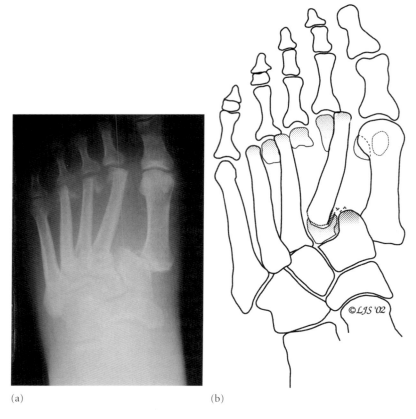

(a)   (b)

Fig. 8.41 Acute Charcot's arthropathy of the left foot. (a) Anteroposterior radiograph reveals fracture-dislocations of the tarsometatarsal joints (Lisfranc's joint), with medial dislocation of the 1st metatarsocuneiform joint, and dorsally displaced fractures of the 2nd, 3rd and 4th metatarsal heads. (b) Illustration of the radiographic findings.

medial dislocation of the 1st metatarsal (Fig. 8.42). Manual reduction of the dislocation was not possible because of soft tissue interposed in the joint. A sagittal power saw was used to resect a wafer of bone from the base of the 1st metatarsal, and to remove the articular cartilage from the medial cuneiform. The metatarsal was then easily relocated and fixed with two 4.0 mm cannulated screws, under C-arm fluoroscopy. A four-hole, 1/3 tubular plate was then placed across the 1st metatarsocuneiform articulation and secured with four 3.5 mm cortical screws. Attention was then directed to the fracture-dislocation of the 2nd metatarsocuneiform joint, where a 6 cm linear incision was made over the dorsum of the foot. The base of the metatarsal was resected and the cartilage removed from the intermediate cuneiform. The 2nd metatarsal was placed in proper alignment, secured with a K-wire, and fixed with a 4.0 cannulated screw. Wounds were irrigated thoroughly with normal sterile saline solution, and two closed suction drains were inserted. Deep closure of the soft tissues was obtained using 3–0 absorbable sutures, and the skin was closed with stainless steel staples.

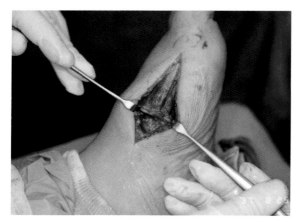

Fig. 8.42 Intraoperative view showing dislocation of the 1st metatarsocuneiform joint.

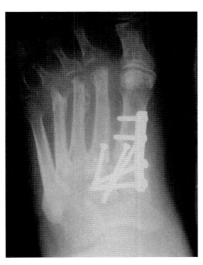

Fig. 8.43 Anteroposterior radiograph reveals satisfactory postoperative realignment of the tarsometatarsal joints.

Postoperative radiographs revealed satisfactory realignment of Lisfranc's joint (Fig. 8.43).

Dressings and postoperative care

Non-adherent petrolatum gauze was applied to the wounds and covered with a fluffy compression dressing, followed by a plaster splint.

The patient was immobilized in fibreglass non-weight-bearing casts for a period of 3 months. Casts were changed every 3 weeks. The patient was then placed in a walking brace for 1 month, and allowed to gradually return to full weightbearing. Custom-moulded shoes were provided. The postoperative recovery for this patient was essentially uncomplicated. The patient remained ambulatory and lived 4 more years, eventually succumbing to cardiovascular and renal complications.

Ankle arthrodesis

Arthrodesis for severe ankle deformity and instability has traditionally been reported to have a high incidence of non-union and pseudoarthrosis in patients with neuroarthropathy. Recent reports, however, are more encouraging, with authors reporting success rates ranging from 66% to 100%. In cases where solid ankle fusion is not achieved, there may still be an acceptable outcome with fibrous ankylosis, when the foot is satisfactorily aligned beneath the leg. Failure to obtain fusion may be due to postoperative infection, deficiency of the arthrodesis, refracture through the site of fusion or hardware failure. The following case illustrates the surgical treat-

ment for severe destruction and instability of the ankle in a patient whose deformity could not be braced or accommodated in custom footwear. The surgical procedure was a tibiocalcaneal fusion with autogenous bone graft and intramedullary nailing. The goal of surgery was to realign the calcaneus under the tibia, in a plantigrade weightbearing position.

CASE STUDY
Tibiocalcaneal fusion with autogenous bone graft and intramedullary nailing

A 74-year-old man, with type 2 diabetes of 17 years' duration, presented for initial consultation to the diabetic foot clinic with the chief complaint of swelling and deformity of his left ankle that developed suddenly and unexpectedly following an ankle sprain 6 months earlier. The patient had previously been treated elsewhere with a walking brace. Physical examination revealed marked deformity of the left ankle, characterized by swelling and displacement of the foot lateral to the leg. Pitting oedema extended up the leg to the level of the knee. There was a shallow ulcer 1.0 cm diameter on the medial malleolus that appeared to be caused by the brace. Skin temperature was elevated over the entire limb. Neurological examination revealed absent deep tendon reflexes at the ankle. Vibratory sensation was diminished below the knee, and absent below the malleoli. Loss of protective sensation was noted, with the patient unable to feel the Semmes–Weinstein 6.10 (90 g) monofilament. Pedal pulses were not palpable due to the swelling of the foot and ankle. Initial conservative management consisted of cast immobilization and non-weightbearing. Despite these efforts, over the course of several months, ankle deformity and instability progressed, with disintegration of the talus (Fig. 8.44a). The patient was given the option of a salvage procedure, a tibiocalcaneal fusion vs. major amputation of the leg, and he opted for ankle fusion in the hope of saving his leg.

Technique

A standard medial incision was made over the medial malleolus, under fluoroscopic guidance, and the distal medial aspect of the tibia was exposed. The entire talus was noted to be destroyed and the foot was dislocated lateral to the leg. The distal tibia was then exposed subperiosteally and circumferentially and the bone was cut parallel to the standing alignment. A small portion of the talus was present laterally and this was planed down flat. Detritus was removed from the ankle. A filet guide pin

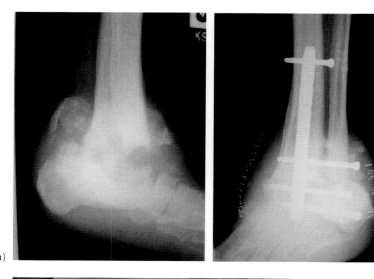

(a)

(b)

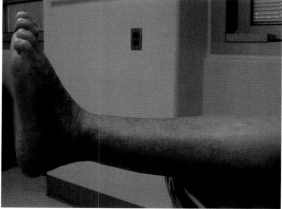

(c)

Fig. 8.44 (a) Lateral radiograph reveals extensive destruction of the left ankle joint with disintegration of the talus and fragmentation of bone. (b) Postoperative radiograph of the left ankle following tibiocalcaneal fusion with the intramedullary nail and interlocking screws in place. (c) Long-term follow-up. Clinical appearance of the left foot and ankle 5 years after surgery.

was placed through the centre of the heel up through the calcaneus and up through the centre of the tibia. Sequential reamers were then utilized and reamed up to 12.5 mm. An 11 mm × 15 cm intramedullary nail was then selected and placed without difficulty. Two interlocking screws were placed in the calcaneus and then the nail was impacted into the distal tibia. The rotation was set with the tibial tubercle and then distal tibial interlocking screws were placed sequentially. A 45-mm cross-linking screw was placed proximally. All screws were checked on the radiograph and were noted to be within the nail (Fig. 8.44b). The previously resected bone from the distal tibia was then morselized and packed with bone graft posteriorly and laterally. The wounds were copiously irrigated, a Hemovac drain was placed and wounds were closed with sutures and staples. The patient recovered on

the acute surgical service for 1 week, was placed in a short-leg cast and was then transferred to the physical medicine and rehabilitation inpatient service for generalized conditioning exercise and ambulation training, non-weight-bearing on the left lower extremity. The patient recovered uneventfully and remains ambulatory after nearly 7 years (Fig. 8.44c). He has experienced recurrent ulceration on the plantar aspect of his heel, requiring local wound care, oral antibiotics, and total-contact casts. He is now ambulating with a Charcot restraint orthotic walker (CROW).

External skeletal fixation in management of the Charcot foot

External skeletal fixation is a widely accepted surgical approach to the management of acute lower extremity trauma as well as for the correction of chronic severe foot and ankle deformities. Circular external fixators are applied proximal and distal to the surgical site (osteotomy or arthrodesis) and maintain alignment during healing. However, the application of external fixation frames is controversial with respect to the surgical management of the diabetic Charcot foot. This approach is not yet routine nor is it the standard of care. Treatment is lengthy, the frames are cumbersome and complication rates are high. This is especially problematic in a uniquely vulnerable population of patients with diabetes and multiple comorbidities. The threat of complications is significant for these patients who have cardiovascular risk factors, peripheral neuropathy, nutritional deficiency and who may also be immunocompromised. There is limited peer reviewed literature on the use of external fixation in the treatment of the Charcot foot. Most published studies are small, anecdotal, short term and retrospective. Long-term outcomes including functional evaluations and quality of life studies comparing alternative methods of treatment are lacking.

Elomrani and colleagues reported on 55 adult patients who were treated with circular external fixation, for chronic severe foot and ankle deformities, at an academic referral centre in Sheffield, UK. In this retrospective analysis of patients treated between 1992 and 2000, the mean time spent in external fixation frames was 2.1 (range 1 to 12) months. The mean time to begin partial weightbearing was 4.1 (range 1 to 8) months and full weightbearing 5.2 (range 1 to 10) months. Foot frames were removed within 2 to 16 (mean 6.7) months. The leg was immobilized in a cast after frame removal for 6 to 30 (mean 5.6) weeks. Complications were common, with wire-related infection being the most common. There were 1.2 infections per deformity correction. Five patients had below-knee amputations. One of these patients had a voluntary below-knee amputation because of depression, 14 months after frame application.

Farber and Juliano at the Pennsylvania State University College of Medicine published a retrospective review of 11 patients who underwent operative treatment for mid-foot Charcot neuroarthropathy with external skeletal fixation. The average age of their patients was 55 (range 41 to 66) years. Ten patients had diabetes and one patient had end-stage renal disease. Eight of the 11 patients had a rocker-bottom deformity, and all were facing limb amputation secondary to severe ulceration of the foot or ankle. Average time in the external fixator was 57 (range 12 to 113) days, followed by total-contact casting for an average 131 (range 52 to 271) days and then to therapeutic footwear. Average follow-up was 24 months. Four of 11 feet developed a bony union of the osteotomy. The remaining seven patients were noted to have a fibrous union. The authors did not discuss the incidence of complications.

Indications, advantages and disadvantages for external fixation

External skeletal fixation is indicated as a surgical option for arthrodesis of the unstable Charcot foot with deformity of the mid-foot or hindfoot that is frequently associated with ulceration. This option may also be appropriate for the surgical management of a stable Charcot foot with chronic deformity, e.g. rocker-bottom deformity, that cannot be accommodated by a shoe or a brace. The deformity presents a serious and predictable risk for the development of ulceration. Chronic recurrent ulceration with infection will ultimately result in extension of the infection to bone (osteomyelitis), systemic sepsis and amputation. The goal of surgical management is to provide a stable plantigrade foot free from ulceration that can be fitted in a shoe or brace.

Advantages of external fixation
- Can be used in the presence of an open wound or infection when internal fixation is contraindicated
- Can be used to supplement or provide primary stabilization for arthrodesis of the mid-foot
- Can be adjusted postoperatively, to allow for gradual correction of deformity
- Fine wire ring fixation can be used in osteopaenic bone.

Disadvantages of external fixation
- Damage to neurovascular structures during frame application
- Pin tract infections
- Deep soft tissue infections
- Osteomyelitis or septic arthritis
- Cumbersome and difficult for the patient
- Prolonged application up to 3 months, followed by an extended period of immobilization.

CASE STUDY
External fixation with circular frame

A 53-year-old man, a mechanical engineer, had type 2 diabetes of 8 years' duration and peripheral sensory neuropathy, height 70″ tall and weight 200 pounds with a BMI of 28.7. Four months prior to surgery he injured his right foot while stepping off a ladder at

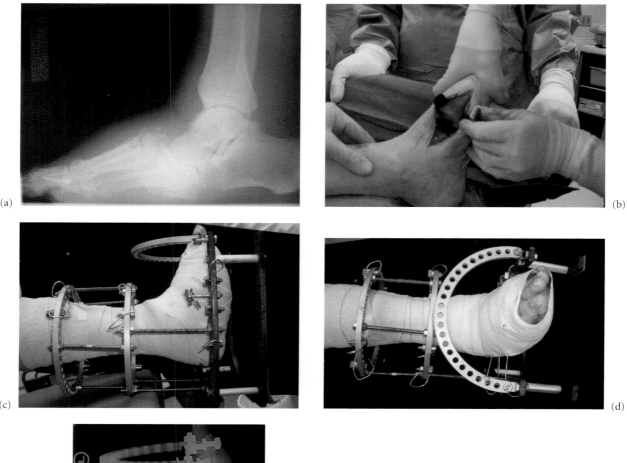

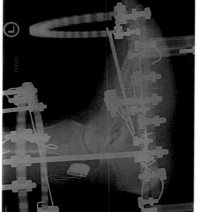

Fig. 8.45 External ring fixation. (a) Lateral radiograph of the left foot demonstrates fracture dislocation of the tarsometatarsal and navicular cuneiform joints (Sanders Patterns II and III). There is collapse of the mid-foot with rocker-bottom deformity. (b) Plantarly based wedge resection at the level of the tarsometatarsal joint. (c, d) Postoperative photos with circular frame in place. There are two tibial rings and a foot plate. Thin Ilizarov wires were used. Olive wires were placed in the lateral tibia, as well as in the medial and lateral calcaneus. (e) Postoperative lateral radiograph with circular frame in place. An implantable bone stimulator is seen in Kager's triangle.

work. He noticed mild swelling of his foot, however because he had only minimal pain he continued to work with uninterrupted physical activities. He was initially seen by his family physician who appropriately ordered X-rays. The initial radiographs were interpreted as nor-mal with no evidence of fracture or dislocation. Over the next month the patient noticed that his right foot was changing shape. He consulted with an orthopaedic surgeon who ordered repeat radiographs. These X-rays revealed fracture dislocation of the tarsometatarsal joints with total mid-foot collapse and rocker-bottom deformity (Fig. 8.45a). The patient subsequently presented to a specialized diabetic foot clinic, where he received a comprehensive evaluation. He was placed in an instant total-contact cast (iTCC) and kept non-weightbearing on a Roll-A-Bout. He was prescribed intranasal calcitonin along with supplemental calcium and vitamin D. Serial skin temperature measurements were performed. At presentation the skin temperature on the affected foot was 6°C warmer than the uninvolved foot. After 4 weeks of immobilization the difference in skin temperature was less than 3°C. Computerized gait analysis demonstrated abnormally high peak plantar pressure beneath the cuboid. Surgical options were discussed with the patient and he opted for reconstructive foot surgery with external fixation. Surgery was performed in the operating room under general anaesthesia. Achilles tenotomy was carried out, followed by a plantarly based wedge resection at the level of the tarsometatarsal joint (Fig. 8.45b). An implantable bone stimulator was inserted in Kager's triangle and the leads were placed in the fusion site. A pre-built external fixator with two tibial rings and a foot plate were applied with thin Ilizarov and olive wires (Fig. 8.45c,d,e). A second foot plate was added to the device after application to avoid plantar foot pressure during a seated position or from the foot board of a hospital bed. The patient was admitted to the hospital for rehabilitation for 4 weeks postoperatively. He was then discharged to home non-weightbearing in a wheelchair. The external fixator remained in place for 11 weeks, followed by non-weightbearing in a Charcot restraint orthotic walker (CROW).

Key points
- Long-term outcomes are lacking
- Prolonged treatment is required
- Complication rates are high
- Close follow-up is essential

Complications of surgery

Infection, non-union, delayed union, pseudoarthrosis, progressive bone and joint destruction, pathological fractures, hardware failure, recurrent deformity and delayed wound healing have all been reported following surgery on patients with Charcot's joint disease. Attention to detail, targeted antibiotic coverage, meticulous surgical technique and postoperative non-weightbearing immobilization will help to minimize these complications.

Prospective studies comparing alternative methods of treatment are needed to assess long-term surgical outcomes, function and quality of life in order to determine the most beneficial approach to management of the diabetic foot.

ACKNOWLEDGEMENTS

Lee Sanders would like to recognize the invaluable research assistance provided by Barbara E. Deaven, medical librarian, and Dorothy Melan, library technician, VA Medical Center, Lebanon, Pennsylvania.

Photos courtesy of Drs. David Armstrong, Lee Rogers and Nicholas Bevilaqua, Center for Lower Extremity Ambulatory Research (CLEAR), Dr. William M. Scholl College of Podiatric Medicine at Rosalind Franklin University of Medicine and Science.

FURTHER READING

The diabetic foot

Armstrong DG, Lavery LA, Stern S *et al.* Is prophylactic diabetic foot surgery dangerous? *J Foot Ankle Surg* 1996; **35**: 585–9.

Joslin EP. The menace of diabetic gangrene. *N Engl J Med* 1934; **211**: 16.

Levin ME, Pfeifer MA, Bowker J (eds). *The Diabetic Foot*, 6th edn. Mosby Inc., St Louis, USA, 2001.

Achilles tendon lengthening

Armstrong DG, Stacpoole-Shea S, Nguyen H, Harkless LB. Lengthening of the Achilles tendon in diabetic patients who are at risk for ulceration of the foot. *J Bone Joint Surg* 1999; **81A**: 535.

Grant WP, Sullivan R, Sonenshine DE *et al.* Electron microscopic investigation of the effects of diabetes mellitus on the Achilles tendon. *J Foot Ankle Surg* 1997; **36**: 272–8.

Hatt RN, Lamphier TA. Triple hemisection: a simplified procedure for lengthening the Achilles tendon. *N Engl J Med* 1947; **236**: 166–9.

Sanders LJ. Transmetatarsal and midfoot amputations. *Clin Podiatr Med Surg* 1997; **14**: 741.

Amputation surgery

McKittrick LS, McKittrick JB, Risley T. Transmetatarsal amputation for infection or gangrene in patients with diabetes mellitus. *Ann Surg* 1949; **130**: 826.

Mueller MJ, Sinacore DR. Rehabilitation factors following transmetatarsal amputation. *Phys Ther* 1994; **74**: 1027.

Murdoch DP, Armstrong DG, Cacus JB *et al.* The natural history of great toe amputations. *J Foot Ankle Surg* 1997; **36**: 204–8.

Sanders LJ. Amputations in the diabetic foot. *Clin Podiatr Med Surg* 1987; **4**: 481.

Sanders LJ. Transmetatarsal and midfoot amputations. *Clin Podiatr Med Surg* 1997; **14**: 741–62.

Sanders LJ, Dunlap G. Transmetatarsal amputation: A successful approach to limb salvage. *J Am Podiatr Med Assoc* 1992; **82**: 129.

Sanders LJ. Ray and Transmetatarsal Amputations, Chapter 209. In Fischer JE (ed). *Mastery of Surgery* (2 vols), 5th edn. Lippincott Williams & Wilkins, Philadelphia, USA, 2007, pp. 2193–207.

Vitti MJ, Robinson DV, Hauer-Jensen M *et al.* Wound healing in forefoot amputations: the predictive value of toe pressure. *Ann Vasc Surg* 1994; **8**: 99.

Warren R, Crawford ES, Hardy IB, McKittrick JB. The transmetatarsal amputation in arterial deficiency of the lower extremity. *Surgery* 1952; **31**: 132.

Calcanectomy

Bollinger M, Thordarson DB. Partial calcanectomy: an alternative to below the knee amputation. *Foot Ankle Int* 2002; **23**: 927–32.

Smith DG, Stuck RM, Ketner L *et al.* Partial calcanectomy for the treatment of large ulcerations of the heel and calcaneal osteomyelitis. An amputation of the back of the foot. *J Bone Joint Surg* 1992; **74A**: 571–6.

Charcot's joint disease

Baravarian B, Van Gils CC. Arthrodesis of the Charcot foot and ankle. *Clin Podiatr Med Surg* 2004; **21**: 271–89.

Charcot J-M. On some arthropathies apparently related to a lesion of the brain or spinal cord (orig. January 1868). Translated and edited by Hoché G and Sanders LJ. *J Hist Neurosci* 1992; **1**: 75–87.

Herbst SA. External fixation in Charcot arthropathy. *Foot Ankle Clin N Am* 2004; **9**: 595–609.

Johnson JE. Charcot neuroarthropathy of the foot: surgical aspects. In Levin ME, Pfeifer MA, Bowker J (eds). *The Diabetic Foot*, 6th edn. Mosby Inc., St Louis, USA, 2001, pp. 587–606.

Pinzur MS. The role of ring external fixation in Charcot foot arthropathy. *Foot Ankle Clin N Am* 2006; **11**: 837–47.

Sanders LJ. Jean-Martin Charcot (1825–1893): The man behind the joint disease. *J Am Podiatr Med Assoc* 2002; **92**: 375–80.

Sanders LJ, Frykberg RG. The Charcot foot (Pied de Charcot). In Pfeifer MA, Bowker J (eds). *Levin & O'Neal's The Diabetic Foot*, 7th edn. Elsevier, Philadelphia, USA, 2007.

Simon SR, Tejwani SG, Wilson DL *et al.* Arthrodesis as an early alternative to non-operative management of Charcot arthropathy of the diabetic foot. *J Bone Joint Surg AM* 2000; **82A**: 939–50.

Diabetic foot infections

Lipsky BA, Berendt AR, Deery HG *et al.* Diagnosis and treatment of diabetic foot infections. *Clin Infect Dis* 2004; **39**: 885–910.

Great toe ulceration

Dannels E. Neuropathic foot ulcer prevention in diabetic American Indians with hallux limitus. *J Am Podiatr Med Assoc* 1989; **79**: 447–50.

Downs DM, Jacobs RL. Treatment of resistant ulcers on the plantar surface of the great toe in diabetics. *J Bone Joint Surg AM* 1982; **64A**: 930–3.

Lin SS, Bono CM, Lee TH. Total contact casting and Keller arthroplasty for diabetic great toe ulceration under the interphalangeal joint. *Foot Ankle Int* 2000; **21**: 588–93.

Rosenblum BI, Giurini JM, Chrzan JS, Habershaw GM. Preventing loss of the great toe with the hallux interphalangeal joint arthroplasty. *J Foot Ankle Surg* 1994; **33**: 557–60.

Lesser metatarsal osteotomies

Barouk LS. Weil's metatarsal osteotomy in the treatment of metatarsalgia. *Orthopäde* 1996; **25**: 338–44.

Fleischli JE, Anderson RB, Davis WH. Dorsiflexion metatarsal osteotomy for treatment of recalcitrant diabetic neuropathic ulcers. *Foot Ankle Int* 1999; **20**: 80–5.

O'Kane C, Kilmartin TE. The surgical management of central metatarsalgia. *Foot Ankle Int* 2002; **23**: 415–19.

Vandeputte G, Dereymaeker G, Steenwerckx A, Peeraer L. The Weil osteotomy of the lesser metatarsals: a clinical and pedobarographic follow-up study. *Foot Ankle Int* 2000; **21**: 370–4.

Sesamoidectomy

Giurini JM, Chrzan JS, Gibbons GW, Habersahw GM. Sesamoidectomy for the treatment of chronic neuropathic ulcerations. *J Am Podiatr Med Assoc* 1991; **81**: 167–73.

Subject Index

Notes:
Page numbers in **bold** refer to tables.
Page numbers in *italics* refer to figures.
Page numbers suffixed by cs refer to case studies.
Index entries are arranged in letter-by-letter alphabetical order.
Readers are advised to refer to the end of each chapter for practice points and further reading references.